Manipal
Prep Manual of
Medicine
for Dental Students

As per the syllabus prescribed by the
Dental Council of India

with

Multiple Choice Questions (MCQs)

Manipal
Prep Manual of
Medicine
for Dental Students
with **Multiple Choice Questions (MCQs)**

As per the syllabus prescribed by the
Dental Council of India

Manthappa M

MBBS, MD (General Medicine)

Associate Professor
Department of Medicine
JSS Medical College, JSSAHER
Mysuru, Karnataka

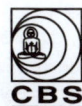

CBS

CBS Publishers & Distributors Pvt Ltd

New Delhi • Bengaluru • Chennai • Kochi • Kolkata • Mumbai
Bhopal • Bhubaneswar • Hyderabad • Jharkhand • Nagpur • Patna
Pune • Uttarakhand • Dhaka (Bangladesh) • Kathmandu (Nepal)

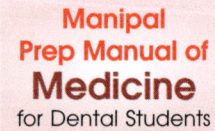

ISBN: 978-93-89261-74-5

Copyright © Author and Publisher

First Edition: 2020

Published by Satish Kumar Jain and produced by Varun Jain for

CBS Publishers & Distributors Pvt Ltd

4819/XI Prahlad Street, 24 Ansari Road, Daryaganj, New Delhi 110 002, India.
Ph: 23289259, 23266861, 23266867   Fax: 011-23243014   Website: www.cbspd.com
                                                                                                              e-mail: delhi@cbspd.com; cbspubs@airtelmail.in.
Corporate Office: 204 FIE, Industrial Area, Patparganj, Delhi 110 092
Ph: 4934 4934   Fax: 4934 4935   e-mail: publishing@cbspd.com; publicity@cbspd.com

Branches

- **Bengaluru:** Seema House 2975, 17th Cross, K.R. Road,
  Banasankari 2nd Stage, Bengaluru 560 070, Karnataka
    Ph: +91-80-26771678/79   Fax: +91-80-26771680   e-mail: bangalore@cbspd.com
- **Chennai:** 7, Subbaraya Street, Shenoy Nagar, Chennai 600 030, Tamil Nadu
    Ph: +91-44-26680620, 26681266   Fax: +91-44-42032115   e-mail: chennai@cbspd.com
- **Kochi:** 68/1534, 35, 36, Power House Road, Opp. KSEB, Kochi 682018, Kerala
    Ph: +91-484-4059061-65   Fax: +91-484-4059065   e-mail: kochi@cbspd.com
- **Kolkata:** 6/B, Ground Floor, Rameswar Shaw Road, Kolkata 700 014, West Bengal
    Ph: +91-33-22891126, 22891127, 22891128   e-mail: kolkata@cbspd.com
- **Mumbai:** 83-C, Dr E Moses Road, Worli, Mumbai 400018, Maharashtra
    Ph: +91-22-24902340/41   Fax: +91-22-24902342   e-mail: mumbai@cbspd.com

Representatives

Bhopal	0-8319310552	Bhubaneswar	0-9911037372	Hyderabad	0-9885175004
Jharkhand	0-9811541605	Nagpur	0-9421945513	Patna	0-9334159340
Pune	0-9623451994	Uttarakhand	0-9716462459		
Dhaka (Bangladesh)	01912-003485	Kathmandu (Nepal)	977-9818742655		

Printed at India Binding House, Noida, UP, India

Preface

After teaching dental students for more than 18 years, I realized that many dental students struggle to understand the concepts of general medicine. General medicine is a subject which overlaps with all other areas of dental and medical practice. Hence, general medicine is also called mother of all subjects. I strongly felt a need for a book in general medicine which is very easy to undesrstand without unnecessary details. The result is this book which is in front of you now. This book is very easy to understand and it contains only that much information which dental students require as per the syllabus of Dental Council of India. This book is especially useful for the students to prepare for the examination as the content is presented in Question–Answer style. Last chapter contains multiple choice questions (MCQs) which are being asked commonly nowadays as part of the theory paper in most of the universities. I am sure this book will help the dental students gain the required knowledge on general medicine and also prepare for their general medicine examination without any struggle and confusion.

Manthappa M

Contents

Preface   v

1. Infections   1

2. Respiratory System   26

3. Gastrointestinal System   50

4. Cardiovascular System   75

5. Hematology   115

6. Renal System   147

7. Nutritional Disorders   156

8. Nervous System   163

9. Endocrinology   177

10. Critical Care   201

11. Multiple Choice Questions   211

Index   227

General Medicine: Theory

1. **Introduction:** Aims of medicine, definitions of signs, symptoms, diagnosis, differential diagnosis, treatment and prognosis.

2. **Infections:** Enteric fever, approach to patient with fever, AIDS, herpes simplex, herpes zoster, syphilis, diphtheria, infectious mononucleosis, mumps, measles, rubella, malaria

3. **GIT:** Stomatitis, gingival hyperplasia, dysphasia, acid peptic disease, jaundice, hepatmegaly
   - Acute and chronic hepatitis, cirrhosis of liver, ascites, diarrhea, dysentery, amoebiasis, malabsorption

4. **CVS:** Acute rheumatic fever, rheumatic valvular heart disease, hypertension, ischemic heart diseases, infective endocarditis, common arrhythmias, congenital heart disease, congestive cardiac failure

5. **RS:** Pneumonia, COPD/emphysema, pulmonary TB, bronchial asthma, lung abscess, pleural effusion, pneumothorax, bronchiectasis

6. **Hematology:** Anemias, bleeding and clotting disorders, leukemias, lymphomas, agranulocytosis, splenomegaly, oral manifestations of hematologic disorders, generalized lymphadenopathy.

7. **Renal system:** Acute nephritis, nephrotic syndrome, renal failure

8. **Nutrition:** Avitaminosis, balanced diet, PEM, vitamin C, vitamin A,D,E,K, B-complex vitamins

9. **CNS:** Facial palsy, facial pain including trigeminal neuralgia, epilepsy, headache including migraine, meningitis, examination of comatose patient, examination of cranial nerves

10. **Endocrines:** Diabetes mellitus, acromegaly, hypothyroidism, thyrotoxicosis, calcium metabolism and parathyroids, Addison's disease, Cushing's syndrome

11. **Critical care:** Syncope, cardiac arrest, CPR, shock, acute LVF, ARDS

General Medicine: Clinical

The student must be able to take history, do general physical examination (including build, nourishment, pulse, BP, respiration, clubbing, cyanosis, jaundice, lymphadenopathy, oral cavity) and be able to examine CVS, RS and abdomen and facial nerve.

Infections

Definition of Fever

Fever is elevated body temperature or an elevation above a person's known normal daily value. Oral temperature of >37.2°C (>98.9°F) is called fever. Body temperature varies from morning to evening (diurnal variation). Lowest level is in the early morning and highest temperature is in the evening. This variation is about 0.5°C.

Pathophysiology

- Body temperature is maintained within a narrow range by a balance between mechanisms which produce heat and mechanisms which promote heat loss. Mechanisms which produce heat are metabolic reactions in the tissues particularly liver and muscles. Shivering also increases heat production. Mechanisms which promote heat loss are sweating and vasodilation. All these mechanisms are coordinated by the thermoregulatory center of hypothalamus.
- Fever results when the hypothalamic set point for temperature is set to a higher level. This happens due to release of endogenous pyrogens (e.g. IL-1, tumor necrosis factor [TNF]-α, interferon-γ, IL-6), by microbial products which raise the hypothalamic set point. This activates mechanisms which increase heat production such as peripheral vasoconstriction and shivering. Temperature rises till the hypothalamic set point is reached. Resetting the hypothalamic set point downward (e.g. with antipyretic drugs) initiates heat loss through sweating and vasodilation.
- Elevated body temperature that is not caused by a resetting of the temperature set point in the hypothalamus is called hyperthermia.

Causes of Fever

- *Infections (most common cause):* All infections can produce fever. Some of the common infections are: Upper and lower respiratory tract infections, GI infections, urinary tract infection, skin infection, etc.
- *Malignancies:* Leukemia, lymphoma, etc.
- *Inflammatory conditions (rheumatic diseases):* Systemic lupus erythematosus, rheumatoid arthritis, etc.

Consequences of Fever

- Most adults tolerate mild to moderate fever well. In fact, fever helps the body fight the infection in a better way. However, extreme temperature elevation (temperature >41°C) may be damaging. At this temperature, protein denaturation occurs, and inflammatory cytokines that activate the inflammatory cascade are released leading to multiorgan damage and death.

- Fever increases the BMR by about 10 to 12% for every 1°C increase over 37°C. This can cause additional load for a diseased heart and lung. Fever can also worsen mental status in patients with dementia. Hence, fever should be carefully monitored in such patients. Fever can reduce the threshold for seizures especially in children (febrile seizures).

APPROACH TO A CASE OF FEVER

History

- Ask about the magnitude and duration of fever. Ask about rigors (involuntary shivering). Presence of rigors usually indicates infection.
- Pain in a particular area can suggest infection in that area. Patient should be asked about pain in the ears, head, neck, teeth, throat, chest, abdomen, flank, rectum, muscles, and joints.
- Other localizing symptoms include nasal congestion and/or discharge (suggests rhinitis or influenza as the cause of fever), cough (suggests respiratory tract infection), diarrhea (intestinal infections), and urinary symptoms (frequency, urgency, dysuria; all these suggest urinary tract infection).
- Enquire about any rash. Some fevers such as measles, chickenpox are associated with rashes.
- Illicit use of injection drugs (predispose to endocarditis, hepatitis, septic pulmonary emboli, and skin and soft-tissue infections)
- *Past history:* Recent surgery (suspect wound or surgical site infection). History of rheumatic heart disease (infective endocarditis may develop and cause fever), HIV infection (prone to develop varieties of infections), diabetes (more prone for infections).
- *Travel history:* Important to suspect diseases endemic in some areas. For example, a person travelling to India may develop typhoid, malaria or tuberculosis.

- *Treatment history:* Some drugs can cause fever. Some drugs can predispose to increased risk of infection by suppressing immune system (e.g. corticosteroids, anticancer drugs).
- *Family history:* Many infections spread from one person to another person. For example, tuberculosis, malaria, dengue, etc. may spread among family members. Hence, if a family member already has an infection and another family member develops fever, it is likely that same infection has developed in that person.

Physical Examination

Vital Signs (temperature, pulse, BP, and respiratory rate)

- Record the temperature. Oral or axillary temperature is routinely measured.
- Check pulse rate, respiratory rate, and blood pressure. Pulse rate usually increases by 10 per degree Celsius rise in temperature. Relative bradycardia (i.e. pulse rate does not correspond to the raise in temperature) may be seen in enteric fever, brucellosis and some viral infections. Relative tachycardia, i.e. pulse rate more than expected to the raise in temperature may be seen in myocarditis, sepsis, hypovolemia and thyrotoxicosis. High respiratory rate usually points to some respiratory pathology such as pneumonia, empyema, ARDS, etc. Blood pressure may be low in cases of fever with septic shock.

General Examination

- General appearance (may appear sick and weak in severe infections).
- Inspect the skin for any rash, particularly petechial or hemorrhagic rash (seen in fevers with rash such as measles, dengue, etc.).
- Lymphadenopathy (suspect infectious mononucleosis, HIV, tuberculosis, etc.).
- Examine ears, nose and throat for any signs of infection such as tenderness, discharge, etc.

- Look for any neck stiffness (seen in meningitis).

Respiratory system: Look for signs of pneumonia (crepitations, bronchial breath sounds, increased vocal resonance).

CVS: Look for any murmurs (suggests possible endocarditis).

Abdomen: Hepatosplenomegaly is seen in many infections. Presence of tenderness indicates intra-abdominal infections such as peritonitis, liver abscess, etc.

Nervous system: Look for any altered mental status (seen in encephalitis, brain abscess, etc.).

Musculoskeletal system: All major joints are examined for swelling, erythema, and tenderness (suggesting a joint infection or rheumatologic disorder).

Investigations

- *Complete blood count:* Total leukocyte count and ESR is elevated in most of the infections. Neutrophilic predominance suggests bacterial infections and lymphocytic predominance suggests viral or chronic infections.
- *Liver function tests* (LFT) and *renal function tests* (urea and creatinine)
- *Tests to identify common infections* are malaria-QBC (to detect malarial parasite in the blood), WIDAL test (positive in cases of typhoid fever), blood culture (to identify the infecting organism), urine microscopy and culture (to identify urinary tract infection), etc.
- *Chest X-ray* (tuberculosis, pmeumonia).
- *Special tests* are ordered based on the history and examination findings. Examples are Paul-Bunnell test for infectious mononucleosis, HIV-ELISA, lumbar puncture and CSF analysis, if meningitis is suspected.

Treatment

- Treatment depends on the underlying cause. For example, antimalarials for

malaria, antibiotics for bacterial infection, etc.
- Until a diagnosis is made, it is better to use only symptomatic treatment. Blind antibiotic therapy may make diagnosis of an occult infection more difficult. Fever can be reduced by giving antipyretic agents such as paracetamol. Paracetamol is given in a dose of 500 to 650 mg three to four times daily.
- Tepid sponging can be used along with paracetamol to reduce temperature when fever is very high.

Q. Enteric fever (typhoid fever).

Etiology

- Typhoid is a systemic infection caused by *Salmonella typhi* or *paratyphi*.
- Salmonellae are gram-negative bacilli. Salmonellae are present worldwide but cause disease only where poor hygiene and overcrowding exist.

Pathogenesis

- Humans are the only reservoir of *Salmonella typhi*. Organisms originate from patients with typhoid, or from carriers excreting organisms in their stools. Human hands, flies, or insects then transfer these organisms to food or drink. Since *S. typhi* survive freezing and drying, infection can also occur through ice or canned food. Shellfish from polluted waters may transmit the disease.
- Once salmonellae reach the small intestine, the bacteria penetrate and traverse through the intestinal wall through phagocytic cells that reside within Peyer's patches. After crossing the epithelial layer of the small intestine, *S. typhi* and *S. paratyphi* are phagocytosed by macrophages.
- Once phagocytosed, salmonellae disseminate throughout the body in macrophages via the lymphatics and colonize reticuloendothelial tissues (liver, spleen, lymph nodes, and bone marrow) where

they start multiplying. Patients have relatively few or no signs and symptoms during this initial stage.

- Once the number of bacteria reaches a critical stage, they invade bloodstream and rest of the body. At this stage, signs and symptoms, such as fever and abdominal pain appear. Peyer's patches can get enlarged and necrosed due to mononuclear cell infiltration. Bacteria also reach gall-bladder via bloodstream and multiply there. From the gallbladder, bacteria reach the intestine and are excreted in the stool which can spread to others via con-taminated foods. Some patients become chronic carriers carrying the bacteria in their gallbladder and are responsible for much of the transmission of the organism. While asymptomatic, they may continue to shed bacteria in their stool for decades.

Clinical Features

- The incubation period averages 10 to 14 days.
- The onset of the disease is insidious, with headache, malaise, anorexia and fever. The fever is continuous (does not touch the baseline) sometimes increasing in a step-like manner (step ladder fever) to reach a peak towards the end of the first week. Thereafter it plateaus and remains for two to three weeks. Accompanying chills are common but frank rigors are rare. Headache is often present.
- Abdominal discomfort with mild bloating and constipation usually occurs, but diarrhea can also occur. Stools may have a 'pea soup' appearance.
- Hepatosplenomegaly may develop by the end of the first week. Mild jaundice may be present.
- The typical rash of typhoid (rose spots) develops in the second week but is seldom seen in Indian patients. 'Rose spots' are macules, 2–3 mm in size, occur in small crops on the chest and abdomen, blanch on pressure and last for 2–3 days.

Investigations

- The diagnostic 'gold standard' for enteric fever is culture of *S. typhi* or *S. paratyphi*. Blood cultures are usually positive in the first week of infection. Cultures of stool and urine may also be positive. Bone marrow culture is highly sensitive and may remain positive even with up to 5 days of antibiotic therapy.
- The Widal test is very helpful in diagnosis. The test is positive, if O antigen titer is more than 1:160. Titres against the flagellar (H) antigen are less specific. Usually it becomes positive after the 1st week of illness.
- Relative bradycardia and leukopenia may be present.
- LFT may show mild elevation of AST and ALT.

Treatment

- Third generation cephalosporins are currently the drugs of choice. Ceftriaxone (1 to 2 g intravenously or intramuscularly) for 10 to 14 days is the treatment of choice in severe typhoid.
- Other antibiotics effective against typoid are ofloxacin, levofloxacin and azithro-mycin.
- Paracetamol is given to control fever, headache and myalgia.
- Other supportive measures include good nutrition and hydration. Soft and bland diet should be given because of inflamed intestines.
- Some patients become chronic carriers of typhoid bacilli. They can be a source of infection to others. Carrier state can be treated with oral amoxicillin or trime-thoprim-sulphamethoxazole or cipro-floxacin. Antibiotics should be given for 6 weeks.

Complications

- Complications are uncommon now due to availability of effective antibiotics.
- *Intestinal bleeding:* Erosion of blood vessels in necrotic Peyer's patches or in the intestinal wall can initiate bleeding.

- *Intestinal perforation:* Typhoid ulcers can perforate. Usually, happens in 3rd week of illness.

- Typhoid can affect almost all the organs. Hence, pneumonia, meningitis, nephritis, cholecystitis, hepatitis, myocarditis, osteomyelitis, encephalitis can occur.

- Involvement of the central nervous system can present as stupor, delirium, convulsions, encephalitis, cerebellar ataxia, extrapyramidal signs, myopathy and deafness.

- Acute renal failure and disseminated intravascular coagulation are rare complications.

Prevention

- Both oral and injectable typhoid vaccines are available now for the prevention of typhoid. Vaccination against typhoid is recommended for persons traveling to developing countries and people who have intimate or household contact with a case or chronic carrier.

- Vaccines provide protection for 3 to 5 years.

Q. Typhoid carrier.

- A person who excretes *Salmonella* organism in stool for more than 12 months after the acute infection is called chronic carrier.

- About 1 to 6% patients become chronic carriers after *Salmonella typhi* infection, and the rate is higher in patients with cholelithiasis or other biliary tract abnormalities.

- Chronic carriers do not develop recurrent symptomatic disease. They develop high level systemic immunity so that they do not develop clinical disease but excrete large numbers of organisms in the stool.

- Chronic carriers act as source of infection to others, particularly if involved in food preparation. Hence, eradication of carrier state should be done, if such individuals are identified.

Treatment

Fluoroquinolones are the drugs of choice to eradicate carrier state (e.g. ciprofloxacin or ofloxacin for 4 weeks). Cholecystectomy should be considered, if there is any abnormality such as cholelithiasis.

Q. Dicuss the etiology, pathogenesis, clinical features, investigations and treatment of diphtheria.

Diphtheria is a localized infection of mucous membranes or skin characterized by a *characteristic pseudomembrane* at the site of infection.

Etiology

- Diphtheria is caused by *Corynebacterium diphtheriae*, a gram-positive bacillus. *C. diphtheriae* appear like *Chinese letter patterns* on *Albert's stain* (Fig. 1.1).

- There are 3 strains of *C. diphtheriae*—mitis, intermedius and gravis. Gravis causes the most severe disease.

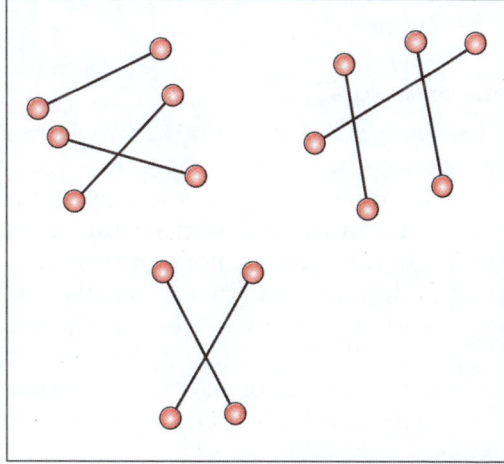

Fig. 1.1: Diphtheria bacilli

Epidemiology

- Diphtheria affects people all over the world. It is mainly a disease of children. It is more common during winter, but now it is uncommon due to immunization practices.

- Humans are the main reservoir of *C. diphtheriae*. Spread occurs in close-contact settings through respiratory droplets or by direct contact with respiratory secretions or skin lesions.

Pathogenesis

- Diphtheria is initiated by entry of *C. diphtheriae* into the nose or pharynx. It multiplies locally without bloodstream invasion.
- It produces a powerful exotoxin which causes local tissue necrosis, and formation of a tough, adherent *pseudomembrane*, composed of a mixture of fibrin, dead cells, and bacteria. The membrane usually begins on the tonsils or posterior pharynx and can spread to fauces, soft palate, and into the larynx, which may result in respiratory obstruction. Toxin entering the bloodstream causes tissue damage at distant sites, particularly the heart (myocarditis), nerves (demyelination), and kidneys (tubular necrosis).
- Nontoxigenic strains may cause mild local respiratory disease, sometimes including a membrane.

Clinical Features

- The faucial (pharyngeal) form is most common. After an incubation period of 1 to 7 days, the illness begins with a sore throat, malaise, and mild to moderate fever. Grayish membrane may be present that is tightly adherent and bleeds on attempted removal. In severe cases, the patient appears toxic. Cervical lymphadenopathy and soft tissue edema may occur, resulting in the typical *bull-neck appearance* and stridor.
- Nose infection presents as a chronic serosanguineous or seropurulent discharge. A whitish membrane may be observed on the septum.
- Laryngeal involvement presents as hoarseness, stridor, and dyspnea.
- Myocarditis presents with signs of low cardiac output and congestive heart failure.

Conduction disturbances, ST-T wave abnormalities, arrhythmias, and heart block can occur.
- Neurologic involvement manifests as cranial nerve palsies and peripheral neuritis. Palatal and/or pharyngeal paralysis occurs during the acute phase.
- Cutaneous diphtheria lesions are classically indolent, deep, punched-out ulcers, which may have a grayish white membrane.

Investigations

- Gram's stain: A presumptive diagnosis of *C. diphtheriae* can be made by identifying gram-positive rods in a 'Chinese letter' distribution on Gram's stain.
- Cultures from beneath the membrane, from the nasopharynx, and from suspicious skin lesions.
- Toxigenicity testing should be performed on all *C. diphtheriae* isolates.
- Polymerase chain reaction test may allow both detection of the organism and determination of toxigenicity.
- ECG may show abnormalities.

Treatment

The goals of treatment are to neutralize the toxin, eliminate the infecting organism, provide supportive care, and prevent further transmission.

Antitoxin

- Diphtheria antitoxin is a hyperimmune antiserum produced in horses, which inactivates the diphtheria toxin.
- The antitoxin is only effective before toxin enters the cell and thus must be administered as early as possible.
- There is risk of allergic reactions to antitoxin since it contains horse serum. Hence, a test dose should be given before administration.
- The dose of antitoxin depends upon the site and severity of infection. 20,000 to 40,000

units for pharyngeal/laryngeal disease, 40,000 to 60,000 units for nasopharyngeal disease, and 80,000 to 120,000 units for severe disease with 'bull-neck'. The dose should be administered intravenously over 60 minutes.

Antibiotics

- They decrease toxin production indirectly by killing the organisms.
- Penicillin is the drug of choice. Penicillin is given intravenously initially followed by oral therapy for a total of 2 weeks.
- Erythromycin is an alternative.

Diphtheria Toxoid

Patients should be given diphtheria toxoid immunization during their convalescence since natural infection does not induce immunity.

Prevention

- Isolate the patient.
- Non-immunized contacts should be given both antibiotics and diphtheria antitoxin.
- Immunized contacts are given a booster dose of diphtheria toxoid.

Q. Syphilis.

- Syphilis is a sexually transmitted disease caused by the spirochete *Treponema pallidum*.
- It is characterized by episodes of active disease interrupted by periods of latency.

Etiology

- Syphilis is caused by *Treponema pallidum* which belongs to spirochete group.
- It is spiral in shape. Live organisms can only be seen under dark-ground illumination because of poor resolution with conventional light microscopy. *Treponema* organisms have characteristic to-and-fro, undulating, corkscrew-like and angulating movements.

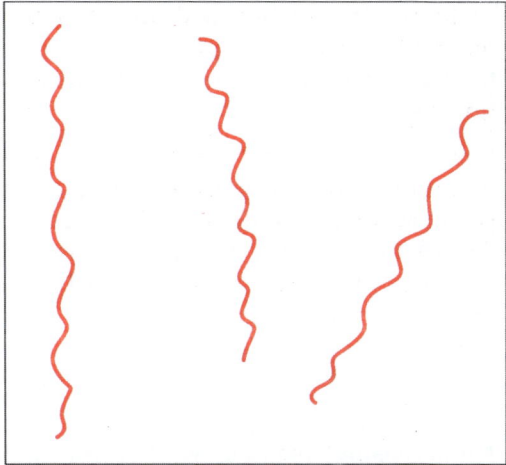

Fig. 1.2: *Treponema pallidum*

Syphilis is becoming a rare disease now after the discovery of penicillin. However, efforts to eradicate this disease have been unsuccessful.

Pathophysiology

- The only known natural host for *T. pallidum* is man.
- Almost all cases of syphilis are acquired by sexual contact. Less commonly it is acquired by nonsexual personal contact, infection *in utero* (congenital syphilis), and blood transfusion. 1 in 2 persons exposed to infection gets infected.
- Acquired syphilis has predictable stages though there may not be clear cut demarcation between the stages. Four stages can usually be recognized and include: 1. *Primary*, 2. *secondary*, 3. *latent*, and 4. *tertiary* syphilis.
- *Primary syphilis:* In acquired syphilis, after exposure, *T. pallidum* penetrates intact mucous membranes or dermal abrasions and enters the lymphatics and blood to produce systemic infection. Primary syphilis is characterized by the development of a painless chancre at the site of entry after an incubation period of 3–6 weeks. The lesion has a punched-out base and rolled edges and is highly infectious. Histologically, the chancre is characterized

by local inflammation with infiltration by macrophages and lymphocytes. Whether treated or not, healing occurs with residual fibrosis.

- *Secondary syphilis* develops several weeks or months after the appearance of the primary lesion. During this stage, the spirochetes multiply and spread throughout the body. Secondary syphilis has numerous clinical manifestations. Common manifestations include malaise, fever, myalgias, arthralgias, lymphadenopathy, and rash.

- *Latent syphilis* is characterized by resolution of skin lesions and other clinical manifestations. However, serologic tests are positive for *T. pallidum*.

- *Tertiary or late syphilis* develops years after the initial infection (5–10 years later) and can involve any organ system. The most dreaded complications are neurosyphilis and involvement of the aortic valve and root. Initially syphilis mainly involves meninges and vasculature of CNS (meningovascular syphilis), later the parenchyma of brain and spinal cord is involved.

- Regardless of the stage of disease and location of lesions, histopathologic hallmarks of syphilis are endarteritis and a plasma cell-rich infiltrate. The syphilitic infiltrate is actually a delayed-type hypersensitivity response to *T. pallidum*, and can result in gummatous ulcerations and necrosis seen in tertiary syphilis. Antigens of *T. pallidum* induce treponemal antibodies and nonspecific reagin antibodies.

Clinical Features

Primary Syphilis

The typical lesion is a primary chancre which begins as a single painless papule that rapidly becomes eroded and usually becomes indurated. It has a firm consistency. In heterosexual men, the chancre is usually located on the penis, whereas in homosexual men, it is often found in the anal canal or rectum, in the mouth, or on the external genitalia. In women, it is usually found on the cervix and labia. Regional lymphadenopathy is usually seen. Lymph nodes are firm, nonsuppurative, and painless.

Secondary Syphilis

- Secondary syphilis has protean manifestations. These include skin and mucous membrane lesions and generalized painless lymphadenopathy. The healing primary chancre may be still present in some cases. The skin lesions are macular, papular, papulosquamous rashes, and occasionally pustules. The rashes may be very subtle and may be missed. Initial lesions are bilaterally symmetric, pale red or pink, nonpruritic, discrete, round macules that measure 5 to 10 mm in diameter and are distributed on the trunk and proximal extremities. After many days or weeks, red papular lesions appear. These lesions may progress to pustular lesions.

- In warm and moist areas like perianal area, vulva, scrotum, etc., papules can enlarge and become eroded to produce moist, pink or gray-white, highly infectious lesions called condylomata lata. Mucosal lesions include erosions, called mucous patches and occur on lips, oral mucosa, tongue, palate, pharynx, vulva and vagina, glans penis. The mucous patch is painless with a red periphery.

- Constitutional symptoms may accompany secondary syphilis and include fever, weight loss, malaise, anorexia and headache. Meningitis can occur rarely.

- Less commonly there can be hepatitis, nephropathy, arthritis, periostitis, iritis and uveitis.

Latent Syphilis

In latent syphilis, serologic tests for syphilis are positive but there are no clinical manifestations. In latent syphilis, *T. pallidum* is present in the body. Latent syphilis can get transmitted to the fetus *in utero* and to others through blood transfusion.

Tertiary Syphilis

Tertiary syphilis is characterized by a persistent low-level burden of pathogens, against which a potent and self-destructive immune response is mounted. It is usually very slowly progressive and noninfectious. Any organ of the body may be involved, but three main types are: *Neurosyphilis, cardiovascular syphilis* and *gummatous (late) syphilis.*

Neurosyphilis

- Neurosyphilis can be meningeal, meningovascular, and parenchymatous syphilis. The last category includes general paresis and tabes dorsalis. Meningeal syphilis occurs usually within one year after infection, meningovascular syphilis occurs 5 to 10 years after infection, general paresis after 20 years, and tabes dorsalis after 25 to 30 years.

- Meningeal syphilis presents with typical signs and symptoms of meningitis like headache, nausea, vomiting, neck stiffness, and alteration of mental status.

- Meningovascular syphilis involves meninges and also blood vessels leading to stroke.

- General paresis happens due to widespread brain parenchymal damage and includes abnormalities corresponding to the mnemonic PARESIS—**p**ersonality disturbances, **a**ffect abnormalities, **r**eflex hyperactivity, **e**ye abnormality (Argyll Robertson pupils), **s**ensorium changes, **i**ntellectual impairment and **s**lurred speech.

- In tabes dorsalis, there is demyelination of the posterior columns, dorsal roots, and dorsal root ganglia. Symptoms include ataxic wide-based gait, paresthesia, bladder disturbances, impotence, areflexia, loss of joint position, deep pain, and temperature sensations. Argyll Robertson pupil can be seen in both tabes dorsalis and general paresis. It reacts to accommodation but not to light.

Cardiovascular syphilis: Cardiovascular manifestations are due to endarteritis obliterans of the vasa vasorum, which provide blood supply to large vessels. This results in weakening of tunic media and formation of aneurysm, aortitis (with linear calcification of the ascending aorta on chest X-ray), aortic regurgitation, or coronary ostial stenosis. Symptoms usually appear 10 to 40 years after infection. The most common finding on cardiovascular examination is a diastolic murmur with a tambour quality, secondary to aortic dilation with valvular insufficiency.

Gummatous syphilis (late syphilis): Gummas are nothing but areas of granulomatous inflammation with a central area of necrosis. Gummas may be single or multiple and size varies from microscopic to many centimeters. The most commonly involved sites are skin, mucous memebranes and skeletal system. Gummas of the skin produce painless and indurated nodular lesions which may breakdown to form punched-out ulcers with vertical edges. The ulcer heals in the middle with an atrophic tissue-paper scar and spreads peripherally. The base of the lesion is dull red and appears like 'wash-leather'. Nocturnal bone pain may occur due to bone involvement.

Congenital Syphilis

- Transmission of *T. pallidum* from a syphilitic woman to her fetus across the placenta may occur at any stage of pregnancy, but the lesions in fetus develop after the fourth month of gestation.

- Treatment of the mother before 4th month of gestation can prevent fetal damage. Untreated maternal infection may lead to abortion, stillbirth, prematurity, neonatal death, or nonfatal congenital syphilis.

- Among infants born alive, congenital syphilis may or may not be clinically apparent.

- All women should be screened for syphilis in early pregnancy. In areas of high prevalence serologic screening should be repeated in the third trimester and at delivery.

- The manifestations of congenital syphilis can be divided into three types:

  1. *Early manifestations:* Appear within the first 2 years of life. These are due to infection of various organs by *Treponema pallidum* and resemble secondary syphilis in the adult. These include rhinitis (snuffles), bullae (syphilitic pemphigus), vesicles, petechiae, papulosquamous lesions, mucous patches, and condylomata lata. The most common early manifestations are bone changes including osteochondritis, osteitis, and periostitis. Hepatosplenomegaly, lymphadenopathy and jaundice are also common.

  2. *Late manifestations:* Appear after 2 years and are noninfectious manifestations. These include interstitial keratitis, eighth-nerve deafness, recurrent arthropathy and bilateral knee effusions known as Clutton's joints. Neurosyphilis and gummatous periostitis can also occur.

  3. *Residual stigmata:* These include Hutchinson's teeth (centrally notched, widely spaced, peg-shaped upper central incisors) and 'mulberry' molars (molars with multiple, poorly developed cusps). There can be abnormal facies like frontal bossing, saddle nose, and poorly developed maxillae. Saber shins, characterized by anterior tibial bowing, are rare. Rhagades are linear scars at the angles of the mouth and are caused by healing of early facial eruption.

Diagnosis

The diagnosis of syphilis is suspected based on history and clinical features. Since the clinical features are protean, lab confirmation of diagnosis is required.

Dark-Field Microscopy

This is the most specific technique for diagnosing syphilis and can demonstrate *Treponema pallidum* in samples taken from chancre and condylomata lata. But dark-field microscopy is not widely available.

Non-Treponemal Tests

- These include venereal disease research laboratory (VDRL) test and rapid plasma reagin (RPR) test.
- Syphilitic infection leads to the production of non-specific antibodies that react to cardiolipin. This reaction is the basis of VDRL and rapid plasma reagin (RPR) test. Nontreponemal tests are widely used for syphilis screening.

Treponemal-specific Tests

- Treponemal-specific tests detect antibodies to antigenic components of *T. pallidum*. These tests are used primarily to confirm the diagnosis of syphilis in patients with a positive nontreponemal test.
- Treponemal-specific tests include the EIA (enzyme-linked immunoassay) for anti-treponemal IgG, the *T. pallidum* hemagglutination (TPHA) test, the microhemagglutination test with *T. pallidum* antigen, and the fluorescent treponemal antibody-absorption test (FTA-ABS).

Treatment

- *Primary syphilis:* The treatment of choice is parenteral long-acting penicillin such as benzathine penicillin, given in a single dose of 2.4 million units in equally divided portions in each buttock deep IM. For penicillin allergic patients, doxycycline 100 mg BD for 1 month should be given. Doxycycline is contraindicated in pregnant women and children. In such cases, penicillin should be administered after desensitization. Ceftriaxone 1 g daily IM/IV for 8 to 10 days is an alternative. At 6 and 12 months after treatment, patients with primary syphilis should be reexamined and undergo repeat serologic testing.
- *Secondary syphilis:* Treatment and follow up is same as primary syphilis.

- *Latent syphilis:* Early latent syphilis is treated in the same way as primary syphilis. Late latent syphilis is treated with 2.4 million units of benzathine penicillin given IM once a week for three weeks.
- *Tertiary syphilis:* Treatment for gummatous and cardiovascular syphilis is the same as that of late latent syphilis. Neurosyphilis should be treated with intravenous penicillin G (3 to 4 million units IV Q 4h for 10 to 14 days) followed by benzathine penicillin 2.5 million units deep IM once a week for 3 weeks. Cetriaxone 2 g daily IV or IM for 10–14 days is an alternative.
- *Congenital syphilis:* A single dose of 50,000 units of penicillin per kg should be given.

Q. VDRL (venereal disease research laboratory) test.

- VDRL is a nontreponemal antibody test to diagnose syphilis. It is quite sensitive but not very specific for syphilis. VDRL is reactive in 78% of patients with primary syphilis. It becomes positive within 4 to 6 weeks after infection or 1 to 3 weeks after the appearance of the primary lesion. Thus, these tests can be negative in early syphilis. VDRL can also be negative in some untreated patients in late syphilis. Hence, VDRL cannot be relied on for diagnosis in very early or late stage of syphilis.
- False positive VDRL test can occur in infections (TB, HIV, Lyme disease, infectious mononucleosis, malaria), pregnancy, connective tissue diseases, liver disease, and malignancy.
- Because of frequent false positive and false negative VDRL test, all positive tests and and all negative tests in patients in whom syphilis is strongly suspected clinically, should be verified by a specific treponemal test.
- The nontreponemal tests are quite useful for monitoring the patient's response to treatment, because the titers reflect disease activity.

Q. Discuss the transmission, pathogenesis, clinical features, investigations and management of human immunodeficiency virus (HIV) infection (AIDS).

Q. Enumerate the AIDS (acquired immunodeficiency syndrome) indicator conditions.

Q. Opportunistic infections in AIDS.

- Human immunodeficiency virus (HIV) is a single-stranded RNA virus belonging to retroviridae family. It is spherical in shape and has a lipid membrane lined by a matrix protein that is studded with glycoprotein (gp)120 and gp41 spikes surrounding a cone-shaped protein core. The core contains two copies of the single-stranded RNA genome and viral enzymes.

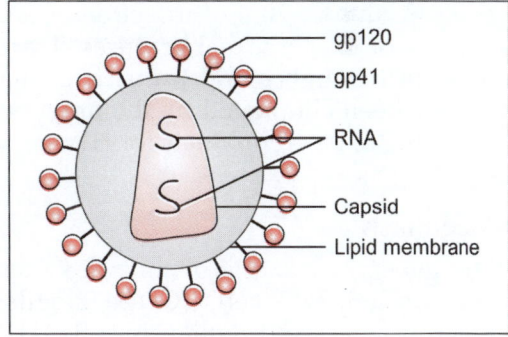

Fig. 1.3: HIV

- HIV infection leads to AIDS (acquired immunodeficiency syndrome), a condition in which the immune system begins to fail, leading to life-threatening opportunistic infections. Immune deficiency is due to destruction of CD4 lymphocytes. Most of the AIDS cases are caused by HIV-1. HIV-2 causes a similar illness to HIV-1 but is less aggressive and is seen mainly to western Africa.
- AIDS was first recognized in the United States in 1981 in male homosexuals. Since

then, it has grown to become a major pandemic in the world. It has become the second leading cause of disease burden world-wide and the leading cause of death in Africa. Two-thirds of these cases are in developing countries, mainly sub-Saharan Africa and Southeast Asia.

- Most AIDS cases occur in adults aged 25–49 years (70% of cases).

Transmission of HIV

- Transmission of HIV occurs through almost any body fluid such as blood, semen, vaginal fluid, or breast milk. Within these bodily fluids, HIV is present as both free virus particles and virus within infected immune cells.

- The four major routes of transmission are unsafe sex, contaminated needles, breast milk, and transmission from an infected mother to her baby at birth (vertical transmission). >70% of infections occur because of unsafe sexual practices. Transmission through blood transfusion has largely been eliminated by the universal screening of blood products for HIV.

Pathogenesis

- HIV infects mainly cells of immune system such as helper T cells (CD4+ T cells), macrophages, and dendritic cells. HIV enters into these cells by binding to CD4 receptor through its gp120 molecule. The virus replicates itself by generating a DNA copy by reverse transcriptase. Viral DNA becomes incorporated into the host DNA, enabling further replication.

- HIV infection leads to fall in CD4+ T cells. When CD4+ cell count declines below a critical level, cell-mediated immunity is lost. Progressive failure of immune system leads to development of AIDS characterized by development of opportunistic infections and malignancies. The speed of progression of HIV infection to AIDS is variable depending on viral load, host, and environmental factors. Most will progress to AIDS within 10 years of HIV infection.

Clinical Stages and Natural History of HIV Infection

Clinical HIV infection undergoes three distinct phases—acute seroconversion, asymptomatic infection, and AIDS.

Acute Seroconversion (Primary Infection, Acute HIV Infection)

- This stage is characterized by rapid viral replication leading to an abundance of virus in the peripheral blood. There is a marked drop in the numbers of circulating CD4+ T cells. It usually occurs 2 to 6 weeks after exposure to HIV and lasts an average of 28 days. The immune system responds to the replication of virus by activation of CD8+ T cells, and antibody production against the viral antigens. Hence, this phase is also called seroconversion phase.

- Most people develop flu-like illness during this stage. Common symptoms are fever, lymphadenopathy, pharyngitis, rash, myalgia, malaise, aphthous ulcers, hepatosplenomegaly, oral candidiasis, and weight loss. All these signs and symptoms are not specific for HIV infection and can be seen in many other infectious diseases. Hence, diagnosis may be missed at this stage.

Asymptomatic Infection

During this stage (category A disease in CDC classification), strong immunity reduces the viral load and patient may remain asymptomatic except for the possible presence of persistent generalized lymphadenopathy (PGL, defined as enlarged lymph nodes at ≥ 2 extra-inguinal sites). But HIV remains active within lymphoid organs, and also as free viral particles. Patient remains infective during this stage also. CD4 count decreases usually at a rate between 50 and 150 cells/year. Asymptomatic infection lasts for a variable period (can last from 2 weeks to 10 years or more).

AIDS Stage

This stage (category C in CDC classification) is characterized by signs and symptoms of various opportunistic infections. The CD4 count is usually below 200/mm^3.

CDC Classification System for HIV-infected Adolescents and Adults

This system is based on three ranges of CD4+ cell counts and clinical conditions associated with HIV (Table 1.1).

Clinical Categories of HIV Infection

Category-A: Consists of one or more of the conditions listed below in an adolescent or adult (>13 years) with documented HIV infection. Conditions listed in categories B and C must not have occurred.
- Asymptomatic HIV infection
- Persistent generalized lymphadenopathy
- Acute (primary) HIV infection with accompanying illness or history of acute HIV infection

Category-B: Consists of symptomatic conditions in an HIV-infected adolescent or adult that are not included among conditions listed in clinical category C and that meet at least one of the following criteria: (1) The conditions are attributed to HIV infection or are indicative of a defect in cell-mediated immunity; or (2) the conditions are considered by physicians to have a clinical course or to require management that is complicated by HIV infection. Examples include, but are not limited to, the following:
- Bacillary angiomatosis
- Oropharyngeal candidiasis (thrush)
- Vulvovaginal candidiasis, persistent or resistant
- Pelvic inflammatory disease (PID)
- Cervical dysplasia (moderate or severe)/cervical carcinoma *in situ*
- Hairy leukoplakia, oral
- Herpes zoster (shingles), involving two or more episodes or at least one dermatome
- Idiopathic thrombocytopenic purpura
- Constitutional symptoms, such as fever (>38.5°C) or diarrhea lasting >1 month
- Peripheral neuropathy

Category C (AIDS indicator conditions)
- Candidiasis of bronchi, trachea, or lungs
- Candidiasis, esophageal
- Cervical cancer, invasive
- Coccidioidomycosis, disseminated or extrapulmonary
- Cryptococcosis, extrapulmonary
- Cryptosporidiosis, chronic intestinal (>1 month's duration)
- Cytomegalovirus disease (other than liver, spleen, or nodes)
- Cytomegalovirus retinitis (with loss of vision)
- Encephalopathy, HIV-related
- Herpes simplex: chronic ulcer(s) (>1 month's duration); or bronchitis, pneumonia, or esophagitis
- Histoplasmosis, disseminated or extra-pulmonary
- Isosporiasis, chronic intestinal (>1 month's duration)
- Kaposi's sarcoma
- Lymphoma, Burkitt's (or equivalent term)
- Lymphoma, primary, of brain

Table 1.1: CDC classification for HIV-infected patients			
CD4 cell categories	A– asymptomatic, PGL or acute	B–symptomatic (not A or C) HIV infection	C–AIDS indicator condition
>500/mm^3	A1	B1	C1
200–499/mm^3	A2	B2	C2
<200/mm^3	A3	B3	C3

- *Mycobacterium avium* complex or *M. kansasii*, disseminated or extrapulmonary
- *Mycobacterium tuberculosis*, any site (pulmonary or extrapulmonary)
- *Mycobacterium*, other species or unidentified species, disseminated or extrapulmonary
- *Pneumocystis jirovecii* pneumonia
- Pneumonia, recurrent
- Progressive multifocal leukoencephalopathy
- *Salmonella* septicemia, recurrent
- Toxoplasmosis of brain
- Wasting syndrome due to HIV

Investigations

- HIV ELISA and western blot test
- CD4 count
- Viral load
- Hepatitis B surface antibody (HBsAg)
- Hepatitis C IgG antibody
- Hepatitis A IgG antibody
- Toxoplasma antibody
- Cytomegalovirus (CMV) IgG antibody
- Treponema serology (VDRL and TPHA)
- Chest X-ray

MANAGEMENT OF HIV INFECTION

Management of HIV infection can be broadly divided into following categories:

1. Treatment of the HIV infection itself with ART (antiretroviral therapy)
2. Prophylaxis for opportunistic infections
3. Treatment of opportunistic infections and complications of HIV.
4. Rreduction of HIV transmission (mother-to-child and person-to-person).

Treatment of the HIV Infection Itself

- The aims of HIV treatment are to decrease viral load to an undetectable level (<50 copies/mL) for as long as possible and improve the CD4 count to above 200 cells/mm^3.
- The availability of antiretroviral agents has drastically improved the prognosis of HIV-infected patients. Patients who receive successful ART have stabilization or improvement of their clinical condition, improved life expectancy and decrease in AIDS-related complications.

When to Initiate ART (Antiretroviral Therapy)

- Latest guidelines recommend that ART should be started for all people with a confirmed HIV diagnosis and a CD4 count of 500 cells/mm^3 or less.
- It is also recommended to initiate ART in people with active TB disease, all pregnant and breastfeeding women with HIV, regardless of CD4 cell count.

First-line ART Regimens

- First-line ART should consist of two nucleoside reverse transcriptase inhibitors (NRTIs) plus a non-nucleoside reverse-transcriptase inhibitor (NNRTI). **T**enofovir + **L**amivudine (or **E**mtricitabine) + **E**favirenz (remember TLEE) as a fixed-dose combination is recommended as the preferred option to initiate ART.
- If the above regimen is contraindicated or not available, one of the following options is recommended:
- Zidovudine + Lamivudine + Efavirenz (ZLE)
- Zidovudine + Lamivudine + Nevirapine (ZLN)
- Tenofovir + Lamivudine (or Emtricitabine) + Nevirapine (TLEN)
- Second-line ART for adults should consist of two nucleoside reverse-transcriptase inhibitors (NRTIs) + a ritonavir-boosted protease inhibitor (PI).

Prophylaxis for Opportunistic Infections

Prophylaxis of opportunistic infections are usually based on the CD4 count. If the CD4 count increases above the levels that are used to initiate prophylaxis—prophylactic therapy can be discontinued (Table 1.2).

Table: 1.2: Prophylaxis for opportunistic infections		
Opportunistic infection	*Indication for prophylactic therapy*	*Prophylactic regimen*
Pneumocystis jirovecii pneumonia	CD4 counts below 200 cells/μL	Trimethoprim-sulfamethoxazole, one double-strength tablet (960 mg) daily or dapsone 50–100 mg daily
Mycobacterium avium complex infection	CD4 counts below 75–100 cells/μL	Azithromycin (1200 mg orally weekly) or clarithromycin (500 mg orally twice daily)
M. tuberculosis infection	All HIV-infected patients with positive PPD reactions (defined as >5 mm of induration for HIV-infected patients)	
Toxoplasmosis	Patients with a positive IgG toxoplasma serology and CD4 counts below 100 cells/μL	Isoniazid, 300 mg daily, plus pyridoxine, 50 mg orally daily, for 9–12 months
CMV infection	CD4 counts below 50 cells/μL and positive serum CMV IgG antibody	Trimethoprim-sulfamethoxazole (one double-strength tablet daily) Ganciclovir (1000 mg orally three times daily)

Treatment of Opportunistic Infections and Complications of HIV

Table 1.3: Treatment of opportunistic infections and complications of HIV	
Opportunistic infection or complication	*Treatment*
Pneumocystis jirovecii infection	Trimethoprim-sulfamethoxazole
Mycobacterium avium complex infection	Clarithromycin with ethambutol
Toxoplasmosis	Pyrimethamine combined with sulfadiazine
Cryptococcal meningitis	Amphotericin B
Cytomegalovirus infection	Valganciclovir or ganciclovir or foscarnet
Esophageal candidiasis or recurrent vaginal candidiasis	Fluconazole
Herpes simplex infection and herpes zoster	Acyclovir or famciclovir or valacyclovir or foscarnet.
Kaposi sarcoma	Observation or intralesional vinblastine for limited cutaneous disease. Combination chemotherapy (e.g. daunorubicin, bleomycin, vinblastine) for extensive or aggressive disease

Reduction of HIV Transmission (Mother-to-Child and Person-to-Person)

Prevention of Mother-to-Child Transmission

During antenatal period, zidovudine (ZDV) 300 mg twice daily should be given starting at 14 to 34 weeks gestation and continued throughout the pregnancy. During labor, intravenous administration of ZDV, 2 mg/kg loading dose, followed by a continuous infusion of 1 mg/kg per hour until delivery should be given. After delivery, the neonate should be given 2 mg/kg ZDV syrup orally four times daily for the first 6 weeks of life, beginning at 8–12 hours after birth.

Prevention of Person-to-Person Transmission

- Precautions regarding sexual practices and injection drug use.
- Universal screening of donor blood and blood products for HIV.
- Infection control practices in the health care setting.
- Vaccines are under development.
- Post-exposure prophylaxis, if there is accidental exposure to a known source of HIV.

Q. Post-exposure prophylaxis (PEP) for HIV.

- *Immediate decontamination*: Wash the area with soap and water. Small wounds and punctures may be cleansed with an antiseptic such as alcohol, iodophors, or chlorhexidine. For mucous membrane exposure, irrigate the area with water or sterile saline.
- *Testing of source of exposure:* Voluntary testing for HIV antibody, hepatitis C virus antibody, and hepatitis B surface antigen (HBsAg); if HIV test is positive, confirmatory Western blot and CD4 count. If the source patient's rapid HIV test is negative but there has been a risk for HIV exposure in the previous 6 weeks, plasma HIV RNA testing is recommended.
- *Testing of exposed person*: Testing for HIV antibody, HCV antibody, HbsAg, and hepatitis B surface antibody (HBsAb); in females of child-bearing age, pregnancy testing.
- *Recommended regimen*: Three-drug PEP regimens are now the recommended regimens for all exposures due to the safety and tolerability of new HIV drugs. The preferred 3-drug PEP regimen is as follows: **Tenofovir (TDF)** combined with either **lamivudine (3TC)** or **emtricitabine (FTC)** as preferred backbone drugs. The recommended third drug is **raltegravir** 400 mg

PO twice daily. The duration of treatment is 28 days.

- PEP should be initiated as soon as possible, ideally within 2 hours of exposure; a first dose of PEP should be offered to the exposed worker while the evaluation is underway.
- Repeat HIV testing should be done at 4 and 12 weeks post-exposure.

Q. Herpes simplex.

Herpes simplex viruses are ubiquitous and cause a wide variety of diseases. There are two types: Herpes simplex virus type 1 (HSV-1) and type 2 (HSV-2). HSV-1 usually causes gingivostomatitis, herpes labialis, and herpes keratitis. HSV-2 usually causes genital lesions.

Pathogenesis

- Transmission of HSV results from close contact with a person who is actively shedding virus.
- After the initial infection, HSV remains dormant in nerve ganglia, and can get activated during stress such as febrile illness, overexposure to sunlight, physical or emotional stress, immunosuppression, etc.

Diseases Caused by Herpes Simplex

- **Herpetic gingivostomatitis:** It is usually caused by HSV-1, typically in children. Rarely HSV-2 can also involve gingiva and oral cavity through oral-genital contact. Lesions consists of clusters of small vesicles on an erythematous base. Leisons are usually painful and after a few days, rupture leaving behind yellowish crust. Healing occurs 8 to 12 days after onset. Local infection can spread systemically in immunocompromised patients. After resolution, the virus resides dormant in the trigeminal ganglion and can get reactivated later.
- **Herpes labialis:** It is usually a secondary outbreak of HSV. It develops as ulcers (cold sores) on the lip or as ulcerations of the mucosa of the hard palate.

- **Herpetic whitlow:** It is a swollen, painful, erythematous lesion of the distal phalanx which results from inoculation of HSV through the skin.
- **Genital herpes:** It is a sexually transmitted disease. It is usually caused by HSV-2, although a small number of cases are caused by HSV-1. Lesions consist of vesicles which can break and form ulcers. Lesions occur on the genitals. They may occur around the anus and in the rectum in men or women who engage in receptive rectal intercourse. Healing of ulcers may leave behind scaring.
- **Herpes simplex keratitis:** Infecton of the cornea is called keratitis. HSV infection of the corneal epithelium causes pain, tearing, photophobia, and corneal ulcers.
- **Neonatal herpes simplex:** Infection develops in neonates transmitted during birth through contact with vaginal secretions containing usually HSV-2. It usually develops between the 1st and 4th week of life, often causing mucocutaneous vesicles or CNS involvement.
- **CNS infection:** Herpes encephalitis occurs sporadically and may be severe. Patients often present with seizures and altered conscious level. There may be speech disturbances.

Investigations

- Tzanck test (a superficial scraping from the base of a freshly ruptured vesicle stained with Wright-Giemsa stain) often reveals multinucleate giant cells in HSV infection.
- Viral culture for serious disease
- Serological tests
- PCR of CSF in cases of encephalitis
- MRI brain for HSV encephalitis

Treatment

- Antiviral drugs such as acyclovir, valacyclovir, or famciclovir are used to treat herpes simplex infections. Intravenous acyclovir is given for herpes encephalitis.
- For keratitis, topical trifluridine is used.

Q. Varicella (chickenpox) (HHV-3).

Q. Herpes zoster (shingles).

- Varicella-zoster virus (VZV; human herpes virus-3) is a DNA virus and belongs to Herpesviridae family.
- It produces two clinical entities—varicella (chickenpox) and herpes zoster (shingles).
- Chickenpox is the primary infection, and usually occurs in childhood. Chickenpox rarely occurs twice but the virus remains latent in the dorsal root and cranial nerve ganglia. Years later it may be reactivated to cause vesicular eruption in the relevant sensory dermatomes which is known as herpes zoster (shingles). Sometimes the virus may affect a motor nerve such as the facial nerve to produce facial palsy.

Varicella (Chickenpox)

- Chickenpox affects children commonly.
- Incubation period is 10 to 21 days.
- There may be a prodrome of low grade fever, headache and malaise lasting 1 to 2 days before the onset of rash.
- Rashes appear first on the face and trunk and then spread to other parts of the body. Lesions can also be found on the mucosa of the pharynx and vagina. To start with rashes are maculopapular and in a few hours become vesicles. Vesicles become pustules which later form crusts. New lesions continue to appear for 2 to 4 days so that all stages of the eruption are present simultaneously (pleomorphic rash). Rashes usually heal without scarring. Lesions can get secondarily infected with bacteria.
- Complications include CNS involvement in the form of cerebellar ataxia, meningitis, encephalitis, transverse myelitis, Guillain-Barre syndrome, varicella pneumonia, myocarditis, nephritis, hepatitis and arthritis. Reye's syndrome (hepatic encephalopathy), another complication, is associated with aspirin therapy.
- The clinical diagnosis can be confirmed where necessary by isolation of virus in

tissue culture, demonstrations of high titres of antibodies or the detection of VZV DNA by PCR. Tzanck smear made by scraping of the base of the lesions may show multi-nucleated giant cells.

- Most people recover with supportive treatment. Antibiotics may be used for secondary skin infection. Antiviral agents like acyclovir, famciclovir and valacyclovir are recommended for adolescents and adults with chickenpox of ≤24 hours duration.

Herpes Zoster (Shingles)

- Herpes zoster is the consequence of reactivation of latent VZV from the dorsal root ganglia.
- The first symptom is severe burning or shooting pain in the affected dermatome followed by erythematous maculopapular eruption in 2 to 3 days. These eruptions turn into vesicles and start crusting. The skin eruption is unilateral.
- The total duration of disease is generally between 7 and 10 days.
- The dermatomes from T3 to L3 are commonly affected.
- In ophthalmic herpes, the trigeminal ganglion is affected and the ophthalmic branch of the trigeminal nerve is involved. Lesions develop on the nose, conjunctiva and cornea of the affected side. Corneal lesions heal leaving behind opacities causing blindness.
- Complications of herpes zoster are post-herpetic neuralgia and CNS involvement. In post-herpetic neuralgia, pain persists even after the lesions have healed. CNS complications include meningoencephalitis and transverse myelitis. Sometimes weakness and wasting in segments supplied by the nerve root may occur due to motor neuritis. Immunocompromised patients can develop severe disease with multiorgan involvement.

Treatment

Antiviral drugs are indicated for the treatment of shingles. Drugs used are same as for varicella (acyclovir, famciclovir and valacyclovir). Herpes zoster causes severe pain which may be difficult to control. NSAIDs, opioid analgesics can be used along with neuron modulator drugs such as carbamazepine, gabapentin, amitriptyline and lidocaine patches to control pain.

Q. Infectious mononucleosis (glandular fever).

Etiology

- Infectious mononucleosis (IM) is a disease caused by Epstein-Barr virus (EBV). EBV is a DNA virus belonging to the family Herpesviridae. EBV also causes many tumors in human beings like nasopharyngeal carcinoma, Burkitt's lymphoma, Hodgkin's disease, and B cell lymphoma.
- Infectious mononucleosis (IM) is also known as *glandular fever* or *kissing disease*. Later it was called infectious mononucleosis because it is characterized by atypical mononuclear cells in the blood.
- It is characterized by a triad of fever, pharyngitis, and lymphadenopathy.

Pathogenesis

- In humans, it spreads commonly through saliva ('the kissing disease') and rarely by blood transfusion.
- After entry into the body, the virus multiplies primarily in B lymphocytes but also may replicate in the epithelial cells of the pharynx and parotid duct. Infected B cells are responsible for the dissemination of infection throughout the lymphoreticular system, i.e. liver, spleen, and peripheral lymph nodes. Infected B lymphocytes produce antibodies against the virus. Cytotoxic T cells are also produced by the body against the EBV-infected B lymphocytes.

Clinical Features

- Incubation period is 4–8 weeks. Infectious mononucleosis is a disease of childhood, adolescence and low socioeconomic groups.

- Initially, there is a prodrome of fatigue, malaise, and myalgia.
- Prodrome is followed by typical features such as fever, sore throat, and lymphadenopathy.
- Fever is usually low grade. Lymphadenopathy most often affects the posterior cervical nodes but may be generalized. Rarely hepatosplenomegaly may be found.
- A generalized maculopapular rash is occasionally seen. Rash may develop, if ampicillin is taken.
- IM should be suspected in an adolescent or young adult with fever, sore throat and lymphadenopathy (especially posterior cervical lymphadenopathy).
- The illness usually lasts 2–4 weeks but weakness can persist for a long time.
- Complications include splenic rupture, thrombocytopenia, autoimmune hemolytic anemia, meningitis, encephalitis, and GB-syndrome.

Investigations

- Blood tests show raised leukocyte count with atypical lymphocytosis.
- Liver enzymes may be raised but jaundice is rare.
- Paul-Bunnell test and monospot test (detect heterophile antibodies) are usually positive.
- Demonstration of antibodies to viral capsid antigen (i.e. VCA-IgG and VCA-IgM).

Differential Diagnosis

- Other infections which produce fever and lymphadenopathy: Streptococcal pharyngitis, cytomegalovirus, acute HIV, or toxoplasma.
- Lymphoma.

Treatment

- There is no specific treatment for infectious mononucleosis. Antiviral drugs do not have much benefit.

- Supportive measures, rest and antipyretics are given as required.
- Ampicillin should be avoided in suspected infectious mononucleosis because it causes rash.

Q. Measles (rubeola).

Measles (also known as rubeola) is an acute viral exanthematous disease.

Etiology

Measles is caused by measles virus which is an RNA virus belonging to the family of paramyxoviruses.

Epidemiology

- It most commonly affects preschool children. Incidence of measles has come down after the introduction of measles vaccine.
- Measles virus is transmitted by inhalation of respiratory droplets. It can also spread through direct contact with larger droplets.
- The virus is present in nasopharyngeal secretions, blood, and urine during the prodromal period and for a short time after the rash appears.
- Patients are contagious from 1 or 2 days before the onset of symptoms until 4 days after the appearance of the rash. Infectivity is maximum during the prodromal phase.

Clinical Features

- Incubation period is 10 to 14 days.
- Measles starts with a prodrome of malaise, cough, lacrimation, nasal discharge, and fever. At this stage, it resembles influenza.
- Just before the onset of the rash, Koplik's spots appear as 1 to 2 mm blue-white spots on a bright red background. Koplik's spots are usually seen on the buccal mucosa alongside the second molars. They are characteristic of measles because they are not seen in any other disease. The spots disappear after the onset of rash.

- Rash appears 3–4 days after the onset of fever. Rash begins first at the hairline and behind the ears, and then spreads to the trunk and limbs. Rashes do not spare the palms and soles, are erythematous, non-pruritic, and maculopapular. Rash is mono-morphic, i.e. all rashes have similar mor-phology. Rash begins to fade by the fourth day, in the order in which it appeared.
- The entire illness lasts about 10 days. The disease tends to be more severe in adults than in children.

Diagnosis

- Diagnosis is mainly by clinical features.
- Serum anti-measles IgM antibody is detec-table three days after the appearance of rash. Anti-measles IgG antibody appears 7 days after the appearance of rash.
- Demonstration of measles antigen by immunofluorescent staining of a smear of respiratory secretions.
- Measles virus can be cultured and isolated from respiratory secretions or urine.
- PCR for measles virus RNA can also diagnose measles.

Treatment

- There is no specific treatment for measles.
- Patient should be isolated.
- Most people recover spontaneously and only supportive treatment is necessary.
- Ribavirin may be considered for use in immunocompromised individuals.
- Administration of vitamin-A has been shown to prevent complications especially in malnourished children.
- Secondary bacterial complications are treated with appropriate antibiotics.

Complications

- *Respiratory tract complications:* Laryng-itis, croup, or bronchitis, otitis media, pneumonia.
- *CNS complications:* Encephalitis, trans-verse myelitis, subacute sclerosing pane-

ncephalitis (SSPE). SSPE is a chronic, rare form of measles encephalitis. It is common in children who have measles before the age of 2 years. SSPE is now rare due to widespread vaccination against measles. Clinical features are progressive dementia which evolves over several months.
- *Gastrointestinal complications:* Hepatitis, appendicitis, and mesenteric adenitis.
- *Others:* Myocarditis, glomerulonephritis, postinfectious thrombocytopenic purpura and reactivation of tuberculosis.

Prevention

- Immediate protection can be obtained by giving immunoglobulin within 6 days of exposure to the disease. Measles vaccine given within 72 hours of exposure may also protect against disease.
- Active immunization with measles vaccine is included in the national immunization programme. A single dose of vaccine is given at 8 to 9 months of age. It provides lifelong immunity. Giving MMR vaccine at 15 to 18 months takes care of occasional failure of measles vaccine given at 8 to 9 months of age. However, if there is an epidemic of measles, vaccination may be given at 6 months of age followed by another dose or MMR vaccine at 15 months.

Q. Mumps.

Mumps is a systemic viral infection whose most distinctive feature is swelling of parotid glands. It can involve other salivary glands, meninges, pancreas, and the gonads.

Etiology

Mumps is caused by mumps virus which is a member of the paramyxovirus group. It is an RNA virus.

Epidemiology

- Mumps occurs worldwide but the inci-dence has decreased after the introduction of mumps vaccine (MMR).

- Mumps occurs mainly during winter and spring. It is mainly a disease of childhood, but nowadays adults are getting affected more commonly. Both sexes are affected equally.
- Epidemics occur in close populations, such as in schools and military services.
- Mumps is highly infectious and spreads rapidly among susceptible people living in close quarters.
- Mumps virus is transmitted by droplet nuclei, saliva, and fomites. Fomites contaminated by infected saliva and possibly also by urine transmit the infection. Transmission of infection occurs a day before the appearance of the parotid swelling and for about three days after the swelling disappears.
- One attack of mumps or vaccination confers lifelong immunity.

Clinical Features

- Incubation period is 2–3 weeks.
- Mumps starts with a prodrome of fever, malaise, myalgia, and anorexia.
- Parotitis may develop within the next 24 h or may be delayed up to a week. Parotitis is usually bilateral, although sometimes only one side is affected. Parotid glands are involved most commonly and submaxillary and sublingual glands are involved rarely. Parotid gland becomes swollen and tender. Gland swelling increases for a few days and then gradually subsides within a week.
- Other than parotitis, orchitis is the most common manifestation. Testis becomes swollen, painful and tender. Testicular atrophy develops in half of the affected men. However, since orchitis is usually unilateral and other testis remains unaffected, sterility is rare. Oophoritis can occur in women but less common than orchitis and does not lead to sterility.
- Aseptic meningitis is a common manifestation of mumps in both children and adults. Rarely, encephalitis can occur. Other CNS problems occasionally seen are cerebellar ataxia, facial palsy, transverse myelitis, and Guillain-Barré syndrome.
- Other clinical manifestations are pancreatitis, myocarditis, mastitis, thyroiditis, nephritis, arthritis, and thrombocytopenic purpura.

Differential Diagnosis

Mumps has to be differentiated from other causes of parotid gland swelling, such as:
  o Influenza, parainfluenza and coxsackie virus infections
  o Bacterial parotitis
  o Obstruction of Stenson's duct by a calculus
  o Parotid tumor
  o Sarcoidosis
  o Sjögren's syndrome

Diagnosis

Diagnosis is mainly by clinical features.
- Serological detection of IgM antibodies.
- Virus islolation by culturing appropriate clinical specimens.
- PCR

Treatment

- Symptomatic treatment; analgesics and antipyretics for fever and pain, cold compresses for parotid swelling.
- Patients with meningitis or pancreatitis may require hospitalization for intravenous fluids.
- Patients with orchitis are also treated symptomatically with bed rest, non-steroidal anti-inflammatory agents, support of the inflamed testis and ice packs.

Prevention

- Patients should be isolated to prevent transmission to others.
- Passive immunization using immunoglobulin is not effective to prevent infection in close contacts and is not recommended.
- Active immunization is routinely given as MMR vaccine (measles, mumps, rubella)

subcutaneously at 15 months of age or later; repeat dose may be necessary after 5–10 years. MMR vaccine is also recommended for susceptible older children, adolescents, and adults, particularly adolescent males who have not had mumps. Vaccine should not be given to pregnant women, immunosuppressed patients, or persons with advanced malignancies.

Q. Rubella (German measles).

- Rubella is an acute viral exanthematous disease caused by rubella virus, an RNA virus.
- It is also known as German measles because it was first recognized to be different from measles in Germany.

Epidemiology

- Humans are the only natural hosts for rubella infection.
- It spreads by respiratory droplets or is maternally transmitted to the fetus causing congenital infection.
- The peak incidence of the disease is in children of 5–12 years of age.

Clinical Manifestations

- The incubation period is usually 2–3 weeks.
- The disease is characterized by fever, rash, and lymphadenopathy.
- It is more severe in adults than children.
- There is usually a prodrome of low grade fever, malaise, anorexia and sore throat, followed by lymphadenopathy and appearance of skin rash. Rash often begins on the face and spreads down the body. It is maculopapular but not confluent. It disappears in the same order. Lymphadenopathy usually affects suboccipital, cervical and post-auricular nodes but rarely axillary nodes can also be involved. Complications are rare and include arthritis (in women), encephalitis and thrombocytopenia.

Congenital Rubella

Maternal infection in early pregnancy can lead to fetal infection, leading to teratogenic effects and congenital rubella. Sensorineural hearing loss is the most common manifestation of congenital rubella syndrome. Other signs of congenital rubella are cataract, heart disease (patent ductus arteriosus), deafness, and many other defects like mental retardation, microcephaly, and thrombocytopenic purpura. Infection in the first trimester leads to more severe congenital rubella in the fetus.

Investigations

- Most cases are mild and are difficult to diagnose on clinical grounds.
- Rubella can be diagnosed by specific IgM rubella antibody and also by virus isolation.

Treatment

- Isolate the patient for 7 days after the onset of rash to prevent infection to others.
- There is no specific treatment. Most cases recover spontaneously.
- Antipyretics, like paracetamol, can be used to treat fever.

Prevention

- Presently all infants are routinely immunized against rubella by giving MMR vaccine at 12–15 months of age.
- Vaccine is administered in a single dose of 0.5 mL subcutaneously. Immunity wanes after 10–15 years and hence the vaccine may have to be repeated at 10–15 years of age.
- Live rubella vaccine is contraindicated during pregnancy and it is recommended that pregnancy be avoided for at least 3 months after rubella vaccination.

Q. Malaria.

Malaria is a protozoan disease caused by *Plasmodium* species of protozoa.

Etiology

Five species of *Plasmodium* namely, *Plasmodium vivax*, *P. falciparum*, *P. ovale*, *P. malariae* and *P. knowlesi* are responsible for almost all human infections. Out of these, *P. falcifarum* causes severe infection and is responsible for most of the deaths due to malaria.

Epidemiology

Malaria is the most important of the parasitic diseases of humans. It has been eliminated from the United States, Canada, Europe, and Russia. Malaria is very common in tropical countries such as Africa, Asia, New Guinea, and Hispaniola.

Pathogenesis and Life Cycle of Malarial Parasite (Fig. 1.4)

- It is transmitted by the bite of infected Anopheles mosquitoes.
- It affects mainly the hepatocytes and RBCs and manifests clinically as fever and splenomegaly.
- Human infection begins when a female anopheline mosquito bites man and inoculates sporozoites into the blood. These sporozoites are motile forms of the malarial parasite and are carried via the bloodstream to the liver.

- In the liver, sporozoites invade hepatic parenchymal cells and start multiplying there to produce merozoites (asexual cycle). This is known as pre-erythrocytic schizogony or merogony. In *P. vivax* and *P. ovale* infections, some sporozoites become hypnozoites and do not multiply. These hypnozoites can remain dormant for up to a year or longer before starting multiplication. These dormant forms are the cause of the relapses in vivax and ovale.
- After 8–14 days, the swollen liver cell containing merozoites bursts, releasing motile merozoites into the bloodstream. Each merozoite can invade an RBC and start multiplying there.
- Inside the RBCs, merozoites become trophozoites and appear as 'ring forms' in the early stages of development. As the trophozoite grows, the parasite assumes an irregular or ameboid shape. The fully grown trophozoite occupies most of the RBC and is called a schizont. This schizont contains many merozoites. When the RBC ruptures, merozoites are released, each capable of invading a new RBC and repeating the cycle.

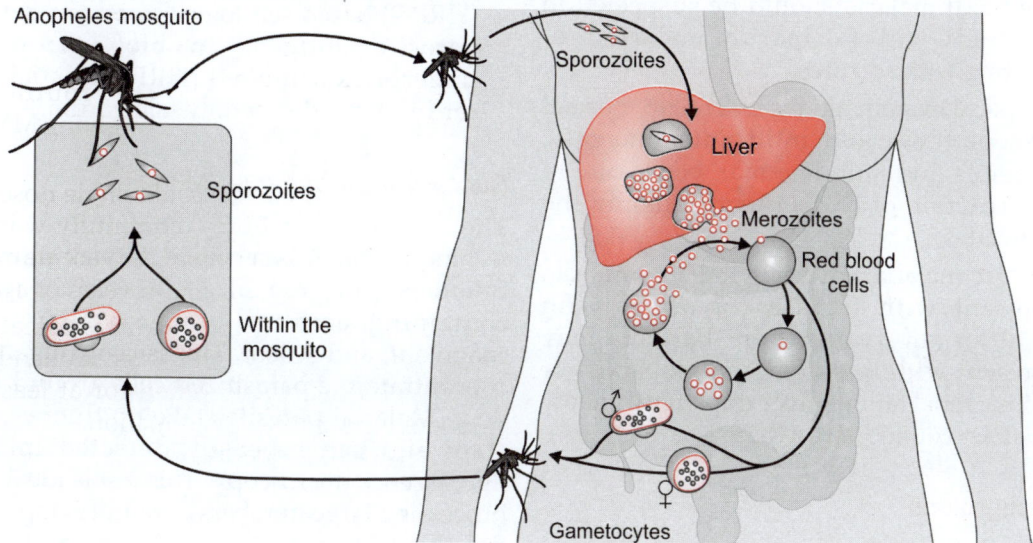

Fig. 1.4: Malarial parasite—life cycle

- Some of the merozoites after release from liver or RBCs develop into gametocytes (sexual forms) which are picked up by mosquitoes when they bite human beings. Inside the mosquito, male and female gametocytes join and develop into motile sporozoites, which are inoculated into man during mosquito bite.
- Malaria can also develop after blood transfusion without any incubation period.

Clinical Features

- The incubation period for vivax, ovale and falciparum infection is 8–24 days. For *P. malariae*, it is 15–30 days.
- The initial symptoms of malaria are non-specific and include malaise, nausea, vomiting, headache, fatigue, body ache and fever. Some cases may also have abdominal pain, arthralgia, or diarrhea. Classic malarial symptoms with intermittent fever, chills, and rigors are usually seen with *P. vivax* or *P. ovale* infection but not in all cases.
- Fever in vivax and ovale comes once in 3 days (tertian malaria) and once in 4 days in *P. malariae* (quartan malaria). In falciparum, fever comes daily and does not follow any pattern.
- Cerebral malaria should be suspected in anybody with falciparum malaria presenting with seizures.
- Physical examination is essentially normal except fever and mild splenomegaly. Anemia and jaundice may occur due to destruction of RBCs (hemolysis) by the parasites.
- Severe malaria, especially falciparum, can present with features of sepsis with multiorgan dysfunction. Patients may present with impaired consciousness or coma, renal failure, liver impairement, low platelet counts, and ARDS.

Investigations

- It is difficult to diagnose malaria clinically with accuracy; hence treatment should be started on clinical grounds pending laboratory confirmation.

Peripheral Smear

The diagnosis of malaria can be easily made by demonstration of asexual forms of parasites in the peripheral blood smear. If initial smears are negative, repeat smears should be made preferably at the time of fever. Thick and thin smears are made and stained with Giemsa stain.

Rapid Diagnostic Tests (RDT)

- These antigen detection tests are rapid and almost as sensitive as thick smear.
- A drop of blood is placed on the dipstick or card, which is then immersed in washing solutions. If malarial antigen is present in the blood, it is captured by the antibody which appears as a colored band. One band is genus specific (all malarias), and the other is specific for *P. falciparum.*
- *Plasmodium LDH-based tests:* The pLDH-based assays specifically detect the parasite lactate dehydrogenase enzyme using a panel of monoclonal antibodies. Different species can be identified. Example is OptiMAL test.
- *HRP-2-based tests:* Histidine-rich protein-2 (HRP-2) based serologic assays can detect parasite antigens in blood from a fingerprick sample. PfHRP2 dipstick or card test can detect only falciparum.

Fluorescent Technique (MP-QBC)

The quantitative buffy coat (QBC) is a technique that is as sensitive as thick smears. Blood is collected in a glass micro-tube containing acridine orange stain, anti-coagulant, and a float. This is centrifuged to concentrate the parasitized cells around the float. Malarial parasites take up fluorescent stain and can be easily detected under fluorescence microscopy. This test is ideal for processing large numbers of samples rapidly. But this test cannot identify the species of malaria.

Other Laboratory Findings

There may be anemia, increased WBC count, neutrophilia, and increased ESR. In severe falciparum malaria, there may be metabolic acidosis, increased bilirubin, elevated liver enzymes, thrombocytopenia, increased urea, creatinine, and hypoglycemia.

Treatment

Chloroquine-sensitive Strains

- Chloroquine **or** Amodiaquine for 3 days.
- In addition to above, primaquine should be given for 14 days to prevent relapse in vivax malaria.

Severe Falciparum Malaria

Artesunate **or** artemether **or** quinine injection.

Supportive Measures

Include IV fluids, antipyretics, blood transfusion to correct severe anemia, and bed rest.

Prevention of Malaria

Decreasing the Mosquito Population

- Spraying of insecticides
- Biological methods such as use of mosquito larva eating fish in water reservoirs.

Personal Protection

Use of clothes extending up to the wrists and ankles when outdoors and mosquito nets when indoors to avoid mosquito bites. Application of insect-repellant creams on the exposed body surfaces like legs and hands.

Chemoprophylaxis

- Recommended for nonimmune visitors to endemic areas and to pregnant women living in endemic areas.
- Travelers should start taking antimalarial drugs at least 1 week before visiting the area and continue for 4 weeks after returning from the endemic area.
- Chloroquine 500 mg per week or mefloquine 250 mg orally per week or doxycycline 100 mg orally once daily can be used for prophylaxis.

Malaria Vaccine

Efforts are under way to develop a vaccine against *P. falciparum*.

Complications of Malaria

Complications usually happen in severe falciparum malaria. These are:

- o Cerebral malaria
- o Renal failure
- o Acute respiratory distress syndrome (ARDS), and respiratory failure
- o DIC (disseminated intravascular coagulation)
- o Hemoglobinuria
- o Jaundice

Respiratory System

Q. Describe the etiopathogenesis, clinical features, differential diagnosis and treatment of bronchial asthma.

- Asthma is a chronic inflammatory disease of airways characterized by increased responsiveness of the tracheobronchial tree to multiple stimuli.
- It is characterized by episodic airflow obstruction, which is reversible.
- Clinically, asthma presents as episodes of dyspnea, wheezing and cough. In between the episodes, the person is usually normal.

Incidence and Prevalence

About 10% of the world's population are affected by asthma. It can occur at any age, but commonly starts before the age of 10 years. In childhood, there is 2:1 male/female preponderance, but the sex ratio equalizes by the age of 30.

Etiology

Asthma is a heterogeneous disease with both endogenous and environmental factors playing a role. Several risk factors have been implicated.

- *Genetic predisposition:* The familial association of asthma and a high degree of concordance for asthma in identical twins indicate a genetic predisposition to the disease.

Risk factors involved in asthma	
Genetic predisposition	Early viral infections
Atopy	Indoor and outdoor
Obesity	allergens
Airway	Diet
hyper-responsiveness	Air pollution
Ethnicity (common in	Occupational sensitizers
Europeans)	Respiratory infections

- *Atopy:* Atopy refers to genetic predisposition to develop an allergic reaction (as allergic rhinitis, asthma, or atopic dermatitis) and produce elevated levels of IgE upon exposure to an environmental antigen. Atopy is the major risk factor for asthma, and nonatopic individuals have a very low risk of developing asthma.
- *Airway hyper-responsiveness:* Airway hyper-responsiveness is due to chronic inflammation of the airways, which leads to bronchospasm and typical symptoms of wheezing, shortness of breath, and coughing after exposure to allergens, environmental irritants, viruses, cold air, or exercise.
- *Ethnicity:* Asthma is more common in industrialized western countries.
- *Obesity:* Obese individuals seem to be at higher risk of developing asthma.
- *Allergens:* Inhaled allergens are common triggers of asthma symptoms and have also

been implicated in allergic sensitization. Exposure to house dust mites in early childhood is a risk factor for allergic sensitization and asthma. Domestic pets, particularly cats, have also been associated with allergic sensitization.

- *Diet:* The role of dietary factors is controversial. Observational studies have shown that diets low in antioxidants such as vitamin C and vitamin A, magnesium, selenium, and omega-3 polyunsaturated fats (fish oil) or high in sodium and omega-6 polyunsaturates are associated with an increased risk of asthma. Vitamin D deficiency may also predispose to the development of asthma.

- *Air pollution:* Air pollutants such as sulfur dioxide, ozone, and diesel particulates may trigger asthma symptoms.

- *Occupational sensitizers:* Exposure to chemicals such as toluene diisocyanate and trimellitic anhydride, may lead to sensitization independent of atopy. Individuals may also be exposed to allergens in the workplace such as small animal allergens in laboratory workers and fungal amylase in wheat flour in bakers.

- *Respiratory infections:* Many viral illnesses (rhinovirus, respiratory syncytial virus) have been known to trigger asthma attack. Many patients with asthma have coexistent sinusitis.

Pathogenesis

- Basically, asthmatics have bronchial hyper-responsiveness compared to normal people. Hence, stimuli that do not produce any clinical response in normal individuals can produce clinical symptoms in asthmatics.

- Bronchial hyper-responsiveness is due to persistent subacute inflammation of the airways. The airways are edematous and infiltrated with eosinophils, neutrophils, and lymphocytes. The inflammatory cells present in airways release mediators on provocation which produce broncho-constriction, vascular congestion, edema

formation, increased mucus production, and impaired mucociliary transport.

- Provocating factors include allergens like pollen, house-dust, mite, drugs like NSAIDs, exercise, inhalation of cold air, infections of the respiratory tract, air pollution, cigarette smoke, strong scents and perfumes, etc.

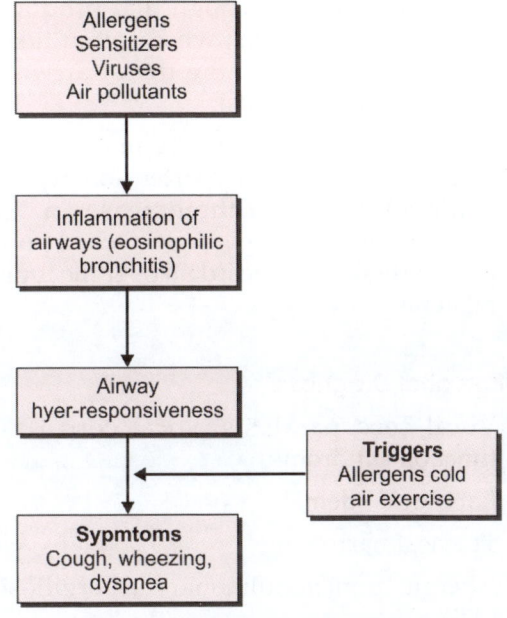

Fig. 2.1: Pathogenesis of asthma

Types

Asthma can be classified into two types—extrinsic and intrinsic asthma (Table 2.1).

Table 2.1: Classification of asthma		
	Extrinsic (atopic)	*Intrinsic*
Etiology	Allergic	Idiopathic
Hereditary predisposition	Yes	No
Onset	Early in life	Late in life
Serum IgE levels	Elevated	Normal
Symptoms	Usually seasonal	perennial
History of allergy	Yes	No

Clinical Features

- The symptoms of asthma consist of a triad of intermittent and reversible attacks of dyspnea, cough, and wheezing. All three symptoms coexist in a typical attack of asthma.

- Asthma usually worsens at night especially early morning. The end of an attack is usually marked by cough that produces thick, stringy mucus, which often takes the form of casts of the distal airways (Curschmann's spirals).

- Examination shows tachypnea, tachycardia, mild systolic hypertension, hyperrinflated lungs, with increase in AP diameter of the thorax. High-pitched polyphonic rhonchi are heard all over the lungs bilaterally.

Differential Diagnosis

- Vocal cord paralysis, vocal cord dysfunction syndrome
- Laryngeal edema
- Tracheal narrowing
- Allergic bronchopulmonary aspergillosis (ABPA)
- Endobronchial disease such as foreign-body aspiration, neoplasm, or bronchial stenosis
- Acute left ventricular failure (cardiac asthma)
- COPD
- Eosinophilic pneumonias

Investigations

- Blood examination may show increased eosinophils.
- Total serum immunoglobulin E levels are frequently elevated.
- *Chest X-ray* may show hyperinflation.
- Pulmonary function tests show a decrease in the forced vital capacity (FVC), peak expiratory flow rate (PEFR) and forced expiratory volume in one second (FEV_1). The FEV_1/FVC ratio is usually less than 75%. The diagnosis of asthma is established by demonstrating reversible airway obstruction. Reversibility is traditionally defined as a ≥15% increase in FEV_1 after two puffs of a β_2-adrenergic agonist.

- Arterial blood gas analysis shows respiratory alkalosis and in severe attacks hypoxia. However, in respiratory failure, CO_2 retention causes respiratory acidosis.

- Skin prick tests are done to identify the allergen in case of allergic or atopic asthma.

Treatment

Controlling Trigger Factors

Avoidance of asthma 'triggers' is important in successful asthma management. It will prevent frequent attacks and also the requirement of medications. Common asthma triggers include: Allergens, respiratory infections, inhaled irritants such as tobacco smoke and air pollutants, exposure to cold air, and emotional stress. Drugs such as beta-blockers and NSAIDs can precipitate an attack and should be avoided.

Drug Treatment

Drugs used in the treatment of asthma can be divided into two categories.

1. First category is drugs that relax the smooth muscle (called 'quick relief medications'). Quick relief medicines are used to treat an acute attack. They can be used as and when required basis. These include β-adrenergic agonists, methylxanthines, and anticholinergics.

2. Second category is drugs that prevent and/or reverse inflammation (called 'long-term control medications'). These medicines prevent or decrease the attacks of asthma. Usually, they are used on a regular basis. These include inhaled glucocorticoids, long-acting β_2-agonists, mast cell stabilizers, and leukotriene modifiers.

Quick relief medications (Table 2.2)

Table 2.2: Quick relief medications	
Drug category	*Mechanism of action*
Adrenergic stimulants Salbutamol, levosalbutamol, terbutaline, adrenaline	They are first-line therapy in acute attack. They act through adrenergic β_2 receptors which mediate smooth muscle relaxation. They can be given orally or by inhalation or by nebulization. Adrenaline and terbutaline can be given parenterally also.
Methylxanthines Theophylline, doxofylline	They act by inhibiting phosphodiesterase enzyme. They are usually used along with β_2-agonists in acute attacks.
Anticholinergics Ipratropium bromide, thiotropium bromide	They have only modest efficacy. They are particularly helpful in patients with heart disease, in whom the use of methylxanthines and β-adrenergic stimulants may be dangerous.

Long-term control medications: These medicines prevent or decrease the number of attacks by preventing or reversing airway inflammation (Table 2.3).

Table 2.3: Long-term control medications	
Drug category	*Mechanism of action*
Inhaled glucocorticoids Beclomethasone Budesonide Flunisolide Fluticasone Triamcinolone	Decrease air way inflammation. Since the drug is directly delivered to lungs, they have less systemic side effects and less pituitary adrenal suppression.
Systemic glucocorticoids Prednisolone Dexamethasone	Decrease in airway inflammation. Especially useful in acute severe attack of asthma but remember that they are not quick relief medications.
Long-acting β_2-agonists Salmeterol Formoterol	Relaxation of bronchial smooth muscle for a long time
Mast cell stabilizers Cromolyn Nedocromil	They inhibit the degranulation of mast cells thus preventing the release of mediators
Leukotriene modifiers Montelukast Zafirlukast Zileuton	Inhibit the synthesis of leukotrienes which mediate airway inflammation

Prognosis

Asthma is a chronic relapsing disorder. Most patients have recurrent attacks but there is no progressive lung damage like COPD.

Q. Acute severe asthma (status asthmaticus).

Acute episodes of bronchial asthma are one of the most common respiratory emergencies. If not treated in time, death may occur due to asphyxia. Patient should be treated in an intensive care unit.

Clinical Features

- Patient appears severely breathless.
- Patient may be restless or drowsy due to hypoxia and hypercarbia.
- There may be cyanosis, paradoxical pulse, use of accessory muscles, inability to speak in sentences, unable to recline, and marked hyperinflation of the chest.
- Severe ronchi are heard bilaterally all over the lung fields.
- A silent chest on auscultation suggests that there is no air movement in and out of lungs due to severe airway obstruction and is a sign of impending respiratory failure.

Investigations

- ECG to rule out MI with pulmonary edema which can also present with dyspnea and wheezing.
- Chest X-ray is usually normal except hyperinflation. It is also helpful to rule out other causes of breathlessness such as pulmonary edema, pneumonia, and pneumothorax, etc.
- ABG and PEFR may be done, if feasible.

Treatment

Supplemental Oxygen

Should be given to maintain adequate oxygenation.

Bronchodilators

- Frequent administration of β_2-agonist through nebulization is the most important measure. Nebulizations are repeated as necessary till the patient feels better. Inhalers also can be used, if the patient can take it.
- Administration of anticholinergic bronchodilators such as ipratropium bromide is also helpful.
- Intravenous aminophylline infusion can also be helpful in addition to nebulized bronchodilators.
- Terbutaline injection can be given subcutaneously, and may be repeated 2–4 hourly depending upon the response.

Systemic Corticosteroids

Methylprednisolone or hydrocortisone or dexamethasone should be given intravenously for 2 days.

Magnesium Sulfate

Intravenous magnesium sulfate may be considered in patients not responding to above therapies. It relaxes bronchial smooth muscle by inhibiting calcium influx.

Mechanical Ventilation

May be required in respiratory failure or impending respiratory failure.

Antibiotics

Antibiotics are indicated, if there is evidence of infection. Sedatives are contraindicated during an acute attack unless the patient is intubated.

Q. Chronic obstructive pulmonary disease (COPD).

Chronic obstructive pulmonary disease is a disease state characterized by slowly progressive airflow obstruction that is not fully reversible. COPD includes:

- *Chronic bronchitis:* It is a condition characterized by chronic cough, sputum production and airway narrowing.

- *Emphysema:* It is a condition characterized by destruction of alveolar walls and enlargement of the alveoli.
- *Small-airways disease:* It is a condition in which small bronchioles are narrowed.

Epidemiology

- COPD occurs all over the world and is a public health problem. Its incidence is expected to increase further.
- In India, COPD is the commonest lung disorder following pulmonary tuberculosis.
- It affects men more commonly than women probably due to smoking habits. But the prevalence is also increasing in women due to increasing smoking habits among them also.
- There is higher prevalence with increasing age probably due to cumulative lung injury.

Risk Factors

- *Smoking:* Cigarette smoking is a major risk factor. 95% of cases are smoking-related, typically >20 pack years (1 pack year is 20 cigarettes smoked per day for 1 year). Passive (second hand) smoking is also a risk factor for COPD.
- *Airway hyper-responsiveness:* Patients with increased airway responsiveness are more likely to develop COPD.
- *Occupational exposures:* Several occupational exposures, like coal mining, gold mining, cotton textile dust, etc., are all risk factors for development of COPD. But their effect is less than cigarette smoking.
- *Air pollution:* It is thought to increase the risk of developing COPD.
- *Genetic factors:* They also play an important role. For example, α_1 antitrypsin (α_1AT) deficiency predisposes to the development of COPD.

Pathology

In COPD, all three components of lungs are affected, i.e. large airways, small airways and lung parenchyma.

- *Changes in large airways:* Changes in large airways include mucous gland enlargement and goblet cell hyperplasia. The Reid index, which indicates the ratio of thickness of the submucosal glands to that of the bronchial wall, is thus increased. There may be squamous metaplasia of mucous membrane which predisposes to cancer development and also impairs mucociliary clearance. These changes produce chronic cough and sputum production.
- *Changes in small airways:* Changes in small airways and alveoli include goblet cell metaplasia, loss of surfactant-secreting Clara cells and smooth-muscle hypertrophy. There is chronic inflammation and fibrosis of small airways. These changes produce airway obstruction.
- *Changes in lung parenchyma:* There is destruction of gas-exchanging air spaces, i.e. the respiratory bronchioles, alveolar ducts, and alveoli leading to emphysema. Recurrent infections may perpetuate airway inflammation. These changes are responsible for luminal narrowing, obstruction and impaired gas exchange.

Clinical Features

- Three most common symptoms of COPD are cough, sputum production, and exertional dyspnea. The duration of these symptoms is usually months to years. Onset of these symptoms is gradual. As COPD advances, dyspnea worsens and in the most advanced stages, patients are breathless doing routine activities or even at rest.
- Episodes of exacerbations occur precipitated usually by upper or lower respiratory tract infections.
- Examination may be normal in early stages of COPD. There may be signs of smoking, like odor of smoke, tobacco staining of teeth or nicotine staining of fingernails.
- Patients with severe COPD may have cyanosis. Accessory muscles of respiration may be active, and patient sits in a characteristic 'tripod' position to facilitate

the actions of accessory muscles. In patients with severe COPD, expiration is prolonged and there is usually expiratory wheezing. Signs of hyperinflation of lungs are present and include a barrel-shaped chest, pushed down diaphragm, and obliteration of cardiac dullness. Tidal percussion reveals decreased movement of diaphragm as it is already pushed down.

- Patients with predominant emphysema are referred to as 'pink puffers', due to lack of cyanosis and pursed-lip breathing. Patients with chronic bronchitis are called 'blue bloaters', due to presence of cyanosis and fluid retention. Usually patients have features of both and cannot be simply classified.
- Patients with advanced COPD have wasting and loss of subcutaneous fat. Such wasting is a poor prognostic sign in COPD.
- In advanced COPD, patient may develop pulmonary HTN and right heart failure, called corpulmonale. Such patients present with peripheral edema, raised JVP, congestive hepatomegaly, etc.

Differences between Chronic Bronchitis and Emphysema (see Table 2.4)

Investigations

- The hallmark of COPD is airflow obstruction. Pulmonary function testing shows reduction in FEV_1 and FEV_1/FVC. DLCO (diffusibility of carbon monoxide across alveolar membrane) may be reduced in emphysema reflecting destruction of alveolar walls. Arterial blood gas analysis and oximetry may show resting or exertional hypoxemia.

- Hematocrit may be high due to chronic hypoxemia.
- ECG may show evidence of right ventricular hypertrophy.
- Chest X-ray may show bullae, flattening of the diaphragm and hyperlucency in emphysema. On lateral film, large retrosternal air space and localised emphysematous bullae may also be seen in emphysema. Increased bronchovascular markings may be seen in chronic bronchitis.
- If the patient is less than 50 years with a strong family history and with a minimal smoking history, serum level of alpha-1 antitrypsin (α_1AT) should be checked.

Treatment

Only smoking cessation and oxygen therapy have been shown to alter the course of COPD. All other treatments are aimed at improving symptoms and decreasing the frequency of exacerbations.

Smoking Cessation

All patients with COPD should be strongly urged to quit smoking. Combining pharmacotherapy with traditional supportive approaches increases the chances of smoking cessation. Two drugs, bupropion, and nicotine

	Chronic bronchitis	Emphysema
Main pathology	Airway inflammation	Destruction of alveolar walls
Main symptom	Cough	Breathlessness
Clinical appearance	Blue bloater	Pink puffer
Sputum production	Copious	Scanty
Cor pulmonale	Common	Only in advanced stage
Respiratory insufficiency	Repeated episodes	Only in advanced stage
Arterial blood gases	Abnormality early in the course of disease	Abnormality only in advanced stage

Table 2.4: Differences between chronic bronchitis and emphysema

are helpful in this regard. Nicotine is available as gum, transdermal patches, inhaler, and nasal spray. All patients should be offered pharmacotherapy, in the absence of any contraindication to treatment.

Oxygen

Domiciliary and ambulatory oxygen therapy decreases mortality in patients with COPD. Oxygen can be given during day or at night at home. Using it for 12 hours or more has been shown to provide significant benefit.

Bronchodilators

These drugs provide symptomatic relief. These include β_2-agonists such as salbutamol, salmeterol, theophylline, ipratopium bromide, etc. Inhaled route is preferred as the incidence of side effects are less. In acute exacerbations, these are given through nebulization.

Glucocorticoids

Inhaled glucocorticoids reduce the frequency of exacerbations. Oral glucocorticoids can be used during exacerbations but long-term use of oral glucocorticoids is not recommended because of more side effects than benefits.

Mechanical Ventilatory Support

This is required in COPD with respiratory failure as happens during exacerbations and advanced stages. Noninvasive positive pressure ventilation (NIPPV) can be given through a tight fitting mask without tracheal intubation.

Other Measures

- All COPD patients should receive the influenza and pneumococcal vaccines since *H. influenzae* and *Pneumococcus* are the causes of frequent infective exacerbations.
- Lung volume reduction surgery can produce symptomatic and functional improvements in selected patients with emphysema.

- Lung transplantation can be an option for advanced COPD.

Prognosis

COPD is a progressive disease. Poor prognostic factors include weight loss, presence of resting hypoxemia and the need for hospital admission for an exacerbation, especially to intensive care unit.

Q. Define pneumonia. How do you classify pneumonia?

Definition

Pneumonia is an inflammation of the lung parenchyma due to acute microbial infection, with at least one opacity on chest X-ray.

Classification

Based on the setting in which pneumonia develops:
- Community-aquired pneumonia (CAP)
- Hospital-aquired (nosocomial) pneumonia:
  - o Ventilator-associated
  - o Non-ventilator-associated

Based on the anatomical distribution of pneumonia:
- Lobar pneumonia
- Bronchopneumonia
- Interstitial pneumonia
- Miliary pneumonia

Q. Discuss the etiology, pathology, clinical features, investigations and management of community-acquired pneumonia.

Definition

- Community-acquired pneumonia (CAP) is defined as an acute infection of the pulmonary parenchyma in a patient who has acquired the infection in the community.
- Community-acquired pneumonia (CAP) is a common and serious illness with considerable morbidity and mortality.

Etiology

- *Bacteria:* Streptococcus pneumoniae, H. influenzae, Moraxella catarrhalis, Mycoplasma pneumoniae, Legionella, gram-negative bacilli, anaerobes, *Mycobacterium tuberculosis, Coxiella burnetii.* Out of these, the first three bacteria (*Streptococcus pneumoniae, H. influenzae, Moraxella catarrhalis*) account for almost 85% of CAP.
- *Viruses:* Influenza virus, parainfluenza virus, respiratory syncytial virus.
- *Fungi: Cryptococcus, Histoplasma capsulatum.*
- Most of the cases are due to bacteria. Nearly 50% of cases of CAP are caused by *Streptococcus pneumoniae* (pneumococcal pneumonia).

Risk Factors for Pneumonia

- Immunocompromised state (such as HIV infection, steroid therapy)
- Uncontrolled diabetes mellitus
- Anatomical defects such as obstructed bronchus, bronchiectasis, or fibrosis
- Chronic alcoholism

Pathogenesis

- Microbial agents reach lungs by aspiration, inhalation, hematogenous spread from a distant site, and direct spread from a contiguous site.
- The most common route is microaspiration of oropharyngeal secretions colonized with pathogenic microorganisms. Aspiration can occur postoperatively and also during seizures and strokes.
- Once microorganisms reach the alveoli, there is inflammatory response against them. This inflammatory response, rather than the proliferation of microorganisms, triggers the clinical syndrome of pneumonia. Inflammatory mediators released by macrophages and neutrophils create an alveolar capillary leak. RBCs can also leak into the alveoli causing hemoptysis. The capillary leak results in a radiographic infiltrate and crepitations heard on auscultation. Alveolar filling also results in hypoxemia.
- Pathologically, pneumonia manifests as four general anatomical patterns: Lobar pneumonia, bronchopneumonia, interstitial pneumonia, and miliary pneumonia.

Lobar Pneumonia

- In lobar pneumonia an entire lobe of lung is involved. Inflammation can involve pleura causing pleuritic chest pain, pleural effusion and pleural rub.
- There are four stages in the course of lobar pneumonia.
  1. Stage of congestion—occurs during the first 24 h and is characterized by vascular congestion and alveolar edema.
  2. The second stage is called red hepatization because the affected part of lung resembles liver in colour and consistency. Microscopically, this stage is characterized by the presence of erythrocytes, neutrophils, desquamated epithelial cells, and fibrin in the alveolar spaces. Erythrocytes give the appearance of red colour.
  3. The third stage is called gray hepatization because the lung is dry, friable, and gray-brown due to fibrinopurulent exudate, disintegration of red blood cells, and presence of hemosiderin. The second and third stages last for 2 to 3 days each.
  4. The last stage is stage of resolution, which is characterized by resolution of above changes by enzymatic digestion of exudates, phagocytosis, and coughing out of debris.

Bronchopneumonia

- This pattern of pneumonia involves one or many lobes, and has patchy distribution. It occurs commonly due to aspiration of oropharyngeal secretions and hence usually involves the dependent parts.
- The consolidated areas are poorly demarcated. The neutrophilic exudate is more in bronchi and bronchioles, with centrifugal spread to the adjacent alveoli.

Interstitial Pneumonia

This pattern of pneumonia involves the interstitium. Inflammation may be patchy or diffuse.

Miliary Pneumonia

- The pattern is so-called because of resemblance of lesions to millet seeds. These lesions are numerous, 2–3 mm in size and diffusely distributed. They result from the spread of the pathogen to the lungs via the bloodstream. The lesions consist of granulomas or foci of necrosis.
- Miliary pneumonia occurs in miliary tuberculosis, histoplasmosis, and coccidioidomycosis.

Clinical Features

- Fever
- Cough (with or without sputum).
- Breathlessness
- Pleuritic type chest pain (in lobar pneumonia)
- General examination shows tachypnea, tachycardia and in severe cases cyanosis.
- RS examination shows dull percussion over the area of consolidation, increased tactile and vocal fremitus, egophony, whispering pectoriloquy, bronchial breath sounds, crepitations and sometimes pleural rub. Crepitations are heard in the stage of congestion and resolution. Bronchial breath sounds are heard in the stage of consolidation in lobar pneumonia. The single most useful sign of the severity of pneumonia is a respiratory rate of >30/min.

Investigations

- *Chest X-ray*: This is the most important investigation. It shows white opacity (pneumonic patch).
- *CT scan of chest* can pick up opacities, even if chest X-ray is normal.
- *Sputum examination*: Sputum should be examined by Gram's stain, AFB stain and culture. Special stains for fungi are useful in selected patients. Sputum culture and sensitivity can clearly identify the organism and also antibiotic susceptibility.
- *Blood culture:* The organism causing pneumonia is sometimes picked up by blood culture due to bacteremia.

Treatment of Pneumonia

Admit the patient, if any one of the following features is there:
- Respiratory rate >28/min
- Hypotension
- New-onset confusion or impaired level of consciousness
- Hypoxemia: PO_2<60 mm Hg while breathing room air or oxygen saturation <90%.
- Unstable comorbid illness (e.g., decompensated congestive heart failure, uncontrolled diabetes mellitus, alcoholism, immunosuppression).
- CURB-65 scoring (Table 2.5) CURB-65 score is used to predict the severity and prognosis of pneumonia. It is very useful to decide whether the patient is to be admitted or not. Each risk factor scores one point, for a maximum score of 5.

Table 2.5: CURB-65 scoring of pneumonia		
Clinical parameter		*points*
C	Confusion	1
U	Urea ≥20 mg/dL	1
R	Respiratory rate ≥30 breaths/min	1
B	Systolic BP <90 mm Hg or Diastolic BP ≤60 mm Hg	1
65	Age ≥65	1

- If the cumulative score is 0 or 1, the risk of mortality is low and patient can be treated as an outpatient.
- If the score is 2 or 3, the risk is moderate and ideally should be treated as inpatient.
- If the score is 4 or 5, the risk of mortality is high and the patient should be treated as inpatient.

Antibiotic Therapy

- Initially empirical antibiotic therapy is started based on clinical judgment till the organism is identified.
- If the patient is admitted, antibiotics should be given intravenously. Injection clarithromycin or levofloxacin or amoxicillin/ clavulanate or ceftriaxone are all good intitial choices. Once the patient starts improving, intravenous antibiotics can be changed to oral antibiotics. Antibiotics should be given for minimum 2 weeks.

General Measures

- IV fluids
- Oxygen
- Addition of bronchodilators and mucolytics may enhance sputum clearance.
- Physiotherapy to teach effective coughing techniques
- Mechanical ventilation may be required in patients with respiratory failure.

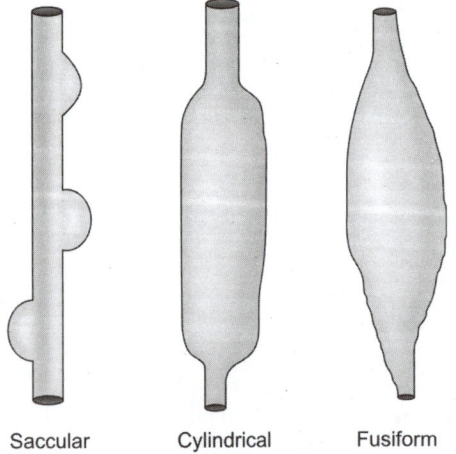

Saccular   Cylindrical   Fusiform

Fig. 2.2: Bronchiectasis

Complications of Pneumonia

- Pleural effusion (common)
- Empyema
- Pneumothorax—particularly with *Staph. aureus*
- Lung abscess
- ARDS

- Sepsis with multiorgan failure
- Ectopic abscess formation (*Staph. aureus*).

Q. Discuss the etiology, pathology, clinical features and management of bronchiectasis.

- Bronchiectasis is an abnormal and permanent dilatation of bronchi.
- It can be congenital or acquired and localized or diffuse.
- It leads to chronic or recurrent infection in the dilated bronchi, copious sputum production and hemoptysis.

Etiopathogenesis

- Development of bronchiectasis is mainly due to two factors—infection and obstruction or both. Infection leads to inflammation and destruction of the bronchial wall, damages respiratory epithelium and impairs mucociliary clearance. This leads to pooling of secretions, and dilatation of bronchi. Dilated bronchi become more susceptible to infection and thus, a vicious cycle results. Pulmonary tuberculosis leads to fibrosis, distorted and dilated bronchi.
- Bronchial obstruction due to any reason can lead to recurrent infections and development of bronchiectasis.
- Some congenital disorders like dyskinetic cilia or mucoviscidosis can also predispose to bronchiectasis.
- A congenital condition, Kartagener's syndrome is characterized by a combination of situs inversus, bilateral bronchiectasis and abnormal cilia lining the respiratory epithelium. This condition leads to stagnant secretions and repeated bronchial infections which lead to bronchiectasis.
- Bronchiectasis usually affects lower lobe bronchi. Upper lobe bronchiectasis is usually due to tuberculosis.
- Three forms of bronchiectasis have been recognized, namely; cylindrical, fusiform, and saccular (cystic).

o In the cylindrical type, there is uniform dilatation of bronchi.

o In the fusiform type, dilatation is irregular with tapering at both ends.

o In saccular type, there are multiple bulgings from side wall of bronchi.

- The bronchial epithelium may be ulcerated with exposure of thin-walled capillaries in the submucosa which are responsible for hemoptysis.

Causes of Bronchiectasis

Bronchial Obstruction

- Foreign body
- Tumor
- Stenosis
- Enlarged lymph nodes
- Impacted secretions

Infections

- Childhood pneumonias in measles, whooping cough
- Pulmonary tuberculosis
- Bronchopulmonary aspergillosis
- Repeated chest infections due to immunodeficient states

Miscellaneous

- Cystic fibrosis
- Kartagener's syndrome
- Alpha-1 antitrypsin deficiency
- Immotile cilia syndrome

Clinical Features

- Persistent or recurrent cough with copious sputum for several years. There is postural variation to cough and sputum quantity depending on which area of the lung is involved. Some patients may have no sputum with cough. This entity is called *bronchiectasis sicca*.
- Sputum is often blood-stained, and occasionally foul-smelling. Haemoptysis can be massive due to erosion of a hypertrophied bronchial artery.

- When there is secondary infection, quantity of sputum increases, becomes more purulent, foul smelling and often more bloody. Patients may also have fever and other constitutional symptoms.
- Physical examination may reveal coarse leathery crepitations, rhonchi, and bronchial breath sounds over the area of bronchiectasis reflecting damaged airways containing secretions and consolidation. Clubbing is usually present. Patients with severe B/L bronchiectasis may have cor pulmonale and right ventricular failure.

Investigations

- *Chest X-ray* may show cystic lesions in cystic bronchiectasis. B/L honeycombing (ring shadows) can occur reflecting end on view of dilated bronchi. When seen longitudinally, the dilated and thickened bronchi appear as 'tram tracks'.
- *Bronchography* is instillation of a radiopaque dye into airways and then taking X-ray images. This can provide excellent visualization of bronchiectatic airways and was once gold standard for the diagnosis of bronchiectasis. But now this technique has been replaced by HRCT.
- *High resolution computed tomography (HRCT)* of the chest is now the preferred method for diagnosis because it is noninvasive. It can pick up even slight abnormalities missed by chest X-ray.
- *Bronchoscopy* may be done, if a foreign body or adenoma is suspected to be the cause of bronchiectasis.
- In diffuse bilateral bronchiectasis with early age of onset, measurement of *sweat chloride levels* to rule out cystic fibrosis.
- *Pulmonary function tests* show both restrictive and obstructive ventilatory dysfunctions. Airway obstruction is due to retention of secretions and bronchial inflammation, whereas the restrictive changes are due to atelectasis and scarring of the lung parenchyma.

Complications

Massive hemoptysis, empyema, respiratory failure, cor pulmonale, pericarditis, metastatic abscesses, and secondary amyloidosis.

Management

- Medical management consists of postural drainage of the secretions, expectorants, bronchodilators and antibiotics. Regular physiotherapy prevents accumulation of secretions and repeated infections. Use of mucolytics like N-acetylcysteine and bromhexine may help in clearing the secretions. If secondary infection is suspected, broad-spectrum antibiotics such as ampicillin, amoxicillin, or trimethoprim-sulfamethoxazole are given till the organism is identified. Bronchodilators relieve airflow obstruction and aid clearance of secretions.
- Surgical resection is considered when bronchiectasis is localized and the morbidity is substantial despite adequate medical therapy.
- Bronchial artery embolization can be considered in patients with recurrent large hemoptysis.

Q. Etiology, clinical features and management of lung abscess.

- Lung abscess is defined as necrosis of the pulmonary tissue and formation of cavity containing necrotic debris or fluid caused by microbial infection. It is usually single and measures >2 cm in diameter.
- Lung abscess may be acute or chronic, single or multiple.

Etiology

- Lung abscess is caused most frequently by bacteria, usually anaerobes. Anaerobes include *Bacterioides fragilis, Fusobacterium* and anaerobic cocci. Common aerobic organisms include *Streptococcus milleri* (member of viridans group), *Streptococcus pyogenes* and *Staphylococcus aureus.*

Common gram-negative organisms are *Klebsiella pneumoniae* and Pseudomonas aeruginosa.

- The routes of infection include inhalation, aspiration, hematogenous, transdiaphragmatic or transthoracic route. Lung abscess can also occur due to secondary infection of a pre-existent cavity, cyst or bulla.
- Aspiration of the oropharyngeal secretions and subsequent abscess formation can occur in patients with altered consciousness, anesthesia, alcohol intoxication, sedative drugs, head injury, cerebrovascular accidents, esophageal stricture, and during seizures. Poor oral hygiene and dental caries is a risk factor for development of abscess.

Pathology

- By definition, a lung abscess is more than 2 cm in diameter and has a wall of variable thickness. The abscess cavity is usually filled with purulent secretions.
- Posterior segments of the right upper lobe and apical segments of the lower lobe of both lungs are affected commonly after aspiration. Abscesses due to other mechanisms may involve any segment. An abscess usually communicates with a bronchus.

Clinical Features

- Patients usually present with high-grade fever with chills and rigors. Cough with purulent sputum, dyspnea and chest pain are usually present. Hemoptysis may also be present.
- Physical examination may show clubbing. There may be cavernous bronchial breath sounds over the cavity. Crepitations and pleural rub may be heard.

Investigations

- Blood count shows increased WBC count.
- X-ray chest shows the abscess cavity with fluid level.

- CT scan may be required to differentiate lung abscess from loculated empyema.
- Sputum examination (Gram stain and culture) can identify the causative organism.
- Bronchoscopy is indicated, if foreign body or tumor is suspected.

Treatment

- Intravenous clindamycin or amoxicillin-clavulanate can be used as initial therapy pending organism identification. Penicillin plus metronidazole is another option, especially if aspiration is susupected.
- Antibiotics should be given for 6 to 8 weeks.
- Physiotherapy in the form of postural drainage can help clear the secretions.
- Chronic abscesses not responding to medical therapy require surgical resection.

Q. Describe the etiology, pathogenesis, clinical features, diagnosis and management of pulmonary tuberculosis.

Q. Describe the etiology, pathogenesis, clinical features, diagnosis and management of post primary (reactivation) pulmonary tuberculosis.

Q. Antituberculous drugs.

Q. Sequelae of tuberculosis.

Tuberculosis is an infectious disease caused by *Mycobacterium tuberculosis*. It is one of the oldest infections known. It usually affects the lungs, although in up to one-third of cases, other organs are involved. Tuberculosis is curable, if properly treated. Untreated disease can be fatal.

Etiology

- *M. tuberculosis* is a rod-shaped, aerobic bacterium. Robert Koch discovered this bacillus.

- It does not take up Gram stain because of the high lipid content, but can be stained by the Ziehl-Neelsen stain. After staining with Z-N stain, it resists decolorization with acid. That is why it is also known as acid-fast bacillus.
- Mycobacteria are rapidly destroyed by sunlight and ultraviolet light. But if protected from sunlight, they can survive for weeks to months. Tubercle bacilli in milk are killed by pasteurization.

Epidemiology

- India has the highest number of tuberculosis cases. It is estimated that about 40% of the Indian population is infected with TB bacteria, the vast majority of whom have latent rather than active TB. Recent data on global trends indicate that incidence is falling in most regions.
- The incidence of tuberculosis is highest during late adolescence and early adulthood due to unknown reasons. The risk increases in the elderly, due to waning immunity and comorbidity.
- Genetic factors also play a role in innate non-immune resistance to infection with *M. tuberculosis*. Hence, susceptibility to tuberculosis differs in different populations.
- Tuberculosis spreads by airborne droplet nuclei produced by patients with active pulmonary tuberculosis. The risk of infection is directly related to the duration and intensity of exposure to air contaminated with infected droplets. Patients whose sputum is smear-positive are highly infectious. Respiratory secretions aerosolized by coughing, sneezing or talking are sufficiently small and can remain suspended for long periods. A cough can produce 3000 infectious droplet nuclei. Talking for 5 minutes can also produce similar number droplets, and sneezing produces more droplets. A single droplet is sufficient to infect a person, if prolonged exposure is there. In hospital wards, six air changes per hour eliminate infectiousness; hence, good ventilation is important to prevent infection.

Pathogenesis

- Majority of inhaled droplet nuclei are trapped in the upper airways and expelled by ciliated mucosal cells. A small fraction reaches the alveoli. There, alveolar macrophages phagocytose the tubercle bacilli. Now two things can happen. Either macrophages kill the bacilli and clear the infection or the bacilli multiply within macrophages and kill the macrophages.

- If bacilli multiply within macrophages, they produce cytokines and chemokines that attract other phagocytic cells, including monocytes, other alveolar macrophages, and neutrophils, which eventually form a nodular granulomatous structure called the tubercle. Tubercles have central caseative necrosis. These lesions may heal by fibrosis and calcification, or undergo further evolution. If the infection is not controlled, the tubercle enlarges and the bacilli spread to local lymph nodes. This leads to local lymphadenopathy. The lesion produced by the expansion of the tubercle into the lung parenchyma with local lymphadenopathy is called the Ghon complex.

- The caseous center of the lesion liquefies and breaks into bronchi. Once the lesion empties into bronchi, cavities are formed. The liquefied caseous material, containing large numbers of bacilli, is brought out as sputumn and infectious to others.

- The bacilli continue to multiply until an effective cell-mediated immunity (CMI) develops. If effective CMI does not develop, the infection continues to spread and destroy the lung. Bacilli may spread hematogenously to produce disseminated TB. Miliary TB is disseminated disease with lesions resembling millet seeds.

- Even after healing, viable bacilli may remain dormant within macrophages or in the necrotic material for many years or throughout the patient's life. Reactivation TB results when the persistent bacteria in a host begin to multiply due to decrease in host immunity. Immunosuppressive conditions associated with reactivation TB include: HIV infection, diabetes mellitus, corticosteroid use and old age.

- When immunity develops to tubercle bacilli, the person also shows reactivity towards PPD skin test. Hence, PPD skin test (Montoux test) positivity suggests *M. tuberculosis* infection.

Clinical Features

- Symptoms begin insidiously and include cough, weight loss, fever and night sweats. Patients may present with only fever and night sweats without cough. Evening rise of temperature is typical. Pleuritic chest pain, dyspnea and hemoptysis are also reported by some patients. Pleuritic chest pain signifies inflammation abutting or invading the pleura. Dyspnea occurs when there is extensive parenchymal involvement, pleural effusion, or a pneumothorax. Pleural effusion can progress to frank empyema.

- Initially, cough may be dry. But as the disease progresses, cough becomes productive with yellow or yellow-green sputum. Frank hemoptysis, due to caseous sloughing or endobronchial erosion, typically is present later in the disease and is rarely massive.

- Physical findings include weight loss, signs of pleural effusion, crepitations and signs of consolidation, if large areas are involved. Amphoric breath sounds may be heard over cavities. Clubbing may be present.

Diagnosis

- *Chest X-ray:* It may show pleural effusion, pulmonary infiltrates, cavities, and fibrosis.

- *Microscopy:* Sputum is stained by Ziehl-Neelsen (ZN) stain. At least three sputum samples should be tested. Demonstration of acid-fast bacilli in sputum indicates tuberculous infection. Cultures of sputum for *M. tuberculosis* is diagnostic. In patients who do not produce sputum or those whose sputum is negative for AFB but still TB is suspected, fibreoptic bronchoscopy can be used to obtain specimens. Through fibreoptic bronchoscopy, bronchial washings are obtained and tested for AFB.

- *Culture:* Tubercle bacilli grow slowly in culture. Hence, it may take 6–8 weeks to grow them in solid media. Once *M. tuberculosis* is grown in culture, drug sensitivity tests also can be done to rule out MDR-TB. Sensitivity testing is done when a treatment regimen is failing, and when sputum cultures remain positive even after 3 months of therapy.

- *Histopathology:* In patients with TB pleural effusions, needle biopsy of the pleura reveals granulomas in 50% of patients.

- *Serologic tests:* Demonstration of IgG antibody against mycobacterial antigens by ELISA. This test is not done routinely.

- *Polymerase chain reaction:* To detect DNA of TB bacilli is a useful test but is expensive. It is used to diagnose CNS tuberculosis like TB meningitis.

- *Adenosine deaminase (ADA):* ADA level of >50 U/L in pleural fluid is highly suggestive of tuberculous pleural effusion.

- *PPD skin testing (Montoux test):* In the absence of a history of BCG vaccination, a positive skin test provides additional support for the diagnosis of tuberculosis.

Treatment

The aim of treatment is not only to cure patients but also to prevent transmission to others.

Antituberculous Drugs

- There are five main first-line drugs for the treatment of tuberculosis: Isoniazid, rifampin, pyrazinamide, ethambutol, and streptomycin (HRZES).
- The treatment regimen usually consists of initial intensive treatment for 2 months followed by 4–6 months of continuation phase. Initial phase includes 4 or more drugs and continuation phase 2 or more drugs.

First-line drugs (*see* Table 2.6)

Second-line drugs: Second line drugs are used when first-line drugs fail to cure tuberculosis. These are:
- Levofloxacin
- Ofloxacin
- Para-aminosalicylic acid (PAS)
- Ethionamide
- Cycloserine
- Thioacetazone
- Kanamycin
- Capreomycin

Table 2.6: First-line antituberculous drugs

Drug	Mechanism of action	Dose/day	Side effects
Isoniazid	Inhibition of mycolic acid synthesis	5 mg/kg	Hepatitis, peripheral neuropathy, drug fever
Rifampicin	Inhibits bacterial DNA-dependent RNA polymerase	10 mg/kg	Hepatitis, flu-like syndrome, thrombocytopenia (rare)
Ethambutol	Exact mechanism unknown. Thought to inhibit the synthesis of arabinogalactan, a mycobacterial cell wall constituent	15–20 mg/kg	Optic neuritis
Pyrazinamide	Inhibits fatty acid synthetase-I (FASI) of *M. tuberculosis*	20–25 mg/kg	Hepatitis, hyperuricemia
Streptomycin	Inhibits bacterial protein synthesis by binding directly to the 30S ribosomal subunits	0.75–1 g	Ototoxicity, vestibular damage, renal toxicity

WHO Guidelines for the Treatment of Tuberculosis

Category	Treatment guidelines
New patients	*Recommended regimen:* 2HRZE/ 4HR (2 months of HRZE daily and 4 months of HR daily)
Previously treated patients	2HRZES/1HRZE/5HRE (2 months of HRZES daily, 1 month of HRZE, 5 months of HRE)

H = Isoniazid, R = Rifampicin, Z = Pyrazinamide,
E = Ethambutol, S = Streptomycin

Monitoring Treatment

- Sputum should be examined monthly until AFB smears and cultures are negative in patients with pulmonary TB. By the end of the second month of treatment, >80% of patients will have negative sputum cultures. By the end of the third month, almost all patients should be culture-negative. AFB smear becomes negative little later than culture due to the presence of dead bacilli in the sputum. If the patient's sputum culture remains positive at ≥3 months, treatment failure and drug resistance should be suspected. If cultures cannot be done, then AFB smear examination should be done at 2, 5, and 6 months. Smears positive after 5 months are indicative of treatment failure.
- During treatment, patients should be monitored for drug side effects. The most important side effect is hepatitis. Baseline LFT should be done for all patients before starting ATT. LFT should be monitored monthly thereafter. For patients with symptomatic hepatitis and those with marked (five- to sixfold) elevations in serum levels of AST, treatment should be stopped and drugs reintroduced one at a time after liver function tests have returned to normal.

Treatment Failure and Relapse

As mentioned above, treatment failure is suspected when a patient's sputum cultures remain positive after 3 months or when AFB smears remain positive after 5 months. In such cases, a drug susceptibility test to first- and second-line agents should be done. Drug susceptibility testing takes a few weeks. Pending the results, same treatment can be continued. However, if the patient's clinical condition is deteriorating, treatment should be changed even before the susceptibility test report becomes available. If so, at least two and preferably three drugs that have never been used and to which the bacilli are likely to be susceptible should be added while continuing isoniazid and rifampicn.

Sequelae of Pulmonary Tuberculosis

- Fibrosis and destruction of the lung
- Bronchiectasis
- Lung abscess
- Aspergilloma (fungal ball)
- Scar carcinoma
- Chronic respiratory failure and cor pulmonale
- Chronic tuberculous empyema and fibrothorax
- Amyloidosis.

Prevention

- *Early diagnosis and treatment:* TB should be diagnosed and treated early in order to prevent deterioration of the disease and spread of the infection.
- *Examination of close contacts:* The close contacts of TB patients, usually the household contacts, should be examined. Tuberculin skin testing and/or chest X-ray examination is done for close contacts.
- *Leading a healthy lifestyle*: Smoking and alcohol intake should be stopped. Balanced diet should be taken. Adequate exercise, enough rest and sleep should be encouraged.
- *Chemoprophylaxis:* For household contacts of TB patients, isoniazid, 300 mg/day for 1 year, can reduce the incidence of tuberculosis.

- *BCG (Bacille Calmette-Guerin) vaccination:* All newborn babies should be vaccinated to protect them against tuberculosis.

Q. MDR tuberculosis.

Q. XDR tuberculosis.

- Multidrug-resistant tuberculosis (MDR-TB) refers to tuberculosis resistant to at least isoniazid and rifampicin, and possibly more drugs.
- Extensively drug-resistant tuberculosis (XDR-TB) refers to tuberculosis resistant to at least isoniazid, rifampin, fluoroquinolones, and either aminoglycosides (amikacin, kanamycin) or capreomycin, or both.
- Primary drug-resistance occurs in a patient who has never received antituberculosis therapy. Secondary resistance refers to the development of resistance during or following chemotherapy, for what had previously been drug-susceptible tuberculosis.

Diagnosis

- Sputum should be sent for culture and sensitivity. If a patient cannot produce sputum, sputum induction should be done by hypertonic saline nebulization. If an adequate sample is still not produced, bronchoscopy may be used to obtain sputum samples or other specimens. In extrapulmonary tuberculosis, samples of involved tissue (e.g. lymph nodes, bone, blood) should be obtained for culture and sensitivity testing as well as pathology.
- Susceptibility testing for first- and second-line agents should be performed at a reliable reference laboratory.

Treatment of MDR- and XDR-TB

- MDR-TB should be managed by medical personnel with expertise and experience in treating such cases. Laboratory facilities to document drug susceptibility and monitor

response should be available. Each dose in an MDR regimen is given as DOT throughout the treatment.
- When MDR-TB is suspected, sputum for culture and drug susceptibility testing (DST) should be sent and patient should be started on empirical MDR regimen till the DST results are available.
- Diagnosis and management of XDR-TB is same as MDR-TB.
- Drugs used for treatment of MDR and XDR tuberculosis are as follows. At least four effective drugs should be chosen from the following drugs.
  o Pyrazinamide
  o Ethambutol
  o Rifabutin
  o Kanamycin
  o Amikacin
  o Capreomycin
  o Streptomycin
  o Levofloxacin
  o Moxifloxacin
  o Ofloxacin
  o Para-aminosalicylic acid
  o Cycloserine
  o Ethionamide
  o Thioacetazone (Thz)

Duration of Treatment

- In MDR-TB treatment, the intensive phase is defined by the duration of treatment with the injectable agent. The injectable agent should be continued for a minimum of 6 months, and for at least 4 months after the patient becomes smear- or culture-negative.
- Total duration of therapy depends on culture conversion. Therapy should be continued for a minimum of 18 months after culture negativity.

Q. DOTS (directly observed therapy short course).

- The WHO-recommended DOTS strategy was launched formally as Revised National TB Control programme (RNTCP) in India in 1997. Since then, it has played an important role in controlling the incidence and prevalence of TB in India. DOTS is the most effective strategy available for controlling TB.

- The key components of DOTS are:
  - o Case detection by sputum smear microscopy examination among symptomatic patients;
  - o Patients are given anti-TB drugs under the direct observation of the health care provider/community DOT provider;
  - o Regular, uninterrupted supply of anti-TB drugs; and
  - o Systematic recording and reporting system that allows assessment of treatment results of each and every patient and of whole TB control programme.
- In DOTS, the responsibility of ensuring regular and complete treatment of the patient lies with the health system.
- In DOTS, the duration of treatment is 6 months, i.e. initial 2 months of intensive phase followed by 4 months of continuation phase. In the intensive phase, H, R, Z and E are administered under a direct supervision daily for 2 months. In the continuation phase, H and R are given daily for 4 months with appropriate supervision.
- Patient should be registered at a local DOTS centre for regular follow-up. Patient should be monitored for regularity of treatment as well as response to treatment. If the patient 'misses' a dose, he must be contacted within a day of the missed dose during an intensive phase and within a week of the missed dose during the continuation phase. In case of drug non-collection due to whatever reasons, the patient and the peripheral health functionary may agree on a mutually convenient location for the drug collection/administration.
- WHO recommends that wherever feasible, daily treatment should be used throughout the course of therapy. In HIV-infected patients, DOTS should not be used.

Q. Enumerate causes of pleural effusion. Give the differential diagnosis, clinical features, investigations and management of pleural effusion.

- A pleural effusion is an abnormal collection of fluid in the pleural space.
- It results from excess fluid production or decreased absorption or both. Normally about 10 to 20 mL of fluid is present in the pleural space which is similar in composition to plasma except low protein (<1.5 g/dL).
- Pleural effusion can be exudative or transudative based on Light's criteria.

Light's criteria to distinguish pleural transudate from exudate

Pleural fluid is an exudate, if one or more of the following criteria are met:
- Pleural fluid protein: Serum protein ratio >0.5
- Pleural fluid LDH: Serum LDH ratio >0.6
- Pleural fluid LDH >two-thirds of the upper limit of normal serum LDH

Causes of Pleural Effusion

Transudative Pleural Effusion

- Congestive heart failure
- Cirrhosis of liver with portal HTN
- Nephrotic syndrome
- Hypoalbuminemia

Exudative Pleural Effusion

- Pneumonia
- Tuberculosis
- Subphrenic abscess
- Malignancy
- Pancreatitis (acute, chronic)
- Pulmonary embolism

Clinical Features

- *Dyspnea:* It is the most common symptom associated with effusion.

- *Cough:* Cough is often mild and non-productive.
- *Chest pain:* Chest pain indicates pleural irritation, and occurs in pleural infection, mesothelioma, or pulmonary infarction. Pain is pleuritic in nature and is typically described as sharp or stabbing and is exacerbated with deep inspiration.
- *Other symptoms:* Symptoms of underlying disease may be present. Lower limb edema, orthopnea, and paroxysmal nocturnal dyspnea may suggest congestive cardiac failure as the cause of pleural effusion. Night sweats, fever, hemoptysis, and weight loss should suggest TB. Hemoptysis also suggests the possibility of malignancy or endobronchial pathology or pulmonary infarction. An acute febrile episode, purulent sputum production, and pleuritic chest pain may suggest effusion associated with pneumonia (synpneumonic effusion).
- Examination shows decreased chest movements, stony dull percussion note, and absent breath sound on the affected side. Vocal fremitus and vocal resonance are decreased. Pleural rub may be heard sometimes. Medastinal shift may be seen in massive pleural effusion. There may be signs and symptoms of underlying disease causing pleural effusion.

Investigations

- *Chest X-ray:* Pleural effusion appears as a homogenous white shadow at the lung base, blunting the costophrenic angle.
- *Ultrasound chest:* It is more accurate than chest X-ray to detect pleural effusion. It can also be used to guide pleural aspiration and pleural biopsy.
- *CT scan:* It is better than both X-ray and ultrasound in showing pleural abnormalities and underlying disease. It is also helpful to distinguish benign from malignant pleural disease.
- *Pleural fluid aspiration and analysis:* If the cause of effusion is obvious (e.g. left ventricular failure), it may not be necessary to do diagnostic pleural aspiration. Colour and texture of fluid can give clue about the possible diagnosis. It is straw coloured in transudates, turbid and purulent in empyema and hemorrhagic in pulmonary infarction or malignancy. A milky, opalescent fluid suggests a chylothorax. Biochemical analysis allows classification into transudate and exudates (see Light's criteria). Measurement of adenosine deaminase level (ADA) in pleural fluid is very helpful in the diagnosis of tuberculosis. ADA level of >50 U/L is highly suggestive of TB. Increased triglyceride and cholesterol levels are seen in chylothorax. Increased amylase level is seen in effusion due to pancreatitis. A low pH suggests infection but may also be seen in rheumatoid arthritis, and ruptured esophagus. Microbiological investigations should be done such as Gram's stain, culture sensitivity and AFB stain. PCR for tuberculosis should be done in most cases of pleural effusion. Cell count, cell type and malignant cytology should also be requested.
- *Pleural biopsy:* Combining pleural aspiration with biopsy increases the diagnostic yield. Pleural biopsy is better obtained under ultrasound or CT guidance.

Management

- Asymptomatic transudative effusions need not be drained.
- *Therapeutic aspiration* should be considered in symptomatic patients (e.g. dyspnea).
- *Tube thoracostomy*: Insertion of intercostal drainage tube (ICD) is required in complicated parapneumonic effusions and empyema.
- *Pleurodesis:* It involves instilling an irritant (such as talc, doxycycline) into the pleural space to cause inflammatory changes that result in bridging fibrosis between the visceral and parietal pleural surfaces, obliterating the pleural space. Pleurodesis is used for recurrent malignant effusions.
- *Treatment of the underlying cause:* For example, heart failure, nephrotic synd-

rome, pneumonia, etc. will often be followed by resolution of the effusion.

Q. Bronchogenic carcinoma (lung cancer).

- The term lung cancer is used for tumors arising from the respiratory epithelium (bronchi, bronchioles, and alveoli).

- Bronchogenic carcinoma can be divided into following types.
  - *Small cell lung cancer (SCLC) (oat cell carcinoma)*
  - *Non-small cell lung cancer (NSCLC)*
    - Adenocarcinoma
    - Squamous cell carcinoma
    - Large cell carcinoma

- NSCLC accounts for approximately 85% of all lung cancers. Identifying the type of cancer is important, because SCLC has a high response rate to chemotherapy and radiation whereas NSCLC can be cured by surgery in certain stages and is not curable by chemotherapy alone.

Incidence and Prevalence

- Bronchogenic carcinoma is the most common cancer in men. It is one of the leading causes of cancer death in both men and women. The incidence of lung cancer peaks between ages 55 and 65 years.

- Males are affected more often than females probably due to smoking habits. However, incidence in females is also increasing because of increased smoking habits in women also.

- Incidence is higher in urban than in rural areas, probably due to air pollution. The precise incidence of lung cancer in India is not known.

Etiology

- Smoking is the main cause of bronchogenic carcinoma. 90% of patients with lung cancer are current or former cigarette smokers. There is a significant dose-response relationship between the risk of lung cancer and the number of cigarettes smoked per day. The risk is increased 60- to 70-fold for a man smoking two packs a day for 20 years as compared with a nonsmoker. Besides the dose, the form of tobacco smoked is also believed to be important. Those who smoke only pipes or cigars have a lower risk. Bidi smoking is equally harmful. The risk of lung cancer is lower among users of filter than non-filter cigarettes. The risk decreases after stopping smoking. Passive smoking can also increase the risk of lung cancer. The risk may be about twice as compared to non-smokers without such exposure.

- Cigarette smoke contains many carcinogenic polycyclic hydrocarbons like 3, 4-benzopyrene. Squamous cell carcinoma and oat cell carcinoma are common in smokers, whereas adenocarcinoma is common in nonsmokers.

- Other risk factors for developing lung cancer include air pollution, ionizing radiation, chromates, metallic iron and iron oxides, arsenic, nickel, beryllium, asbestos, and petrochemicals. Adenocarcinoma can develop in areas of chronic scarring (scar carcinoma).

- Genetic factors like mutations in oncogenes may play an important role in the development of cancer.

Pathology

- Squamous cell carcinoma grows relatively slowly and often presents with local symptoms. Small cell carcinoma grows faster and proves rapidly fatal due to early metastasis. Small cell carcinoma is more often central than peripheral. The classical oat cell type is characterized by round or oval nuclei with scanty cytoplasm. Adenocarcinomas commonly present as mid-zone or peripheral mass lesions. Poorly differentiated adenocarcinomas tend to metastasize early and have a poor prognosis. Large cell carcinomas are made up of large malignant cells with abundant cytoplasm.

Clinical Features

The signs and symptoms of lung cancer are due to local tumor growth, invasion or obstruction of adjacent structures, regional lymph node involvement, metastases and remote effects of tumor products (paraneoplastic syndromes). The patient may be asymptomatic and may be diagnosed incidentally by a chest X-ray.

Symptoms due to Local Growth

- Central or endobronchial tumor may cause cough, hemoptysis, wheeze and stridor, dyspnea, and postobstructive pneumonia. Obstruction of airways can produce wheezing, and unilateral wheezing suggests a localized obstruction.
- Peripheral tumor may cause pain from pleural or chest wall involvement, cough, and dyspnea.

Symptoms due to Local Invasion

- Local spread of tumor into the mediastinum or involvement of mediastinal lymph nodes may cause tracheal compression, dysphagia due to esophageal compression, and hoarseness due to recurrent laryngeal nerve paralysis. Pleural effusion can occur.
- Pancoast syndrome results due to a tumor in the apex or in the superior sulcus of the lung with involvement of the C8 and T1 nerves, cervical sympathetic chain with consequent pain radiating to medial side of arm and forearm, shoulder pain and Horner's syndrome.
- Other problems of local spread include superior vena cava compression, cardiac involvement with resultant malignant pericardial effusion and tamponade, arrhythmia, or cardiac failure.

Symptoms due to Metastases

- Common sites of metastases of lung carcinoma include brain, bone, adrenals, and liver.
- Symptoms are referable to the organ system involved. Brain metastases produce neurologic deficits, bone metastases produce pain and pathologic fractures, liver metastases produce jaundice, and spine metastases produce cord compression.

Paraneoplastic Syndromes

- Paraneoplastic syndromes are clinical syndromes due to nonmetastatic systemic effects of a cancer. These syndromes result from substances produced by the tumor, and they occur remotely from the tumor itself.
- Paraneoplastic syndromes occur in approximately 10% of patients with bronchogenic carcinoma and occasionally are the presenting symptom. Paraneoplastic manifestations include weight loss, fever, hypercalcemia (due to production of parathyroid hormone from the tumor), Eaton-Lambert syndrome, etc.

Physical Signs

Physical examination may reveal clubbing, osteoarthropathy of the wrists and ankles, and lymphadenopathy especially in the supraclavicular regions. RS examination may be normal or show collapse, or consolidation. Pleural effusion may be present. Monophonic wheeze may be heard in localized airway obstruction.

Investigations

Imaging Studies

- Chest X-ray may show an isolated solitary mass lesion. Cavitation or abscess formation may be seen. Pleural and pericardial effusion may be present due to invasion of the pleura and pericardium. Secondary deposits in the ribs and other bones may be present.

- CT scan of the chest is very useful and helps in differentiating malignant leisons from benign ones. It can also pick up mediastinal lymphadenopathy and metastatic disease in the brain, liver, adrenal, kidney and lymph nodes of the abdomen.
- MRI is particularly useful to detect vertebral, spinal cord, and mediastinal invasion.

Bronchoscopy: Fibreoptic bronchoscopy is useful to diagnose and obtain biopsy in case of centrally located and endobronchial tumors.

Cytology: Cytological examination of sputum may show malignant cells. CT-guided FNAC or biopsy from the mass is also helpful for cytological examination.

Mediastinoscopy and thoracoscopy: These are sometimes used to take biopsy from lesions and lymph nodes.

Other diagnostic techniques: Biopsy of involved lymph nodes or of a metastatic nodule in the skin, liver, bone or pleura can help in diagnosis.

Management

Surgical resection: Surgical resection of the primary tumor and regional lymph nodes is the treatment of choice for NSCLC, if the tumor is localized without distant metastases. It is not useful in SCLC.

Radiotherapy: Radiotherapy is used both for curative purposes as well as for palliative therapy. High-dose radiotherapy can produce equal results as that of surgery in squamous cell carcinoma. It is the treatment of choice for unresectable tumors. It can also be used as adjuvant therapy before or after surgery.

Chemotherapy: It is being increasingly used in induction therapy in locally advanced, surgically resectable disease. Combined chemotherapy and radiotherapy is useful in small cell carcinoma. Drugs which are useful include mitomycin-C, ifosfamide cisplatin, carboplatin, and etoposide (remember MICE). Chemotherapy is also of great value in malignant pleural effusion and superior mediastinal compression syndrome.

> **Q. What is pneumothorax? Describe the causes, clinical features and management of pneumothorax.**

Pneumothorax is air in the pleural space. It causes lung collapse.

Causes

- **Spontaneous pneumothorax:** It occurs in patients with or without underlying pulmonary disease. It is thought to be due to spontaneous rupture of subpleural apical blebs or bullae that result from smoking or that are inherited. It most often occurs in patients with severe COPD.
- **Traumatic pneumothorax** is a common complication of penetrating or blunt chest injuries.
- **Iatrogenic pneumothorax** is caused by medical interventions, including transthoracic needle aspiration, thoracocentesis, central venous catheter placement, mechanical ventilation, and cardiopulmonary resuscitation.

Pathophysiology

- Intrapleural pressure is normally negative (less than atmospheric pressure) because of inward lung and outward chest wall recoil. In pneumothorax, air enters the pleural space from outside the chest or from the lung itself. As the air collects in the intrapleural space, lung collapses.
- Tension pneumothorax is a pneumothorax causing a progressive rise in intrapleural pressure which compresses the lung, shifts the mediastinum, and impairs venous return to the heart. Air continues to get into the pleural space but cannot exit. Decreased venous return leads to decreased cardiac output, hypotension, and cardiac arrest.

Tension pneumothorax is an emergency and has to be treated immediately.

Clinical Features

- Small pneumothorax may be asymptomatic.
- Symptoms of pneumothorax include dyspnea and pleuritic chest pain. Dyspnea may be sudden or gradual in onset depending on the rate of development and size of the pneumothorax.
- Physical findings classically consist of absent tactile fremitus, hyperresonance to percussion, and absent breath sounds on the affected side. If the pneumothorax is large, trachea may be shifted to the opposite side. With tension pneumothorax, hypotension can occur.

Diagnosis

- Pneumothorax should be suspected in any patient with sudden onset dyspnea and pleuritic type chest pain.
- Chest X-ray confirms the diagnosis of pneumothorax.

Treatment

- Immediate needle decompression for tension pneumothorax.
- Observation and follow-up X-ray for small, asymptomatic pneumothorax.
- Catheter aspiration for large or symptomatic pneumothorax.
- Tube thoracostomy for secondary and traumatic pneumothorax.
- Oxygen supplementation because O_2 accelerates pleural reabsorption of air.

Gastrointestinal System

Q. Stomatitis.

Stomatitis refers to oral inflammation and formation of ulcers. It can be localized or widespread and is a painful condition.

Etiology

- Recurrent aphthous stomatitis (recurrent aphthous ulcers) (idiopathic).
- Viral infections, particularly herpes simplex and herpes zoster.
- Other infectious agents (*Candida albicans* and bacteria).
- Systemic diseases (Behcet's disease, celiac disease, vitamin B deficiency).
- Trauma.
- Tobacco or irritating foods or chemicals.
- Drugs (antibiotics, anticonvulsants, NSAIDs).
- Chemotherapy and radiation therapy.

Clinical Features

- Stomatitis can be localized or widespread and is a painful condition.
- There may be swelling and redness of the oral mucosa or discrete painful ulcers (single or multiple). Rarely whitish lesions are seen.
- Symptoms hinder eating, sometimes leading to dehydration and malnutrition. Secondary infection occasionally occurs, especially in immunocompromised patients.

Investigations

- Patients with acute stomatitis without any features suggestive of systemic disease do not require any testing.
- If stomatitis is recurrent, viral and bacterial cultures, complete blood count, serum iron, ferritin, vitamin B_{12}, folate, zinc, and endomysial antibody (for sprue) are done. Biopsy is done for persistent lesions that do not have an obvious etiology.

Treatment

- Treat the underlying cause.
- Maintain good oral hygiene.
- Topical agents and rinses (lidocaine rinse, sucralfate plus aluminum-magnesium antacid rinse) can decrease the pain.
- If stomatitis is not due to infection, local application of dexamethasone elixir or triamcinolone oral ointment can be used.
- Chemical or physical cautery can ease the pain of localized lesions.
- A soft diet that does not include acidic, spicy or salty foods is followed.

Q. Gingival hyperplasia.

- Gingival enlargement (also termed gingival overgrowth, hypertrophic gingivitis, gingival hyperplasia, or gingival hypertrophy) is an increase in the size of the gingiva (gums).

Causes

Gingival hyperplasia can be caused by a number of factors as follows.

Inflammatory Enlargement

- Accumulation and retention of plaque due to poor oral hygiene is the chief cause of inflammatory gingival enlargement.
- Physical irritation of the gingiva by improper restorative and orthodontic appliances.

Drug-Induced Enlargement

- Anticonvulsants such as phenytoin, phenobarbital, and lamotrigine.
- Calcium channel blockers, such as nifedipine, amlodipine, and verapamil.
- Cyclosporine.

Enlargement Associated with Systemic Diseases or Conditions

- Pregnancy
- Puberty
- Vitamin C deficiency

Neoplastic Enlargement

- Acute myeloid leukemia
- Fibromas, papillomas, giant cell granulomas, malignant melanoma.

False Enlargement

Due to underlying bony or dental tissue lesion.

Management

- Improvement of oral hygiene so that irritative plaque is removed from around the necks of the teeth and gums.
- Stop the offending drug in cases of drug-induced gum overgrowth.
- Gingivectomy can be done in severe cases not responding to other measures.
- Treatment of any other underlying cause.

Q. Aphthous ulcers.

- These are painful oral ulcers which are localized, shallow, round to oval, with a grayish base.
- Aphthous ulcers are common in childhood and adolescence and become less frequent in adulthood. They usually heal within 10 to 14 days without scarring.

Etiology

- Exact cause of aphthous ulcers is not well known. Alterations in local cell-mediated immunity may play a role in the causation.
- A genetic basis exists for some recurrent aphthous ulcerations. This is shown by a positive family history in about one-third of patients with recurrent aphthous ulcerations.
- Recurrent aphthous ulcers are seen in stress, infections, food allergy, HIV infection, celiac sprue, gluten sensitive enteropathies, inflammatory bowel diseases, Behcet's disease and vitamin and mineral deficiencies (B vitamins, iron, folic acid, and zinc). Drugs like methotrexate may induce oral ulcers.

Treatment

- Local corticosteroid application (triamcinolone gel and hydrocortisone pellets) and other topical analgesics are adequate. These are applied to the ulcer two to four times daily until the ulcer is healed.
- Chlorhexidine gluconate mouth rinses reduce the severity and pain of ulceration but not the frequency.
- Oral corticosteroids are indicated for severe disease.
- Colchicine, dapsone, pentoxifylline, interferon alpha, and levamisole are beneficial in severe recurrent aphthous ulcers.
- Thalidomide is useful for severe recurrent aphthous ulcers especially in patients with HIV infection.

Q. Define dysphagia. What are the causes of dysphagia? How do you approach a case of dysphagia?

- Dysphagia means difficulty in swallowing. Odynophagia is pain while swallowing.
- Swallowing is a process governed by the swallowing center in the medulla, and enteric nervous system in the mid-eso-phagus and distal esophagus by a largely autonomous peristaltic reflex.

Causes of Dysphagia

Congenital
- Congenital stenosis of esophagus
- Congenital web

Acquired
- Esophageal strictures
- Carcinoma esophagus
- Esophagitis (reflux, candida)
- Achalasia cardia
- Plummer-Vinson syndrome
- Scleroderma
- Compression of esophagus from outside (thyroid swelling, malignancy, aortic aneurysm)
- Bulbar palsy
- Pseudobulbar palsy
- Myasthenia gravis

Approach to a Case of Dysphagia

History

- The type of food causing dysphagia gives useful information. Dysphagia only for solids implies a mechanical cause due to partial obstruction. Dysphagia for both solids and liquids occurs in neuromuscular and severe obstructive leisons.
- History of difficulty in initiating swallowing suggests oropharyngeal dysphagia. History of food 'sticking' after swallowing indicates esophageal dysphagia.
- The duration and course of dysphagia is also helpful in diagnosis. Transient dysphagia is usually due to an inflam-matory process. Sudden onset dysphagia occurs due to obstructive foreign bodies. Progressive dysphagia occurs in carcinoma esophagus. Intermittent dysphagia is seen in esophageal spasm.
- Dysphagia with nasal regurgitation is seen in pharyngeal paralysis.
- History of regurgitation of old food and halitosis suggests Zenker's diverticulum.
- Tracheobronchial aspiration with dysphagia is seen in tracheoesophageal fistula.
- Weight loss and progressive dysphagia in elderly is highly suggestive of carcinoma. When hoarseness precedes dysphagia, the primary lesion is usually in the larynx. When hoarseness appears after dysphagia it suggests involvement of the recurrent laryngeal nerve by extension of esophageal carcinoma. A prolonged history of heart burn preceding dysphagia indicates peptic stricture.
- If odynophagia is present, it suggests esophagitis.

Physical Examination

- Pallor is present in Plummer-Vinson syndrome due to iron deficiency.
- Neck should be examined for thyromegaly, lymphadenopathy or any other abnormality.
- Mouth and pharynx should be examined for any local pathology.
- Skin should be examined for evidence of scleroderma.
- Neurological examination should be done looking for evidence of bulbar or pseudobulbar palsy.
- Abdomen should be examined for any distension, mass.
- Cancer spread to lymph nodes and liver may be evident.
- Respiratory system examination may reveal complications of dysphagia such as aspiration pneumonia.

Investigations

- Hemoglobin and peripheral smear for anemia.

- Barium swallow detects tumors as filling defects and strictures as rat tail appearance.
- Endoscopy and biopsy of any lesions.
- Esophageal motility studies.
- Chest X-ray to rule out mediastinal mass or bronchogenic carcinoma.
- CT scan of neck and chest to rule out any mass lesions.

Treatment

Depends on the underlying cause

Q. Acid peptic disease.

Q. Discuss the etiology, clinical features, investigations and management of peptic ulcer.

- Peptic ulcer is a break in the gastric or duodenal mucosa that arises when there is decrease in mucosal defensive factors or increase in ulcerogenic factors such as acid and pepsin.
- Peptic ulcers occur more commonly in duodenum than stomach. They are more common in men than women.
- Duodenal ulcers occur commonly between 30 and 55 years of age, whereas gastric ulcers occur commonly between 55 and 70 years of age.

Etiology of Peptic Ulcer

- *H. pylori* infection (produces mucosal damage)
- NSAIDs and aspirin
- Stress ulcers
- Smoking and alcohol intake
- Gastrinoma (Zollinger-Ellison syndrome)
- Radiation therapy (mucosal damage)
- Carcinoid syndrome
- Crohn's disease
- Renal failure
- Idiopathic

Pathophysiology

- Most cases of peptic ulcer are due to *Helicobacter pylori* infection and use of nonsteroidal anti-inflammatory drugs (NSAIDs).
- Most duodenal ulcer patients have increased acid secretion whereas acid secretion is normal in patients with gastric ulcer. Hence, increased acid may play a role in the causation of duodenal ulcer whereas impaired mucosal defense may play a role in the causation of gastric ulcer (Table 3.1).
- NSAIDs lead to ulcer formation by inhibiting the synthesis of protective prostaglandins which protect mucosa.
- *H. pylori* infection is associated with increased gastric acid secretion and decreased duodenal mucosal bicarbonate secretion. This leads to duodenal ulcer. *H. pylori* also causes chronic inflammation of gastric mucosa and leads to gastric ulcer formation.

Clinical Features

- Epigastric pain (dyspepsia) is the most common symptom of peptic ulcer. However, some patients may have silent ulcers. Pain is well localized, felt in the epigastrium and not severe. It is usually burning type but can also be gnawing, dull, aching, or 'hunger-like'.
- Pain occurs in episodes (periodicity), lasting 1–3 weeks every time, 3–4 times a year. In between, patient is free of pain.
- The typical pain pattern in duodenal ulcer occurs 1 to 3 hours after a meal and is frequently relieved by antacids or food whereas gastric ulcer pain is worsened by intake of food. Pain that awakes the patient from sleep (between midnight and 3 AM) is seen in duodenal ulcer patients.
- Nausea and weight loss are common in gastric ulcer because pain is precipitated by food and hence patient eats less frequently. Weight gain may be present in duodenal ulcer patients because pain relief from food makes them eat more frequently.
- Epigastric pain which becomes constant, and radiates to the back may indicate a penetrating ulcer (pancreas).

- Sudden onset of severe, generalized abdominal pain may indicate perforation.
- Pain associated with vomiting of undigested food suggests gastric outlet obstruction.
- Tarry stools or coffee ground vomitus indicate bleeding from ulcer.
- Physical examination is often normal in uncomplicated peptic ulcer except mild epigastric tenderness. Sometimes pallor may be present due to chronic blood loss from ulcer. In peptic ulcer perforation, board-like rigidity of abdominal wall is found.

Investigations

Blood tests: Anemia may be present due to blood loss from the ulcer. Increased WBC count and increased amylase suggests ulcer penetration into the pancreas. Serum gastrin levels are high in patients with Zollinger-Ellison syndrome.

Endoscopy: Upper GI endoscopy is the procedure of choice for the diagnosis of duodenal and gastric ulcers. Biopsy can also be taken during endoscopy. Gastric ulcers can be malignant and biopsy should be taken whereas duodenal ulcers are virtually never malignant and do not require biopsy.

Barium swallow: Can be used for screening patients with uncomplicated dyspepsia. However, it is less commonly used now because of wide availability of endoscopy.

Tests for *H. pylori*

- Noninvasive tests for *H. pylori* include fecal antigen assay and urea breath test.
- Mucosal biopsies can be obtained during endoscopy for rapid urease test and for histologic examination.

Complications of Peptic Ulcer

- Hemorrhage
- Perforation
- Ulcer penetration
- Gastric outlet obstruction due to scarring.

Treatment

The goal of treatment is to provide relief of symptoms (pain or dyspepsia), promote ulcer healing, and ultimately prevent ulcer recurrence and complications.

General Measures

- Avoid smoking and spicy food.
- Cut down or quit alcohol intake.
- Avoid aspirin and NSAIDs

Antacids

- They relieve the pain by neutralizing the acid. They are mainly used for symptomatic relief of epigastric pain.
- Commonly used antacids are mixtures of aluminum hydroxide and magnesium hydroxide.
- Dose is 15–30 mL 4 to 6 times per day.

Table 3.1: Differences between gastric and duodenal ulcer		
	Gastric ulcer	*Duodenal ulcer*
Age	50–70 years	30–50 years
Sex	Equal in both sexes	More in males
Acid secretion	Normal	Increased
Episodes of pain	Immediately after food	Occur 1 to 3 hours after a meal
Antacids	Inconsistent relief of pain	Prompt relief of pain
Food	Provokes the pain	Relieves the pain
Night pains	Rare	Common
Effect on weight	Weight loss	Weight gain

H₂ Receptor Blockers

- These agents decrease acid secretion. Examples are ranitidine, famotidine, and nizatidine. All are equally effective.
- These agents are given for 4 to 6 weeks.

Proton Pump (H⁺, K⁺-ATPase) Inhibitors

- These agents are the most potent acid inhibitory agents available. They covalently bind and irreversibly inhibit $H^+ K^+$-ATPase which is the final pathway in acid secretion.
- Examples are omeprazole, esomeprazole, lansoprazole, rabeprazole, and pantoprazole.

Mucosal Protective Agents

- Sucralfate forms a viscous paste on coming in contact with stomach acid. This viscous paste forms a coating on ulcers and helps in healing. It does not act in alkaline pH. Hence, giving it along with other acid suppressing agents may render it ineffective.
- Bismuth-containing preparations coat the ulcer and prevent further pepsin-/acid-induced damage.
- Prostaglandin analogues, such as prostaglandin E_1, enhance mucosal defense and repair.

H. pylori Eradication

H. pylori should be eradicated in patients with documented peptic ulcer disease. *H. pylori* eradication prevents the recurrence of peptic ulcer. Commonly used drugs are amoxicillin, metronidazole, tetracycline, clarithromycin, and bismuth compounds. Combination therapy should be used to eradicate *H. pylori*. Treatment should be given for 10–14 days.

Surgical Treatment

- Less commonly used now because of the availability of effective medical therapy.
- Partial gastrectomy for gastric ulcer.
- Vagotomy for duodenal ulcer.
- Emergency surgery is indicated in penetrating or perforating peptic ulcers.

Q. Discuss the etiology, classification, clinical features, investigations and management of malabsorption syndrome.

Q. What are the disorders causing malabsorption? How do you approach a case of suspected malabsorption?

- Malabsorption refers to impaired absorption of nutrients.
- Malabsorption occurs mainly due to diseases of small intestine since this is the major site of absorption of nutrients.
- Fat is the most difficult to absorb and hence most malabsorption syndromes have steatorrhea. A stool test for fat is the best screening test for malabsorption.

Causes of Malabsorption

Disorders of luminal phase
- *Enzyme deficiency*: Chronic pancreatitis, cystic fibrosis.
- *Enzyme inactivation*: Zollinger-Ellison syndrome.
- *Diminished bile salt synthesis*: Parenchymal liver diseases.
- *Impaired bile secretion*: Bile duct obstruction, chronic cholestasis
- *Increased bile salt loss*: Ileal disease or resection
- *Reduced luminal availability of specific nutrients:* Intrinsic factor deficiency in pernicious anemia causing vitamin B_{12} deficiency
- *Bacterial consumption of nutrients*: Bacterial overgrowth causing vitamin B_{12} deficiency

Disorders of mucosal phase
- *Defects in brush border hydrolysis*: Sucrase-isomaltase deficiency, lactase deficiency
- *Defects in mucosal absorption (villous atrophy):* Celiac sprue, tropical sprue, lymphoma, Whipple's disease, radiation enteritis, AIDS, giardiasis, Crohn's disease

Disorders of postabsorptive, processing phase
- *Defects in enterocyte processing*: Abetalipoproteinemia

- *Defects in lymphatic transport:* Intestinal lymphangiectasia, intestinal tuberculosis

Systemic diseases causing malabsorption
- Thyrotoxicosis (rapid transit through gut)
- Hypothyroidism (impaired intestinal motility, bacterial overgrowth)
- Diabetes mellitus (impaired intestinal motility, bacterial overgrowth)
- Scleroderma (impaired intestinal motility, bacterial overgrowth)

Drugs causing malabsorption
- Antibiotics (vitamin B_{12} and vitamin K deficiency)
- Methotrexate (folic acid antagonist, causes inhibition of crypt cell division).
- Cholestyramine (binds bile salts)
- Laxatives (rapid transit through gut. Liquid paraffin causes fat-soluble vitamin deficiency).

Clinical Features

Diarrhea
- Diarrhea is the most common complaint. It is due to the osmotic load received by the intestine because of unabsorbed carbohydrates and solutes.
- Bacterial action producing hydroxy fatty acids from undigested fat also can increase fluid secretion from the intestine, further worsening the diarrhea.

Steatorrhea
- Steatorrhea is due to fat malabsorption.
- The hallmark of steatorrhea is the passage of pale, bulky, and foul smelling stools, which float on top of the toilet water and are difficult to flush. Also, patients find floating oil droplets in the toilet following defecation.

Weight loss and fatigue
- Weight loss is due to protein energy malnutrition from malabsorption.
- Fatigue is due to weight loss plus coexisting anemia.

Flatulence and abdominal distention
- Bacterial fermentation of unabsorbed food substances releases gases, such as hydrogen and methane, causing flatulence.
- Flatulence often causes uncomfortable abdominal distention and cramps.

Edema
- Protein malabsorption causes hypoalbuminemia which causes peripheral edema.
- With severe protein depletion, ascites may develop.

Anemia: Anemia develops due to iron deficiency (microcytic anemia), folic acid or vitamin B_{12} deficiency (macrocytic anemia). Iron deficiency is common in celiac disease.

Bleeding disorders: Bleeding tendency is due to vitamin K malabsorption and decreased production of vitamin K-dependent clotting factors. Ecchymosis is usually seen but patient can also have melena and hematuria.

Bone pain and pathologic fractures
- This is due to vitamin D deficiency causing osteopenia or osteomalacia.
- Malabsorption of calcium can lead to secondary hyperparathyroidism.

Neurologic manifestations
- Electrolyte disturbances, such as hypocalcemia and hypomagnesemia, can lead to tetany, manifesting as Trousseau sign and the Chvostek sign.
- Vitamin malabsorption can cause generalized motor weakness (pantothenic acid, vitamin D) or peripheral neuropathy (thiamine, vitamin B_{12}), a sense of loss for vibration and position (vitamin B_{12}), night blindness (vitamin A), and seizures (biotin).

Summary of Features of Specific Nutrient Malabsorption

Carbohydrates: Watery diarrhea, flatulence, acidic stool pH, milk intolerance.

Protein: Edema, muscle atrophy, amenorrhea.

Fat: Pale, bulky, foul smelling stool which floats on water and difficult to flush. Diarrhea without flatulence. Weight loss.

Vitamins

Vitamin A	Follicular hyperkeratosis, night blindness
Vitamin B$_{12}$	Anemia, neuropathy, subacute combined degeneration of the spinal cord.
Vitamin B$_1$, B$_2$	Cheilosis, painless glossitis, acrodermatitis, angular stomatitis
Folic acid	Megaloblastic anemia.
Vitamin D	Tetany, pathologic fractures due to osteomalacia, muscular irritability.
Vitamin K	Bleeding tendency

Minerals and electrolytes

Iron: Anemia, glossitis, pica

Calcium: Tetany, pathologic fractures due to osteomalacia, muscular irritability.

Zinc: Anorexia, weakness, tingling, impaired taste.

Investigations

Imaging Studies

- *Endoscopy:* Upper GI scopy is helpful to visualize stomach, duodenum and upper jejunum. A cobblestone appearance of the duodenal mucosa is seen in Crohn's disease. Reduced duodenal folds and scalloping of the mucosa may be seen in celiac disease. Small bowel biopsy can also be taken during endoscopy.
- *CT and ultrasound abdomen:* May be helpful in the diagnosis of chronic pancreatitis and other abnormalities in the abdomen.
- *Barium studies:* An upper gastrointestinal series with small bowel follow-through or enteroclysis (a double contrast study performed by passing a tube into the proximal small bowel and injecting barium and methylcellulose) can provide information about the gross morphology of the small intestine. For example, small bowel diverticula and mucosal abnormalities can be identified.
- *Wireless capsule endoscopy:* Wireless capsule endoscopy allows for visualization of the entire small bowel. Because of the risk of retention, it should be avoided in patients with suspected small bowel strictures.

Tests for Fat Absorption

- *Fecal fat estimation:* Increase in stool fat excretion is known as steatorrhea. More than 6 g/day of fat in stool is pathologic.
- *Sudan III stain:* Sudan stain on a spot stool sample can detect more than 90% of patients with steatorrhea.
- Measurement of fat soluble vitamin levels in the blood (A,D,E, K) prothrombin time.
- *Near infrared reflectance analysis (NIRA):* This may become the procedure of choice in future. NIRA can simultaneously measure fecal fat, nitrogen, and carbohydrates in a single sample.

Tests for Carbohydrate Absorption

- *Oral glucose tolerance test:* There will be failure of blood glucose levels to rise after glucose loading.
- *D-xylose test:* Patient ingests 25 g of D-xylose, and urine is tested for the presence of D-xylose. Excretion of lesser amounts of D-xylose suggests abnormal absorption (as in celiac sprue).
- *Lactose tolerance test:* After ingestion of 50 g lactose, blood glucose levels are monitored. Insufficient increase in blood glucose plus the development of symptoms is diagnostic of lactose intolerance.
- *Breath tests:* Breath tests using hydrogen, $14CO_2$, or $13CO_2$ can be used to diagnose specific forms of carbohydrate malabsorption (e.g. lactose, fructose, sucrose isomaltase and others). All of these breath tests rely on bacterial fermentation of nonabsorbed carbohydrate and, therefore, concurrent antibiotic administration often alters the results.

Tests for Protein Absorption

- Serum albumin will be low.
- Intravenous radioactive chromium is used to label circulating albumin. In case of

protein losing enteropathy, radioactivity appears in stools.

- Measurement of nitrogen in the stool will be more than 2.5 g.
- Excretion of alpha-1 antitrypsin in the stool (normally it is absent in the stool).

Tests for Absorption of other Substances

Complete blood count (anemia), serum iron, ferritin, folate, vitamin B_{12} level, Schilling test (for vitamin B_{12} malabsorption), serum calcium, sodium, potassium, β-carotene, and prothrombin time should be obtained in all patients with suspected malabsorption.

Tests for Bacterial Overgrowth

The gold standard for diagnosis of bacterial overgrowth is the direct quantitative measurement of bacterial counts from aspirated intestinal fluid. However, this is invasive and hence the following tests are used more commonly.

- *Hydrogen breath test:* This is used to detect bacterial overgrowth in the intestine. Oral lactulose or glucose is metabolized by bacteria with the production of hydrogen. An early rise in the breath hydrogen indicates bacterial overgrowth in the small intestine.
- *14C-glycocholic acid breath test:* It is rarely done now and has been replaced by the hydrogen breath test. Patient is given radiolabelled bile acid (14C-glycocholic acid) orally. Bacteria in the intestine deconjugate the bile acid, releasing [14C]-glycine, which is metabolized and appears in the breath as $14CO_2$.

Serologic Tests

IgA endomysial antibody and IgA anti-tTG antibody both are found in celiac disease. IgG or IgA antigliadin antibodies are also present in celiac sprue.

Intestinal Mucosal Biopsy and Histopathology

Villous atrophy is seen in celiac disease, and tropical sprue.

Treatment

- Treat the underlying cause.
- Avoid milk and milk products in lactose intolerance.
- Gluten-free diet in celiac disease.
- Pancreatic enzyme supplements in pancreatic insufficiency.
- Reduction of long chain fatty acids and low fat diet in fat malabsorption.
- Antibiotics are the therapy for bacterial overgrowth.
- Corticosteroids, anti-inflammatory agents, such as mesalamine, are used to treat inflammatory bowel disease such as Crohn disease.
- Replacement of specific nutrients which are deficient such as folic acid, iron and vitamin B_{12}, vitamin D, etc.
- Caloric and protein replacement.

Q. Define jaundice. Enumerate the causes of jaundice. How do you approach a case of jaundice?

Jaundice is defined as yellowish discolouration of skin, mucous membranes and sclera due to hyperbilirubinemia. Hyperbilirubinemia may be due to abnormalities in the formation, transport, metabolism, and excretion of bilirubin. Total serum bilirubin is normally 0.3–1 mg/dL. Jaundice is clinically detectable when levels are more than 2.5 mg/dL.

Causes of Jaundice

Prehepatic causes
- Hemolysis, breakdown of hematomas,
- Gilbert's syndrome
- Neonates
- Hyperthyroidism

Hepatic causes
- Acute and chronic hepatitis
- Liver abscess
- Cirrhosis
- Sepsis
- Drugs (antituberculous drugs)

- External pressure on common duct, pancreatitis
- Carcinoma head of pancreas
- Periampulary carcinoma.

Approach to a Case of Jaundice (Fig. 3.1)

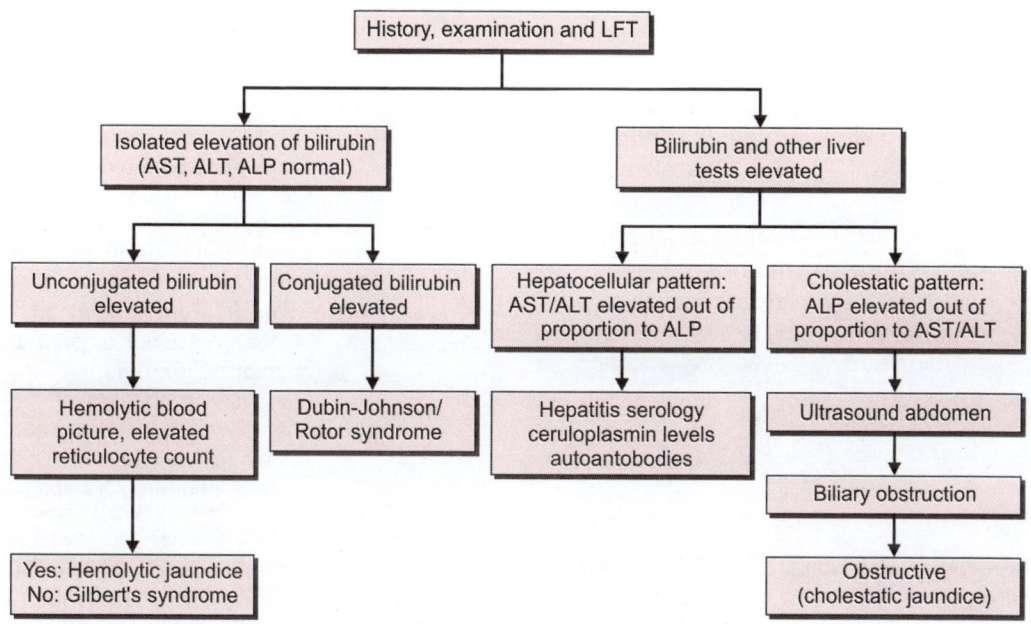

Fig. 3.1: Approach to a case of jaundice

Q. Discuss briefly the congenital hyperbilirubinemic disorders.

Table 3.2: Congenital hyperbilirubinemic disorders				
	Inheritance	Defect	Type of hyperbiliru-binemia	Features
Gilbert's syndrome	Autosomal dominant	Mild deficiency of UDP-glucuronyl transferase	Unconjugated	Benign, asymptomatic jaundice. More common in males. Urobilinogen in the urine is increased but there is no bilirubinuria. Peripheral blood smear, reticulocyte count and haptoglobin are normal (suggesting absence of hemolysis). Hyperbilirubinemia

(Contd.)

Table 3.2: Congenital hyperbilirubinemic disorders *(Contd.)*

	Inheritance	Defect	Type of hyperbiliru-binemia	Features
				increases after fasting. No treatment required (Phenobarbital can increase the activity of UDP-glucuronyl transferase). Prognosis excellent
Crigler-Najjar syndrome type I	Autosomal recessive	Complete absence of UDP-glucuronyl transferase	Unconjugated	Seen in infants. Bilirubin is very high (20 to 25 mg/dL, can be as high as 50 mg/dL). Stool color is normal, but fecal urobilinogen excretion is diminished due to the marked reduction in the conjugation of bilirubin. Peripheral blood smear, reticulocyte count and haptoglobin are normal (suggesting absence of hemolysis). Prognosis poor. Death occurs due to kernicterus, unless vigorously treated
Crigler-Najjar syndrome type II	Autosomal recessive	Partial absence of UDP-glucuronyl transferase	Unconjugated	Usually benign, kernicterus occurs rarely. Hyperbiliru-binemia can be reduced by treatment with phenobarbital.
Dubin–Johnson syndrome	Autosomal recessive	Reduced ability to transport conjugated bilirubin into biliary canaliculi	Conjugated	Benign, asymptomatic jaundice. Gallbladder not visualized on oral cholecystography. BSP (bromsulphalein) test shows reduced clearance. Liver darkly pigmented on gross examination. Biopsy shows centrilobular brown pigment. No treatment required. Prognosis excellent
Rotor's syndrome	Autosomal recessive	Faulty excretory function of hepatocytes	Conjugated	Similar to Dubin–Johnson syndrome, but liver is not pigmented and the gallbladder is visualized on oral cholecystography. Prognosis excellent

Q. Discuss the clinical and laboratory differentiation of different types of jaundice.

Clinical features	Hemolytic jaundice	Hepatocellular jaundice	Obstructive jaundice
• Color of jaundice	Lemon yellow	Orange yellow	Greenish yellow
• Depth of jaundice	Mild	Moderate	Deep
• Pruritus (itching)	Absent	Sometimes	Present
• Bleeding tendency	Absent	Present	Present (late)
• Bradycardia	Absent	Absent	Present
• Pallor	Present	Absent	Absent
• Splenomegaly	Present	Sometimes	Absent
• Features of liver cell failure	Absent	Present	Present (late)
• Stool color	Normal	Normal	Light color (clay color)
• Urine color	Normal	Dark	Dark
Laboratory features			
• Bilirubin	Predominantly unconjugated	Mixed	Predominantly conjugated
• ALT, AST	Normal	Markedly increased	Minimally increased
• Alkaline phosphatase	Normal	Increased	Markedly increased
• Serum albumin	Unchanged	Decreased	Unchanged
• Prothrombin time	Normal	Prolonged and does not respond to parenteral vitamin K	Prolonged in late stages and responds to parenteral vitamin K
• Urine bilirubin	None	Increased	Increased
• Urine urobilinogen	Increased	Increased	Absent

Q. Hepatomegaly

Enlargement of liver is called hepatomegaly. Normal size of liver is 10 to 12 cm.

Causes of Hepatomegaly

- o Viral hepatitis
- o Enteric fever (typhoid)
- o Malaria
- o Cirrhosis of liver (early stages)
- o Fatty liver
- o Lymphoma and leukemias
- o Liver abscesss
- o Hepatocellular carcinoma
- o Congestive cardiac failure.

Q. Describe the etiology, epidemiology, clinical features, laboratory findings and treatment of hepatitis A.

Q. Describe the etiolgy, epidemiology, clinical features, laboratory features and treatment of acute viral hepatitis.

Many viruses can cause viral hepatitis. These are as follows.

- *Hepatitis viruses*: Hepatitis A, B, C, D, E.
- *Other viruses*: Cytomegalovirus, Epstein-Barr virus, herpes simplex virus, yellow fever virus.

HEPATITIS A

Etiology

- Hepatitis A is caused by hepatitis A virus which is an RNA virus.
- Replication occurs in the liver. The virus is secreted into the bile and found in stool. Highest titers are found in stool during the incubation period and early symptomatic phase of illness.

Epidemiology

- It is transmitted almost exclusively by the fecal-oral route and rarely through blood transfusion. Most are due to direct person-to-person exposure and, to lesser extent, to direct fecal contamination of food or water. Consumption of shellfish from contaminated waterways is also a rare source of hepatitis A infection.
- It is more prevalent in low socioeconomic groups in which a lack of adequate sanitation and poor hygienic practices facilitate spread of the infection.

Clinical Features

- Incubation period is 15 to 45 days (mean 30 days).
- Hepatitis A infection usually results in an acute, self-limited illness and only rarely leads to fulminant hepatic failure.
- Illness begins with the abrupt onset of prodromal symptoms including, fatigue, malaise, nausea, vomiting, anorexia, fever, and right upper quadrant pain. Dark urine, jaundice, and pruritus develop in a few days. Prodromal symptoms decrease as the jaundice appears.
- Physical examination shows jaundice and hepatomegaly. There may be splenomegaly, and cervical lymphadenopathy.
- Hepatitis A does not lead to chronic infection, chronic hepatitis, cirrhosis or carrier state.

Laboratory findings

- Serum aminotransferases are markedly elevated (peak levels vary from 400 to 4,000 IU). ALT (SGPT) is more elevated than AST (SGOT). Aminotransferase elevations precede the bilirubin elevation. Bilirubin is elevated (up to 30 mg/dL) and is usually equally divided between the conjugated and unconjugated fractions. ALP is normal or mildly elevated. Other laboratory abnormalities are increased CRP, ESR and immunoglobulins.
- Prothrombin time (PT) may be prolonged and signifies extensive hepatocellular necrosis and worse prognosis.
- IgM anti-HAV antibody appears early in the disease and persists for 4 to 12 months. It can be used for the diagnosis of acute hepatitis A. IgG antibodies also appear early in the course and persists for life. Other viral markers such as HbsAg, anti-HCV and anti-HEV should be done to rule out other causes of viral hepatitis.
- Imaging studies, such as ultrasound abdomen, are done, if there is possibility of an alternative diagnosis. It may show hepatomegaly in acute hepatitis.

Treatment

- The disease is usually self-limited, and treatment is mainly supportive with hydration, vitamins and antipyretics.
- Liver transplantation should be considered for patients who develop fulminant liver failure.

Prevention of Hepatitis A

- Improvement of sanitation, handwashing before eating, heating foods appropriately, and avoidance of water and foods from endemic areas prevent the transmission of virus. Chlorination and household bleach (1:100 dilution) inactivate the virus.
- *Vaccine:* A safe and effective HAV vaccine is available (HAVRIX by GlaxoSmithKline). It is given as two injections 6 months apart (1.0 mL intramuscular). It is recommended for patients at high risk of acquiring hepatitis A such as travelers to endemic areas, children in communities with high rates of infection,

men who have sex with men, injection drug users, patients with chronic liver disease and recipients of pooled plasma products, such as hemophiliacs.

- *Post-exposure prophylaxis:* Vaccine is not effective for post-exposure prophylaxis because antibodies take a few days to develop. Immunoglobulin is recommended for post exposure prophylaxis of household and intimate contacts of persons with acute hepatitis A. The dose is 2 mL given intramuscularly within 2 weeks of exposure. Concurrent HAV vaccination is also appropriate.

Q. Describe the etiology, epidemiology, pathogenesis, clinical features, laboratory findings and treatment of hepatitis B.

Q. Prevention of hepatitis B.

Hepatitis B is an acute systemic infection which primarily affects liver.

Etiology

Hepatitis B is caused by the hepatitis B virus (HBV) which is a DNA virus belonging to the family of Hepadnavirus. It has double-stranded DNA.

Epidemiology

- Incubation period is about 90 days (50–150 days).
- The virus infects only humans and higher apes.
- It is transmitted mainly by parenteral route, and unsafe sexual practices.
- Persons at risk of developing infection include; spouse of an acutely infected person, unprotected sex with multiple partners (especially men who have sex with men), health care workers, injection drug users, receipients of repeated blood transfusions, dentists, prisoners, family members of chronically infected persons,

persons on hemodialysis, being born to an infected mother.

Pathogenesis

The pathogenesis of HBV-related liver disease is largely due to immune-mediated mechanisms resulting in destruction of HBV-infected hepatocytes by cytotoxic T cells. Rarely HBV can cause direct cytotoxic liver injury.

Clinical Features

Clinical features are similar to hepatitis A.

Laboratory Findings

- Liver function tests are same as described in hepatitis A.
- Presence of HBsAg confirms the diagnosis of hepatitis B infection. Presence of IgM anti-HBc (hepatitis B core antigen) indicates acute infection. Presence of serum IgG anti-HBc indicates chronic hepatitis-B infection. Presence of HBeAg is associated with high infectivity. Serum anti-HBsAg indicates immunity and found during recovery from hepatitis B and after vaccination.
- HBV DNA by PCR is helpful when hepatitis B is strongly suspected in spite of negative HBsAg. It is also useful to monitor the disease activity and response to treatment.

Treatment

Same as acute hepatitis A.

Complications

- Serum sickness–like syndrome.
- Glomerulonephritis with nephrotic syndrome.
- Polyarteritis nodosa–like systemic vasculitis.
- Fulminant hepatitis (massive hepatic necrosis).
- Chronic hepatitis B (persistence of HBeAg beyond 3 months or HBsAg beyond 6 months).

- Aplastic anemia.
- Transverse myelitis.

Prognosis

- 95–99% of patients recover completely.
- Fulminant hepatitis: 0.1–1%
- Chronic hepatitis: 1–10%
- Carrier state: 0.1–30%

Prevention

Pre-Exposure Prophylaxis

- Recombinant hepatitis B vaccine (e.g. Engerix-B), 1 mL (20 µg) given IM at 0, 1, and 6 months.
- Alternative schedules have been approved, including accelerated schedules of 0, 1, 2, and 12 months. Vaccine should be given to deltoid and not gluteal region. A booster dose is required after 5 years. Half the dose is given for children.
- Vaccination is indicated for high-risk groups. But nowadays, hepatitis B vaccine is being given to all.

Post-Exposure Prophylaxis

- Hepatitis B immunoglobulin: 0.06 mL/kg IM should be given within 1 week after exposure, followed by a complete course of hepatitis B vaccine started within the first week. After sexual exposure, immunoglobulin can be given up to 14 days.
- For perinatal exposure of infants born to an HBsAg-positive mother, a single 0.5 mL IM dose of immunoglobulin should be given immediately after birth in combination with a complete course of 3 injections of hepatitis B vaccine.

Q. Define chronic hepatitis.

Q. Discuss the causes, pathology, clinical features, investigations and management of chronic hepatitis.

Definition

Chronic hepatitis is hepatitis that lasts >6 months.

Etiology

- Viruses (hepatitis B, C, D).
- Drugs (isoniazid, nitrofurantoin, amiodarone, methotrexate).
- Alcoholic steatohepatitis.
- Nonalcoholic steatohepatitis (NASH).
- Metabolic causes (Wilson's disease, hemochromatosis, alpha-1 antitrypsin deficiency, primary biliary cirrhosis, sclerosing cholangitis).
- Autoimmune hepatitis.
- Cryptogenic hepatitis.

Clinical Features

- Many patients are asymptomatic.
- Some may have malaise, anorexia, fatigue, low-grade fever and nonspecific upper abdominal discomfort.
- Jaundice is usually absent. Signs of chronic liver disease (e.g. splenomegaly, spider nevi, palmar erythema) or complications of cirrhosis (e.g. portal hypertension, ascites, encephalopathy) may be present in advanced cases.

Investigations

- Liver function tests show elevation of liver enzymes such as AST and ALT.
- Viral serologic tests.
- Autoantibodies, immunoglobulins, α_1-antitrypsin level, and other tests.
- Liver biopsy.

Treatment

- Supportive care.
- Treatment of cause (e.g. corticosteroids for autoimmune hepatitis, antivirals for HBV and HCV infection, withdrawal of offending drug in drug-induced chronic hepatitis).

Prognosis

Drug-induced chronic hepatitis often regresses completely when the causative drug is withdrawn. Untreated chronic viral hepatitis can lead to cirrhosis or development of hepatocellular carcinoma.

Q. Discuss the etiology, pathology, clinical features, investigations, complications and management of cirrhosis of liver.

Q. Child-Turcotte-Pugh scoring system.

- Cirrhosis refers to a late stage of progressive hepatic fibrosis characterized by distortion of the hepatic architecture and the formation of regenerative nodules.
- It represents the final common pathway of many types of chronic liver injury.

Causes of Cirrhosis

Infectious diseases
- Hepatitis B, C, D
- Cytomegalovirus
- Epstein-Barr virus
- Schistosomiasis

Drugs and toxins
- Alcohol (Laennec's cirrhosis)
- Amiodarone
- Oral contraceptives
- Pyrrolidizine alkaloids and antineoplastic agents

Inherited and metabolic disorders
- Alpha-1antitrypsin deficiency
- Wilson's disease
- Hemochromatosis
- Galactosemia
- Gaucher's disease
- Glycogen storage disease
- Cystic fibrosis

Biliary disorders
- Primary biliary cirrhosis
- Biliary atresia
- Primary sclerosing cholangitis
- Chronic biliary obstruction

Cardiovascular causes
- Chronic right heart failure (cardiac cirrhosis)

Others
- Nonalcoholic fatty liver disease (NASH)
- Sarcoidosis
- Scleroderma
- Autoimmune hepatitis
- Cryptogenic

Epidemiology

- Alcoholic cirrhosis is the most common type of cirrhosis seen all over the world. Post-hepatitic cirrhosis especially due to hepatitis B or C is the second most common cirrhosis.
- Cirrhosis is more common in males but primary biliary cirrhosis is more common in females.
- Cirrhosis is the most common indication for liver transplantation.

Pathology

- Cirrhosis is the final common pathway of many types of chronic liver injury.
- Irreversible chronic injury of the hepatic parenchyma leads to extensive fibrosis, loss of the normal liver architecture and formation of regenerative nodules. The changes in cirrhosis affect the whole liver. Destruction of the liver architecture causes distortion and loss of the normal hepatic vasculature with the development of portosystemic vascular shunts.
- Activation of the hepatic stellate cell is the central event leading to hepatic fibrosis. When activated, the quiescent fat-storing stellate cells become multifunctional cells, capable of collagen production, contraction and cytokine synthesis.
- Cirrhosis can be classified histologically into two types: (1) Micronodular cirrhosis is characterized by small nodules less than 3 mm in diameter, (2) Macronodular cirrhosis is characterized by larger nodules which are more than 3 mm in diameter. Differentiation between these morphologic types of cirrhosis has limited clinical value.

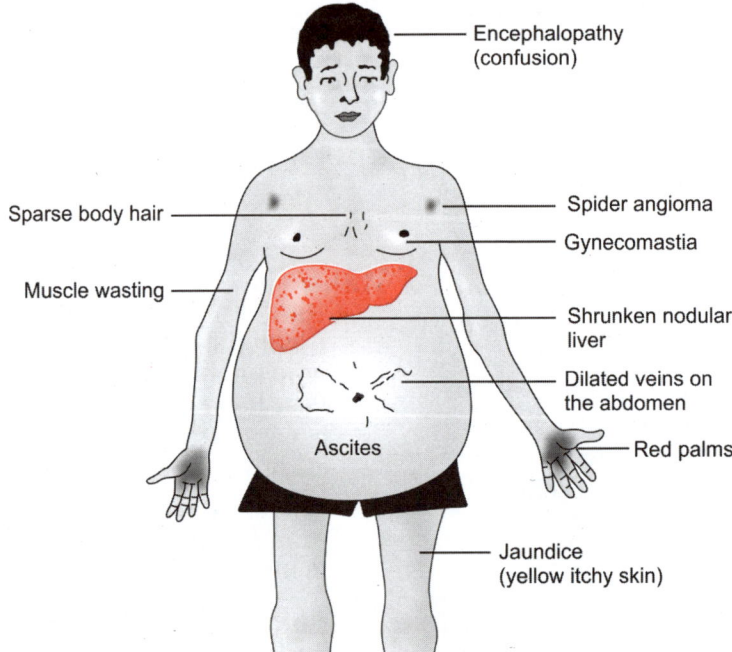

Fig. 3.2: Clinical features of cirrhosis of the liver

Clinical Features (Fig. 3.2)

Symptoms
- May be asymptomatic.
- Anorexia, weight loss, fatigue/weakness.
- Hematemesis, malena due to bleeding esophageal varices.
- Abdominal distension due to ascites.
- Women may report menstrual irregularities due to endocrine alterations.

General Examination
- Muscle wasting
- Pallor due to GI blood loss
- Jaundice
- Spider angiomas
- Bleeding manifestations such as purpura, bruises
- Palmar erythema
- Pruritus
- Decreased body hair
- Gynecomastia
- Testicular atrophy
- Flapping tremors (in hepatic enecephalopathy)
- Parotid gland enlargement
- Edema

Abdomen
- Liver is shrunken, firm and nodular.
- Splenomegaly may be present.
- Ascites as evidenced by bulging flanks, shifting dullness and fluid thrill.
- Caput medusa (dilated veins around the umbilicus).
- Melanosis: Gradual darkening of the exposed areas of the skin.
- Steatorrhea.

CVS
Look for evidence of right heart failure (cardiac cirrhosis) such as raised JVP, right-sided S3, S4, dilated heart, etc.

RS

Pleural effusion (especially right sided) may develop in severe ascites.

NS

Patient can be in altered sensorium in hepatic encephalopathy, electrolyte imbalance, hypoglycemia, etc.

Investigations

Complete Blood Count

Anemia may be present due to blood loss, folate deficiency and hypersplenism. Pancytopenia due to hypersplenism.

Liver Function Tests

Hypoalbuminemia and increased globulin levels (reversal of A:G ratio). Bilirubin level and aminotransferases may be mildly elevated. ALP is mildly elevated. Prothrombin time (PT) may be prolonged.

Urea, Creatinine, Serum Electrolytes

- Urea and creatinine are usually normal unless there is development of hepatorenal syndrome.
- Metabolic disturbances such as hyponatremia, hypokalemia and hypoglycemia may be present. Hypoglycemia is due to impaired gluconeogenesis by the liver.

Investigations to Identify the Underlying Cause

- Hepatitis serologies (HBsAg, anti-HCV, anti-HDV).
- Iron, total iron-binding capacity and ferritin, if hemochromatosis is suspected.
- Antimitochondrial antibody (AMA), if primary biliary cirrhosis is suspected.
- Antinuclear antibody, anti-smooth-muscle antibody, if autoimmune etiology is suspected.
- Serum copper and ceruloplasmin levels, if Wilson disease is suspected.
- Alpha-1 antitrypsin levels, if deficiency is suspected.

Imaging

- Abdominal ultrasound with Doppler may show nodular liver, splenomegaly and dilated portal vein with collateral vessels.
- CT or MRI is rarely required.

Liver Biopsy (Percutaneous, Transjugular, or Open)

This is the test for definitive diagnosis of cirrhosis but not routinely required except in cases of doubt about diagnosis and etiology. It shows regenerating nodules and fibrosis.

Treatment

- Diet should provide adequate calories and protein (1–1.5 g/kg/d). Reduce protein intake to 60–80 g/d, if there is hepatic encephalopathy. Restrict sodium, if there is fluid retention. Benefit of branched-chain amino acids to prevent or treat hepatic encephalopathy is uncertain. Vitamin supplementation is advisable, especially vit-K.
- All patients with cirrhosis should receive the HAV, HBV, and pneumococcal vaccines and a yearly influenza vaccine.
- Portal hypertension can be reduced by nonselective beta blockers such as propranolol or nadolol. Nitrates can be used for patients in whom beta-blockers are contraindicated. Esophageal varices should be treated by endoscopic variceal ligation.
- Ascites and edema is treated by diuretics (spironolactone and frusemide). Correction of hypoalbuminemia by albumin transfusions also helps edema and ascites. Paracentesis is indicated for tense ascites. Transjugular intrahepatic portosystemic shunt (TIPS) is helpful in the treatment of severe refractory ascites.
- Lactulose syrup is used daily (15 mL at night) to pevent hepatic encephalopathy.
- Complications of cirrhosis such as hepatic encephalopathy and variceal bleed should be treated as per standard guidelines.
- Liver transplantation can be considered in suitable patients.

Prognosis

- The overall prognosis in cirrhosis is poor. Only 25% of patients survive 5 years from diagnosis. Prognosis is more favourable, if the underlying cause can be corrected, such as alcohol abuse. Complications such as variceal bleed can cause unexpected death.
- *Indicators of poor prognosis in cirrhosis:* Presence of jaundice, ascites, encephalopathy, renal impairement, hyponatremia (<130 mEq/L), elevated hepatic venous pressure gradient, albumin <3 g/dL, bilirubin >3 mg/dL, cachexia, upper gastrointestinal bleeding.
- The Child-Pugh score is a tool to assess prognosis in cirrhosis.

Child-Turcotte-Pugh scoring system to assess the severity of liver disease			
Parameter	*Points assigned*		
	1	*2*	*3*
Ascites	Absent	slight	Moderate
Bilirubin, mg/dL	<2	2–3	>3
Albumin, g/dL	>3.5	2.8–3.5	<2.8
Prothrombin time	<4	4–6	>6
Seconds over control or INR	<1.7	1.7–2.3	>2.3
Encephalopathy	None	Grade 1–2	Grade 3–4

- A total score of 5–6 is considered grade A (well-compensated disease).
- Score 7–9 is grade B (significant functional compromise).
- Score 10–15 is grade C (decompensated disease).
- These grades correlate with one- and two-year patient survival: Grade A—100 and 85%; grade B—80 and 60%; and grade C—45 and 35%.

Complications

- Portal HTN
- Variceal bleeding
- Spontaneous bacterial peritonitis
- Hepatic encephalopathy
- Hepatorenal syndrome
- Hepatopulmonary syndrome
- Hepatocellular carcinoma

Q. Define ascites. Discuss the causes and approach to a case of ascites.

Q. Discuss the etiology, clinical features, investigations and management of a case of ascites.

Ascites refers to the accumulation of excess fluid in the peritoneal cavity.

Causes of Ascites

- Cirrhosis of liver with portal hypertension
- Cardiac failure
- Renal failure
- Hypoproteinemia (nephrotic syndrome, protein-losing enteropathy, malnutrition)
- Intra-abdominal malignancy
- Pancreatitis
- Abdominal tuberculosis
- Hepatic venous occlusion (Budd-Chiari syndrome, veno-occlusive disease)
- Rare causes (Meigs' syndrome, lymphatic obstruction, vasculitis, hypothyroidism)

Clinical Features

Symptoms

- Abdominal distension.
- Dyspnea and orthopnea due to pushed up diaphragm.
- Epigastric and retrosternal burning sensation due to gastroesophageal reflux due to increased intra-abdominal pressure.
- Low grade fever and weight loss suggests tuberculous etiology.
- Presence of exertional dyspnea, orthopnea and PND suggests heart failure.

Signs

- At least 1 litre of fluid should be present in the abdomen to be clinically detectable.

- Presence of jaundice and dilated veins over the abdomen indicate cirrhosis of liver with portal HTN. Other stigmata of liver disease such as spider naevi, palmar eryrthema, and gynecomastia may be present.
- Diffuse abdominal distension with fullness in the flanks. Skin appears shiny.
- Umbilicus is flush with the skin or everted.
- Shifting dullness present on percussion. Fluid thrill is present in tense ascites.
- Tenderness may be present in the abdomen and points towards an infectious etiology such as tuberculosis or peritonitis.
- Herniae, abdominal striae, divarication of the recti and scrotal edema may be present.
- Pleural effusions may be present in some patients usually on the right side.
- In cases of ascites due to heart failure, signs of congestive heart failure such as raised JVP, basal lung crepitations and third heart sound may be present.
- In cases of malignant ascites, sometimes a mass may be palpable per abdomen.

Investigations

Ultrasound abdomen: This is the easiest and most sensitive test to detect ascites. It can also show the underlying cause of ascites in many cases (such as cirrhosis of liver, intra-abdominal malignancy, portal HTN).

Ascitic fluid analysis

- *Appearance:* Clear or straw colored in case of transudates. Turbid appearance is seen in infections and malignancy. White color appearance is seen in chylous ascites.
- *Cell count:* Normal ascitic fluid contains fewer than 500 WBCs/µL and fewer than 250 polymorphonuclear leukocytes (PMNs)/µL. High WBC count is found in infections. A PMN count of greater than 250 cells/µL is highly suggestive of bacterial peritonitis. Presence of high percentage of lymphocytes indicates tuberculous etiology.
- *Serum-ascites albumin gradient (SAAG):* The SAAG is the best single test for classifying ascites into transudative (SAAG >1.1 g/dL)

and exudative (SAAG <1.1 g/dL) causes. It is calculated by subtracting the ascitic fluid albumin value from the serum albumin value.
- *Total protein:* Total ascitic fluid protein greater than or equal to 2.5 g/dL indicates exudative ascites.
- *Culture/Gram stain/AFB stain:* They are useful to identify the infecting organism in cases of ascites due to intra-abdominal infections.
- *Malignant cytology:* Useful in cases of suspected malignant ascites.
- *Ascitic fluid amylase:* It is typically >1000 mg/dL in pancreatic ascites.
- *Adenosine deaminase (ADA):* It is usally more than 40U/L in tuberculuos ascites.

Chest X-ray: Pleural effusion may be present in cases of massive ascites.

CT abdomen: Useful to diagnose or rule out cirrhosis, malignancy, tuberculosis, etc.

ECG/echocardiogram: To rule out congestive cardiac failure.

Treatment

- Treat the underlying cause.
- Salt restriction and diuretic therapy in cases of transudative ascites.
- Therapeutic paracentesis may be performed in patients who require rapid symptomatic relief for refractory or tense ascites.
- The transjugular intrahepatic portosystemic shunt (TIPS) is useful in cirrhotic patients with refractory ascites.

Q. Define diarrhea, pseudo-diarrhea and fecal incontinence.

Q. What are the causes of acute diarrhea? How do you evaluate and manage a case of acute diarrhea?

- Diarrhea is defined as abnormal increase in stool liquidity, frequency and quantity. Typically a stool weight >200 g/d or frequency more than 3 times per day is considered to indicate diarrhea.

- Depending on the duration, diarrhea may be classified as acute—if <2 weeks, persistent—if 2 to 4 weeks, and chronic—if >4 weeks in duration.
- Diarrhea should be differentiated from pseudo-diarrhea, and fecal incontinence. Pseudo-diarrhea is frequent passage of small volumes of stool. It is seen in irritable bowel syndrome and anorectal disorders such as proctitis. Fecal incontinence is involuntary discharge of fecal matter and is seen in neuromuscular disorders and structural anorectal problems.

Causes of Acute Diarrhea

Bacterial	Viral
• *Staphylococcus aureus*	• Noroviruses
• *Bacillus cereus*	• Rotavirus
• *Vibrio cholerae*	• Cytomegalovirus
• *Clostridium difficile*	**Protozoal**
• *Shigella*	• *Giardia lamblia*
• *Salmonella*	• *Cryptosporidium*
• *Campylobacter jejuni*	• *Cyclospora*
• Enteroinvasive *E. coli* (EIEC)	• *Entamoeba histolytica*

Pathophysiology of Diarrhea

- Diarrhea is the reversal of the normal net absorptive status of water and electrolyte absorption to secretion. Such a derangement can be the result of either an osmotic force that acts in the lumen to drive water into the gut (osmotic diarrhea) or the result of an active secretory state induced in the enterocytes (secretory diarrhea).
- Example of osmotic diarrhea is lactulose induced diarrhea. In secretory diarrhea, the epithelial cells' ion transport processes are turned into a state of active secretion. Example of secretory diarrhea is cholera. Pathogens can induce secretory diarrhea through multiple mechanisms such as production of enterotoxins or cytotoxins, release of cytokines, etc.

EVALUATION OF A PATIENT WITH ACUTE DIARRHEA

History

- Residence (cholera is common in India, *Salmonella* is common in coastal areas).
- Occupational exposure.
- Recent and remote travel (suspect diseases endemic in the area of travel).
- Duration of diarrhea (whether acute or chronic, because the causes are different).
- Frequency and quantity of stools (to assess the severity of diarrhea).
- Appearance of stools: Rice water stool is seen in cholera, pea soup appearance in enteric fever, brown colored in amebiasis.
- Presence of blood and/or mucus (suggests invasive infection. Fresh blood and mucus is seen in large intestinal diarrhea).
- Any associated vomiting (suggests food poisoning or gastroenteritis).
- History of pain abdomen (suggests invasive infection).
- Urine output (to assess dehydration).
- History of fever (suggests infection with invasive organisms).
- Multiple people getting affected after having same food (suggests food poisoning).
- Recent antibiotic use (may suggest antibiotic-induced diarrhea due to *C. difficile*).
- History of immunocompromised state (suspect diarrhea due to unusual organisms such as *Cryptosporidia*, *Isospora belli*, etc).
- History of animal exposure: Exposure to young dogs or cats is associated with *Campylobacter* organisms. Exposure to turtles is associated with *Salmonella* organisms.

Examination

- Look for any signs of dehydration. Assess pulse, BP, postural hypotension, skin turgor, dryness of mucous membranes.
- Assess conscious level as patient can be in altered sensorium due to electrolyte imbalance.
- Examine the abdomen for any distension, tenderness and bowel sounds.

Investigations in Acute Diarrhea

Most cases of acute diarrhea improve spontaneously with supportive treatment and do not require investigations. However, acute diarrhea should be investigated, if it is severe with dehydration, associated with bloody stools, fever, lasts more than 2 days without improvement, new community outbreaks, severe abdominal pain and in immunocompromised patients.

Complete Blood Count (CBC)

Hemoconcentration is commonly seen due to dehydration. High leucocyte count suggests infectious diarrhea.

Urea/Creatinine, Serum Electrolytes

Urea and creatinine may be elevated due to dehydration. Electrolyte disturbances such as hyponatremia and hypokalemia occur in severe diarrhea.

Stool Analysis

Stool should be sent for bacterial and viral cultures, microscopy for ova and parasites, immunoassays for bacterial toxins (*C. difficile*), viral antigens (rotavirus), and protozoal antigens (*Giardia, E. histolytica*). Pathogens can also be identified by detecting their DNA sequences.

Ultrasound Abdomen

Useful, if there is severe abdominal pain or abdominal distension or any mass is felt.

GI Scopy

- If stool analysis does not reveal the cause of diarrhea, then flexible sigmoidoscopy with biopsies and upper endoscopy with duodenal aspirates and biopsies may be indicated.
- Colonoscopy may be indicated to identify any growth, or to exclude inflammatory bowel disease.

CT Scan Abdomen

Is useful in the evaluation of ischemic colitis, diverticulitis, or partial bowel obstruction.

Assessment of Dehydration

Assessment of dehydration is depicted in Table 3.3.

Treatment

Fluid and Electrolyte Replacement

This is very important in acute diarrhea since dehydration is the major cause of death. If the patient is able to take orally, oral fluid replacement (ORS) can be given in mild-to-moderate dehydration. Intravenous rehydration is

Table: 3.3: Assessment of dehydration

Feature	Mild dehydration	Moderate dehydration	Severe dehydration
General	Well	Restless	Lethargic
Oral mucosa	Moist	Dry	Very dry
Skin turgor	Normal	Reduced	Markedly reduced
Capillary refilling	Normal	Slow	Very slow
Eyes	Normal	Sunken	Markedly sunken
Pulse rate	Normal	Tachycardia	Markedly increased
BP	Normal	Postural drop or reduced	Hypotension/shock
Urine output	Normal	Reduced	Markedly reduced
Urine specific gravity	<1.020	>1.020	>1.035
Blood urea	Normal	Normal or high	High

required, if the patient is not able to take orally, in severe dehydration, in infants, and elderly.

Antimotility Agents

Agents like loperamide, diphenoxylate/atropine combination decrease the frequency and quantity of diarrhea. They can be used in diarrhea without fever and without blood in stools. These agents should be avoided in infective diarrhea (febrile dysentery), which may be exacerbated or prolonged by them.

Antisecretory Agents

Example is racecadotril. It inhibits secretion of water and electrolytes into the intestinal lumen and hence decreases the frequency of loose stools. It is useful in acute watery diarrhea.

Antispasmodics

Such as dicyclomine, hyoscine, etc. can be used in patients with crampy abdominal pain.

Antibiotics

- Severe dysentery with fever may be empirically treated with a quinolone, such as ciprofloxacin (500 mg bid for 3 to 5 days).
- Empirical treatment with metronidazole can also be given for suspected giardiasis or amebiasis (400 mg TID for 5 to 7 days).
- Antibiotic therapy may be modified when specific pathogen is identified.
- Antibiotics should also be given to patients who are immunocompromised, have mechanical heart valves or recent vascular grafts, or are elderly, even if the organism is not identified.

Q. Traveler's diarrhea.

- Traveler's diarrhea refers to diarrhea occurring in persons traveling from resource-rich to resource-poor regions of the world. It is common among travelers to developing countries.
- Food and water contaminated with fecal matter are the main sources of infection. Most cases are benign and self-limited, but

occasionally can be severe enough to cause dehydration and other complications.

Causes of Traveler's Diarrhea

Bacteria	Viruses
• *Escherichia coli (E. coli)*	• Rotavirus
• *Campylobacter jejuni*	• Norwalk virus
• *Salmonella*	**Parasites**
• *Shigella*	• *Giardia lamblia*
• *Vibrio cholerae*	• *Entamoeba histolytica*

- These organisms are often transmitted by food and water.
- More than 90% cases are due to bacteria; the most common being enterotoxigenic *Escherichia coli* (ETEC).

Clinical Features

- Most cases occur within first 2 weeks of travel.
- Abdominal cramps followed by sudden onset, watery diarrhea, lasting 2 to 5 days.
- Malaise, anorexia, nausea, vomiting, and fever.
- Diffuse tenderness over abdomen.
- Additional specific features may be present depending on the organism.

Treatment

- *Fluid replacement:* Most cases are self-limited and resolve on their own within 3 to 5 days of treatment with fluid replacement only. Oral fluid replacement is enough in most cases. ORS is especially useful in severe diarrhea.
- *Antibiotics:* Shorten the disease duration to about one day. Antibiotics are indicated in patients with severe diarrhea associated with fever, blood, pus, or mucus in the stool. Ciprofloxacin or norfloxacin may be used.
- *Antimotility agents:* Antimotility agents such as loperamide (imodium) or diphenoxylate (lomotil) can be used to reduce severity of diarrhea. However, caution

should be exercised in using these agents in bloody diarrhea.

Prevention

- *Improving food and drink selection:* Avoid raw food items such as chutney, salads, buttermilk, and curds. Use only boiled or bottled water. Avoid fresh fruit juices with ice.
- *Prophylactic antibiotics:* Not routinely necessary. Quinolones or doxycycline 100 mg/day for a few weeks. Bismuth subsalicylate 60 mL four times a day is an alternative. Rifaximin may prove to be the preferred antibiotic because it is not absorbed and is well tolerated.
- *Probiotics:* Such as *Lactobacillus* and *Saccharomyces boulardii* have been shown to decrease the incidence of diarrhea in travelers.

> **Q. Define chronic diarrhea. What are the causes of chronic diarrhea? How do you investigate and manage a case of chronic diarrhea?**

Chronic diarrhea is defined as diarrhea lasting for more than 4 weeks.

Causes of Chronic Diarrhea

- Inflammatory bowel disease (ulcerative colitis and Crohn's disease)
- Malabsorption syndromes (celiac sprue, tropical sprue, Whipple's disease, chronic pancreatitis)
- Hyperthyroidism
- Irritable bowel syndrome (IBS)
- Chronic infections (intestinal tuberculosis, amebiasis, AIDS-related infections)
- Diabetes mellitus with autonomic neuropathy
- Carcinoid syndrome
- Cancer of colon
- Laxative abuse.

Investigations in Chronic Diarrhea

- In contrast to acute diarrhea, most cases of chronic diarrhea are noninfectious.

- All the tests described for acute diarrhea are required for chronic diarrhea.
- 24-hour stool fat estimation, testing for presence of laxatives, and estimation of stool osmolality (normal osmotic gap in secretory diarrhea, increased in osmotic diarrhea) should be done.
- Intestinal aspirates and quantitative cultures to rule out small bowel bacterial overgrowth.
- If suggested by history or other findings, hormonal excesses should be ruled out by appropriate tests (serum gastrin, VIP, calcitonin, thyroid function tests, etc.).
- Low fecal pH suggests carbohydrate malabsorption; lactose malabsorption can be confirmed by lactose breath testing or by a therapeutic trial with lactose exclusion and observation of the effect of lactose challenge.
- Pancreatic disease should be excluded by secretin-cholecystokinin stimulation test, or by assay of fecal chymotrypsin activity or a bentiromide test.
- Ultrasound abdomen to rule out pancreatitis and malignancy.
- Colonoscopy to rule out ileocecal TB, carcinoma colon, inflammatory bowel disease, etc.
- CT abdomen, if malignancy or pancreatitis or abdominal TB is suspected.

Treatment of Chronic Diarrhea

Treatment of chronic diarrhea depends on the specific etiology. For example, elimination of lactose containing foods in lactase deficiency or gluten in celiac sprue, use of steroids or anti-inflammatory agents in inflammatory bowel diseases, etc.

> **Q. Define dysentery. Describe the etiology, clinical features, investigations and management of dysentery.**

Definition

Dysentery is bloody diarrhea, i.e. any diarrheal episode in which the stools contain visible red blood.

Etiology

- There are two main types of dysentery. The first type, *amebic dysentery*, is caused by *Entamoeba histolytica*. The second type, *bacillary dysentery*, is caused by invasive bacteria such as *Shigella*, *Campylobacter*, *E. coli*, and *Salmonella*. Bacillary dysentery is the most common cause of dysentery.
- Poor hygiene and sanitation increase the risk of dysentery by spreading the parasite or bacteria that cause it through food or water contaminated from infected human feces.

Clinical Features

The main symptom of dysentery is loose stools flecked with blood, mucus, or pus. Other symptoms include fever, abdominal pain, cramps and bloating, flatulence (passing gas) and vomiting. Dehydration can occur in severe dysentery. Signs of dehydration include dry mouth, sunken eyes, and poor skin tone.

Investigations

- Stool sample analysis: Stool culture for bacteria such as *Shigella*, stool micrscopy to look for *Entamoeba histolytica*.

- Detection of serum antiamebic antibody helps in the diagnosis of amebic dysentery.

Treatment

- It is very important to replace the fluids lost from dysentery. Oral rehydration salts are available for this purpose. In mild cases, soft drinks, juices, and bottled water will be enough. Intravenous fluid may be needed in severe cases.
- For bacillary dysentery, antibiotics like ciprofloxacin or azithromycin are used.
- For amebic dysentery, antiparasitic medications such as metronidazole or tinidazole are used.

Prevention

- Dysentery can be prevented to some extent by practicing careful personal hygiene.
- Do not eat any foods cooked in unhygienic circumstances, such as from street vendors. Only eat cooked foods that have been heated to a high temperature. Do not eat raw vegetables. Avoid species of fruits without peels.
- Drink only commercially bottled or boiled water. Do not use ice unless it has been made from purified water.

Cardiovascular System

Q. Discuss the etiology, clinical features, investigations, and treatment of acute rheumatic Fever.

Q. Aschoff nodule.

Q. Erythema marginatum.

Q. Jones criteria.

Rheumatic fever involves the heart, joints, central nervous system, skin, and subcutaneous tissues with varying frequency. Involvement of the heart may lead to rheumatic heart disease, which can lead to heart failure later.

Etiology

- Rheumatic fever is an autoimmune inflammatory process that develops as a sequel of group A beta-hemolytic *Streptococcus* infection.
- Rheumatic fever follows pharyngeal infection with group-A beta-hemolytic *Streptococcus*. It usually occurs two to three weeks after the attack of pharyngitis. However, some patients with rheumatic fever do not give history of preceding pharyngitis.

Epidemiology

- Rheumatic fever is a major health problem in the developing countries of Asia, Africa, Middle East, and Latin America.
- The incidence of rheumatic fever has decreased now because of the availability of antibiotics.
- Outbreaks of rheumatic fever closely follow epidemics of streptococcal pharyngitis or scarlet fever. Patients who have suffered an initial attack of rheumatic fever tend to experience recurrences of the disease following group A streptococcal infections. Adequate treatment of streptococcal pharyngitis markedly reduces the incidence of rheumatic fever. Recurrence is rare beyond age 34.
- Acute rheumatic fever is most common among children in the 5- to 15-year age group.

Pathogenesis

- Molecular mimicry is thought to play an important role in tissue injury. There are shared epitopes between cardiac myosin and streptococcal M protein that lead to cross-reactive humoral and T cell immunity. Epitopes of streptococcal M protein also share antigenic determinants with heart valves, sarcolemmal membrane proteins, synovium, and articular cartilage.

- Host factors may also play a role. Associations between disease and human leukocyte antigen (HLA) class II alleles have been identified. Certain B cell alloantigens are expressed to a greater level in patients with rheumatic fever.
- During active rheumatic carditis, there is T cell and macrophage infiltration of heart valves, and the production of interleukin-1 and interleukin-2 is increased. All these result in scarring and collagen deposition in the valves and destruction of myocytes. There will be exudative and proliferative inflammatory lesions in the connective tissue of the heart, joints, and subcutaneous tissue. All the three layers of the heart are involved (pancarditis).

Pericardium

Pericarditis is common and fibrinous pericarditis is occasionally present. Thick exudates give bread and butter appearance macroscopically. Pericarditis usually heals without any sequelae.

Myocardium

- In the myocardium, there is fragmentation of collagen fibers, lymphocytic infiltration, fibrinoid degeneration and the presence of Aschoff nodules, which are considered pathognomonic of acute rheumatic fever.
- The Aschoff nodule consists of an area of central necrosis surrounded by lymphocytes, plasma cells, and large mononuclear and giant multinucleate cells.

Endocardium

- Endocarditis is responsible for chronic rheumatic valvulitis. Small vegetations, 1 to 2 mm in diameter, are seen on the atrial surface of valve margins and chordae tendineae. There is edema and inflammation of the valve leaflets.
- Healing of the valvulitis leads to fibrosis of the leaflets and fusion of the chordae resulting in valvular stenosis or incompetence.
- The mitral valve is affected most commonly, followed by the aortic valve. Tricuspid and pulmonic valves are rarely affected.

Extracardiac Lesions

Inflammation can affect the joints (rheumatic arthritis), skin (subcutaneous nodules), lung (rheumatic pneumonitis) and brain.

Clinical Features

General

Fever, lassitude, prostration, tachycardia.

Sore Throat

Only two-thirds of patients give history of preceding sore throat.

Cardiac

- Carditis is the only manifestation of acute rheumatic fever that has the potential to cause long-term disability and death. Cardiac failure can occur due to severe mitral regurgitation or severe myocarditis.
- It involves all the three layers of the heart, i.e. endocardium, myocardium and pericardium.
- Various murmurs due to valvular stenosis or regurgitation may be found on cardiac examination.
- Acute congestive heart failure can develop leading to hepatic congestion and right upper quadrant pain and tenderness. Congestive heart failure is usually caused by left ventricular volume overload associated with severe mitral or aortic regurgitation.
- Pericardial friction rub may be heard due to pericarditis. Muffled heart sounds due to pericardial effusion.

Polyarthritis

- Arthritis is the most frequent major manifestation of rheumatic fever (occurs in approximately 75% of patients). Arthralgia is pain in the joints without signs of inflammation.
- It is migratory polyarthritis (joints are involved in quick succession, and each for a brief period of time).

- Usually larger joints such as knees, ankles, elbows, and wrists are involved.
- Small joints and spine are involved rarely.
- Polyarthritis responds dramatically to salicylate therapy.

Subcutaneous Nodules

- It occurs in less than 10% of patients. They are round, firm, painless, freely movable subcutaneous lesions varying in size from 0.5 to 2 cm.
- Common sites of occurrence are over bony surfaces and over tendons such as elbows, knees, and wrists, the occiput and vertebrae.

Erythema Marginatum

- It occurs in less than 10% of patients. This rash is usually found on the trunk and proximal parts of the extremities. Face is spared.
- It appears as erythematous macule or papule with clear centre. Lesions may merge and form serpiginous patterns.
- The rash is transient, migrating from place-to-place without leaving residual scarring. Erythema marginatum has also been reported in sepsis, drug reactions, and glomerulonephritis.

Jones Criteria for the Diagnosis of the Initial Attack of Rheumatic Fever

The presence of two major manifestations or one major and two minor manifestations indicates a high probability of acute rheumatic fever (Table 4.1).

Laboratory Findings

- *Blood count:* Shows increased WBC count, elevated CRP and ESR.
- *Streptococcal antibody tests [antistreptolysin O (ASO)]:* ASO titre is elevated in 80% or more of patients with rheumatic fever. ASO titers greater than 200 Todd units/mL is considered significant.
- *ECG:* Tachycardia, prolongation of the PR interval, AV conduction abnormalities.
- *Echocardiogram:* It shows valvular abnormalities and evidence of cardiac failure.
- *Endomyocardial biopsy:* Shows presence of Aschoff nodules and interstitial mononuclear infiltrates with or without myocyte necrosis.

Treatment

- The patient should be kept at strict bed rest until the fever subsides, and ESR, pulse rate, ECG have all returned to baseline.
- *Antibiotics:* Single dose of benzathine penicillin or a 10-day course of penicillin-V (or erythromycin, if penicillin allergic) to curtail exposure to streptococcal antigens. After completion of the course, secondary prophylaxis should be commenced.
- *Anti-inflammatory drugs:* They provide symptomatic relief of fever and joint pain. Aspirin is very effective for fever and joint inflammation. Corticosteroids are used in

Table 4.1: Jones criteria	
Major manifestations	*Minor manifestations*
• Carditis	• Arthralgia
• Polyarthritis	• Fever
• Chorea	• Elevated ESR or CRP level
• Erythema marginatum	• Prolonged PR interval
• Subcutaneous nodules	• Evidence of preceding group A streptococcal infection—positive throat culture or rapid antigen test result
	• Elevated or rising streptococcal antibody titer

patients with carditis manifest by heart failure and in patients who do not tolerate aspirin.

- Cardiac failure is managed by diuretics, ACE (angiotensin-converting enzyme) inhibitors, and beta-blockers. Mitral valve repair or replacement may be life-saving in acute intractable heart failure.

Q. Rheumatic fever prophylaxis.

Patients who have already suffered an attack of rheumatic fever are at risk of developing recurrent attacks of rheumatic fever. Recurrent attacks lead to progressive cardiac damage. Hence, rheumatic fever patients should be protected from subsequent streptococcal infections by giving continuous antimicrobial prophylaxis. The risk of recurrence decreases as the age advances.

Drugs used for prophylaxis

Inj Benzathine penicillin G 1.2 million units deep intramuscular (buttocks) every month. However, injections every three weeks may be more effective in preventing recurrences of acute rheumatic fever.

OR

Penicillin V 250 mg twice daily oral (for patients who cannot be given IM injection such as patients on anti-coagulation).

OR

Erythromycin 250 mg twice daily oral for patients who are allergic to penicillin.

Recommendations for the duration of secondary prophylaxis are given in Table 4.2.

Q. Discuss the etiology, clinical features, investigations, complications, and management of mitral stenosis.

- In normal adults, the cross-sectional area of the mitral valve orifice is 4 to 6 cm^2. If the orifice is reduced to less than this, it is called mitral stenosis.
- Mitral stenosis is considered mild when valve area is 2.5 to 1.5 cm^2, moderate when 1.5 to 1 cm^2, and severe or critical when less than 1.0 cm^2.

Etiology of Mitral Stenosis

- Rheumatic heart disease (RHD)
- Congenital mitral stenosis
- Carcinoid tumors
- Systemic lupus erythematosus
- Mucopolysaccharidoses (Hurler syndrome)

Rheumatic heart disease is the most common cause of MS, but only 50% patients remember the attack of rheumatic fever. MS is the most common valve lesion due to rheumatic fever. Rheumatic mitral stenosis is more common in women.

Pathophysiology

- When there is mitral stenosis, blood from left atrium cannot flow easily into left ventricle. Hence, blood collects in the left atrium and pressure increases in the left atrium. Because of increased pressure, left atrial hypertrophy and dilatation occur.
- Due to increased left atrial pressure, pulmonary venous, pulmonary arterial

Table 4.2: Recommendations for rheumatic fever prophylaxis	
Type	*Duration of prophylaxis after last attack*
Rheumatic fever with carditis and residual heart disease (persistent valvular disease	10 years or until age 40 years (whichever is longer); lifetime prophylaxis may be needed
Rheumatic fever with carditis but no residual heart disease (no valvular disease)	10 years or until age 21 years (whichever is longer)
Rheumatic fever without carditis	5 years or until age 21 years (whichever is longer)

and right heart pressures also increase. Increase in pulmonary vascular pressure leads to pulmonary edema and pulmonary hypertension.

- Pulmonary hypertension leads to right ventricular hypertrophy, dilatation and failure. Right ventricular dilatation results in tricuspid regurgitation.

Clinical Features

History

- Patients are usually asymptomatic until the valve orifice is moderately stenosed. Patient gradually becomes symptomatic as the severity of mitral stenosis increases. Once the patient becomes seriously symptomatic, death occurs in 2 to 5 years unless the stenosis is corrected.

- Patients complain of dyspnea due to pulmonary venous congestion and development of pulmonary hypertension. Dyspnea is exertional initially, but as the severity of MS increases, it may be present at rest also.

- Orthopnea and paroxysmal nocturnal dyspnea can occur because of increased venous return in supine position and consequent congestion of pulmonary vasculature.

- When RV failure occurs, ascites and edema develop.

- Dilated left atrium may lead to atrial fibrillation, giving rise to symptoms such as palpitations. Atrial fibrillation may result in left atrial clot formation and systemic emboli, most commonly to the cerebral vessels resulting in stroke.

Physical Examination

- Patients may have a typical look called 'mitral facies' or malar flush. This is a bilateral, cyanotic or dusky pink discoloration over the cheeks due to arteriovenous anastomoses and vascular stasis.

- Pulse is low volume and may be irregularly irregular due to atrial fibrillation.

- When right heart failure develops, there may be jugular venous distension, ascites, and pedal edema.

- Cardiac apex is tapping in nature due to palpable first heart sound.

- Parasternal heave may be present due to right ventricular hypertrophy.

- Loud first heart sound and opening snap may be heard on auscultation. A mid-diastolic 'rumbling' murmur is heard over the apex.

- Other findings include, tender hepatomegaly, pleural effusion due to right heart failure.

Complications of Mitral Stenosis

- Atrial fibrillation with clot formation and systemic embolization
- Pulmonary hypertension and right heart failure
- Recurrent chest infections
- Hemoptysis
- Infective endocarditis (rare)

Investigations

Chest X-ray: Chest X-ray shows left atrial enlargement, which produces straightening of the left heart border.

Electrocardiogram (ECG): ECG usually shows a bifid P wave due to left atrial enlargement. Atrial fibrillation is frequently present.

Echocardiogram: This is the most important tool to diagnose and confirm MS. It can assess the mitral valve apparatus, calculate mitral valve area, left atrial and right ventricular size and function.

Treatment

Medical Therapy

- Mild mitral stenosis in sinus rhythm does not require any treatment.
- If the patient develops atrial fibrillation, it should be treated with oral digoxin, or a

β-blocker, or a calcium channel blocker to control heart rate.

- Anticoagulation with warfarin should be done (target INR of 2.5 to 3.5) to prevent clot formation, if there is atrial fibrillation.
- Although infective endocarditis in pure mitral stenosis is rare, antibiotic prophylaxis is advised before any invasive procedures.

Mechanical Correction of the Stenosis

This is done by mitral valvotomy. Mitral valvotomy can be done by two techniques: percutaneous balloon mitral valvotomy and surgical valvotomy.

Percutaneous balloon mitral valvotomy (BMV): Here, a balloon is passed into the mitral valve and inflated briefly to split the fused valve commissures. This procedure is performed under local anesthesia in the cardiac catheter laboratory.

Surgical valvotomy: This procedure is done for patients in whom percutaneous valvotomy is not possible, unsuccessful, or in those with restenosis. Here, the cusps are carefully dissected apart under direct vision. Cardiopulmonary bypass is required for this procedure.

Mitral Valve Replacement

Replacement of the mitral valve is necessary when there is significant mitral regurgitation or the mitral valve is badly damaged and calcified. Either prosthetic valves or bioprosthetic valves can be used to replace the mitral valve.

Q. Discuss the etiology, clinical features, investigations and management of mitral regurgitation.

Mitral regurgitation (MR) is defined as an abnormal reversal of blood flow from the left ventricle (LV) to the left atrium (LA).

Etiology

- Rheumatic heart disease (most common cause)
- Mitral valve prolapse
- Ischemic heart disease(due to papillary muscle dysfunction or rupture of chordae tendinae)
- Infective endocarditis—mitral regurgitation may result from destruction of the mitral valve leaflets
- Myocarditis (due to dilatation of left ventricle)
- Dilated cardiomyopathy (due to dilatation of left ventricle)
- Marfan's syndrome and Ehlers-Danlos syndrome cause mitral regurgitation due to myxomatous degeneration of the valve
- Trauma (after balloon mitral valvotomy and blunt chest trauma)
- Congenital

Pathophysiology

- Regurgitation of blood into the left atrium increases the left atrial pressure and leads to left atrial dilatation. Increase in left atrial pressure leads to pulmonary venous congestion, pulmonary edema and pulmonary HTN.
- Pulmonary HTN leads to right ventricular hypertrophy and right heart failure.
- Regurgitated blood as well as blood coming from pulmonary veins both enter the left ventricle in diastole leading to volume overload. Volume overload of left ventricle leads to left ventricular hypertrophy, dilatation and failure.

Clinical Features

History

- Mild mitral regurgitation can remain silent for many years.
- Patients may complain of palpitations due to increased stroke volume
- Dyspnea, orthopnea and PND can occur due to pulmonary venous congestion, pulmonary edema and left ventricular failure.
- Fatigue and lethargy develop due to reduced cardiac output as the blood

regurgitates back into left atrium during systole.

- Patients complain of peripheral edema in the late stages of the disease due to right heart failure.
- Clot formation in the dilated left atrium leading to systemic emboli can occur but less common than in mitral stenosis.
- Patients may present with fever due to infective endocarditis.

Physical Examination

- Pulse may be irregularly irregular, if there is atrial fibrillation.
- Cardiac apex is displaced laterally and outward due to dilated and hypertrophied left ventricle.
- Palpation may reveal a hyperdynamic, diffuse apex beat and a systolic thrill. Parasternal heave may be present due to right ventricular hypertrophy.
- Auscultation reveals soft S1 due to incomplete opposition of the mitral valve, pansystolic murmur (PSM) due to regurgitation of blood throughout the systole.
- Bilateral basal lung crepitations may be present due to pulmonary venous congestion.
- Signs of right heart failure such as raised JVP, and peripheral edema, congestive hepatomegaly may be present.

Investigations

Chest X-ray: Chest X-ray may show cardiomegaly due to left atrial and left ventricular enlargement. Prominent pulmonary artery and vasculature may be seen due to pulmonary HTN.

Electrocardiogram: The ECG usually shows LV hypertrophy and left atrial enlargement. Atrial fibrillation may be present.

Echocardiogram: This is the investigation of choice to confirm and assess the severity of mitral regurgitation. Echo can also show the cause of regurgitation (like chordal or papillary muscle rupture) and also the complications of mitral regurgitation (like left atrial clot formation, infective endocarditis and pulmonary HTN).

Complications

- Atrial fibrillation
- Systemic embolism
- Infective endocarditis
- Left ventricular failure
- Pulmonary HTN
- Right ventricular failure

Treatment

Medical Therapy

- Mild mitral regurgitation without any symptoms does not require any treatment.
- Infective endocarditis prophylaxis, if indicated.
- ACE inhibitors reduce LV volume and afterload and hence decrease mitral regurgitation.
- Diuretics, beta-blockers and dogoxin are helpful to treat heart failure.
- When atrial fibrillation develops, long-term anticoagulation is required to prevent clot formation.

Surgical Therapy

Mitral valve repair or replacement is indicated, if there is evidence of progressive cardiac enlargement. Most patients with the symptoms of dyspnea, orthopnea, or fatigue should undergo surgery.

> **Q. Classify aortic stenosis (AS). Describe the etiology, clinical features, investigations, and management of aortic stenosis.**

The normal aortic valve area is 3 to 4 cm^2. When the area is less than this, it is called aortic stenosis. In severe aortic stenosis, valve area is less than 1 cm^2.

Etiology

- Congenital bicuspid valve with superimposed calcification.
- Age-related degenerative calcific AS (aortic sclerosis).
- Rheumatic heart disease.

Pathophysiology

- Aortic stenosis causes obstruction to left ventricular outflow into the aorta. Obstruction to left ventricular outflow leads to increased left ventricular pressure and compensatory concentric hypertrophy. The hypertrophied LV muscle mass elevates myocardial oxygen requirements. In addition, coronary vessels may be compressed by increased intraventricular pressure leading to dereased blood flow. Both these factors lead to ischemia of myocardium which increases on exertion.
- Since there is obstruction to LV outflow, cardiac output cannot increase on exertion, which leads to exertional syncope, chest pain, and dyspnea. Syncope and light-headedness is due to decreased cerebral perfusion.
- Ultimately, left ventricle may dilate and fail.

Clinical Features

History

When the AS is moderate to severe, exercise-induced syncope, angina and dyspnea develop. Orthopnea and PND may be present, if there is heart failure.

Physical Examination

- Pulse is slow-rising in nature.
- Apex is diffuse and well sustained.
- A systolic thrill may be felt in the aortic area due to turbulent blood flow through narrowed aortic valve.
- Auscultation shows a classic ejection systolic murmur. It radiates to carotid arteries especially to the left carotid. A systolic ejection click may be heard before the murmur. Left ventricular S3 may be heard in left heart failure.

Investigations

- *Chest X-ray:* Cardiomegaly may be present.
- *ECG:* It shows left ventricular hypertrophy.
- *Echocardiogram:* It shows LV hypertrophy and thickened, calcified, immobile aortic valve cusps.
- *Cardiac catheterization:* Catheterization of the left side of the heart and coronary angiography should be done in patients with severe AS who are being considered for surgery. Aortic valve replacement and CABG can be carried out at the same time, if there is coronary artery disease.

Natural Course of AS

- AS is a progressive disease. Symptomatic patients usually die within 4 years after the onset of symptoms.
- Death usually occurs due to congestive heart failure or arrhythmias.

Treatment

- Patients with severe AS should avoid strenuous physical activity.
- Nitrates can be used for angina.
- Sodium restriction, diuretics and digoxin can be used to treat congestive heart failure.
- HMG-CoA reductase inhibitors (statins) have been shown to slow the progression of leaflet calcification and aortic valve area reduction. Hence, treatment with these agents should be considered for all patients.
- Infective endocarditis prophylaxis.
- *Balloon aortic valvotomy* can be used in children and young adults with congenital, noncalcific AS. It is not recommended for adults because of high restenosis rate.
- *Aortic valve replacement:* Patients with severe aortic stenosis should undergo valve replacement surgery.

Q. Discuss the etiology, clinical features, investigations and management of aortic regurgitation (AR).

Q. Peripheral signs of aortic regurgitation (AR).

Aortic regurgitation (AR) is the leaking of the aortic valve that causes blood to flow in the reverse direction from the aorta into the left ventricle. Aortic regurgitation can be either due to problem in the valve itself or problems in the aortic root. Rheumatic fever and infective endocarditis are the commonest causes of AR.

Etiology of AR

- Bicuspid aortic valve
- Infective endocarditis
- Rheumatic heart disease
- Trauma
- Aneurysm of aorta
- Takayasu's disease
- Marfan syndrome
- Aortic dissection
- Syphilis

Pathophysiology

- In AR, some of the blood pumped into the aorta by the left ventricle comes back into the left ventricle through the aortic valve during diastole. This is also joined by the blood coming from left atrium which leads to volume overload of left ventricle (increase in end diastolic volume). There is increase in stroke volume of left ventricle due to this volume overload.
- Increase in stroke volume causes all the peripheral signs of aortic regurgitation. Chronic volume overload causes eccentric hypertrophy and dilatation of left ventricle, which may ultimately fail.
- Increased stroke volume leads to increase in systolic BP and high volume pulses. Since the blood ejected into the aorta regurgitates back into left ventricle, there is

drop in diastolic BP. Rise in systolic BP and fall in diastolic BP leads to increased pulse pressure
- An early diastolic murmur is produced due to blood regurgitating back into left ventricle from the aorta across aortic valve.

Clinical Features

Symptoms

- Patients may c/o palpitations and head pounding due to increased stroke volume.
- When left ventricular failure occurs, symptoms such as exertional dyspnea, orthopnea, PND and fatigue appear.

Signs

- Aortic regurgitation produces a myriad of signs due to increased stroke volume and hyperdynamic circulation.
- The pulse is bounding or collapsing. Systolic BP is typically high and diastolic BP low leading to wide pulse pressure. Systolic pressure in the upper limb is at least 40 mm Hg or more than the lower limb (Hill's sign).
- Table 4.3 describes the peripheral signs may be present in aortic regurgitation.
- The apex beat is displaced laterally and downwards and is forceful in quality.
- On auscultation, S_1 and S_2 are usually normal. S_2 is followed by an early diastolic murmur heard best along the left sternal border with the patient sitting and leaning forward.
- Because of increased stroke volume, there can be a functional ejection systolic murmur mimicking aortic stenosis. However, absence of slow rising pulse differentiates functional ejection systolic murmur from true AS.

Clinical Assessment of Severity of AR

Presence of one or more of the following features suggests that AR is severe.
   o Peripheral signs
   o Pulsus bisferiens

Table 4.3: Peripheral signs of AR	
Sign	Description
• Corrigan's neck sign or dancing carotids	Prominent carotid pulsations in the neck
• Quincke's sign	Systolic plethora and diastolic blanching in the nail bed when gentle pressure is applied on the nail
• De Musset's sign	Head nodding with each heart beat
• Duroziez's sign	Combined systolic and diastolic bruits created by compression of the femoral artery with the stethoscope. It is seen in severe AR
• Traube's sign (pistol shot femorals)	A sharp bang heard on auscultation over the femoral arteries in time with each heart beat
• Hill's sign	Systolic pressure in the upper limb is at least 40 mm Hg or more than the lower limb.
• Collapsing pulse (water hammer pulse; corrigan's pulse)	This is characterized by rapid upstroke, rapid downstroke and high volume
• Pulsus bisferiens	This is a pulse with double peak. It is seen in severe AR
• Muller's sign	Pulsations of the uvula
• Lighthouse sign	Alternate flushing and blanching of the forehead

o Hill's sign more than 60 mm Hg
o Hyperdynamic apex
o Early diastolic murmur lasting more than two-thirds of diastole
o Presence of Austin Flint murmur

Investigations

Chest X-ray: Chest X-ray shows cardiomegaly due to left ventricular enlargement.

ECG: The ECG shows features of left ventricular hypertrophy.

Echocardiogram: Echo can confirm the diagnosis and cause of AR. It can also assess LV function and the status of other valves.

Cardiac catheterization: It is the most accurate way of confirming and assessing the degree of AR. It can also assess LV function and status of coronary arteries.

Other Tests

• VDRL and TPHA to rule out syphilitic etiology.
• ANA, RA factor, CRP and ESR to rule out connective tissue disease.
• ASO titre and throat swab culture, if rheumatic etiology is suspected.

Treatment

Medical

• For asymptomatic patients with normal LV function, afterload reduction is recommended because it delays or reduces the need for aortic valve surgery. Vasodilators like ACE inhibitors, nitrates, hydralazine and nifedifine are helpful to reduce afterload.

- Digoxin, diuretics, ACE inhibitors and salt restriction are useful, if there is heart failure.
- The underlying cause of aortic regurgitation (e.g. rheumatic, syphilitic or infective endocarditis) requires specific treatment.
- Infective endocarditis prophylaxis is recommended for AR.

Surgical

Surgical aortic valve replacement is necessary after the onset of LV dysfunction but before the development of severe symptoms.

> **Q. Define and classify hypertension. Describe the etiology, pathophysiology, clinical features, diagnosis, and management of essential hypertension.**

- Hypertension (HTN) is defined as a systolic blood pressure (SBP) of 140 mm Hg or more, or a diastolic blood pressure (DBP) of 90 mm Hg or more, or taking antihypertensive medication. Normal BP is less than 140/90 mm Hg.
- Hypertension is a major cause of premature atherosclerosis leading to cerebrovascular events, ischemic heart disease, and peripheral vascular disease.
- Hypertension is very common in the developed world and is present in 20–30% of the adult population. Hypertension rates are much higher in black Africans (40–45% of adults). The risk of mortality or morbidity rises progressively with increasing systolic and diastolic pressures.
- BP should be measured at least twice at different times before classifying a patient as hypertensive. Blood pressure should be measured at least twice after 5 minutes of rest with the patient seated, the back supported, and the arm at heart level. The cuff should not be too small for the arm, and tobacco and caffeine should be avoided for at least 30 minutes before measuring BP.

- When assessing the cardiovascular risk, the average blood pressure at separate visits is more accurate than measurements taken at a single visit.

Types of Hypertension

Primary HTN (essential HTN): Here, a single reversible cause of hypertension cannot be identified. Primary HTN accounts for the majority (95%) of cases of HTN. The term 'essential hypertension' was used earlier because it was thought that progressive increase in blood pressure with advancing age was essential to maintain blood flow through atherosclerotic arteries.

Secondary HTN: Here, a definite reason for hypertension can be found such as renal disease, endocrine problems, etc.

Etiology of Primary (Essential) Hypertension

There are many risk factors for essential hypertension.

Genetic factors: Blood pressure tends to run in families and children of hypertensive parents tend to have higher blood pressure than age-matched children of people with normal blood pressure. Concordance of blood pressure is greater within families than in unrelated individuals, greater between monozygotic than between dizygotic twins. However, the exact genetic loci and mutations are unknown.

Gender and ethnicity: Before age 50, the prevalence of hypertension is lower in women than in men, probably due to a protective action of estrogen. After menopause, the prevalence of hypertension increases rapidly in women and exceeds than in men. African Americans have higher prevalence of hypertension than other races.

Obesity: Fat people are more prone to develop hypetension than thin people. The underlying mechanisms by which obesity leads to hypertension are incompletely understood, but there is mounting evidence for an expanded plasma volume plus sympathetic overactivity.

Alcohol intake: People who consume large amount of alcohol have higher blood pressure than those who do not drink. However, small amount of alcohol intake is actually associated with lower blood pressure.

Sodium intake: High sodium intake is associated with hypertension. Studies of the restriction of salt intake have shown a beneficial effect on blood pressure.

Stress: Acute stress can temporarily raise blood pressure. However, the relationship between chronic stress and blood pressure remains to be proven.

Humoral mechanisms: Abnormalities in the autonomic nervous system, and renin–angiotensin system have also been implicated in the pathogenesis of essential HTN.

Insulin resistance: Insulin resistance and/or hyperinsulinemia have been suggested as being responsible for the increased arterial pressure in some patients with hypertension.

Pathophysiology

- If hypertension remains uncontrolled for a long time, many changes take place in blood vessels and various organs.
- The resistance vessels (the small arteries and arterioles) show structural changes in the form of increased wall thickness and reduced lumen diameter. The number of these resistance vessels may also decrease. These changes result in an increased peripheral vascular resistance.
- In large arteries, there is thickening of the media, increase in collagen and deposition of calcium. Over a period of time, atherosclerotic changes develop in large arteries due to mechanical stress and endothelial injury.
- Left ventricular hypertrophy develops due to increased left ventricular load (increase in afterload). Left ventricular failure can happen in long-standing uncontrolled HTN.
- Thickening and atherosclerotic changes in blood vessels supplying various organs results in damage to those organs. Changes

in the renal vasculature lead to a reduced renal perfusion, reduced glomerular filtration rate and, finally, a reduction in sodium and water excretion. Changes in blood vessels of brain may lead to stroke. Changes in blood vessels of heart may lead to myocardial infarction.

Clinical Manifestations

Symptoms

- Hypertension has been termed the 'silent killer', because it hardly produces any symptoms. If it is undetected in this long asymptomatic phase, it damages the heart, brain, kidneys, and blood vessels.
- Headache may be a complaint in hypertension, but usually rare.
- Sometimes patients may experience epistaxis when BP is very high.
- Breathlessness may be present due to left ventricular hypertrophy, diastolic dysfunction, or heart failure.
- Angina and leg claudication may be experienced due to atherosclerotic narrowing of coronary and lower limb arteries.
- Malignant hypertension may present with severe headache, vomiting, visual disturbances, seizures, altered sensorium, or symptoms of heart failure.

Signs

- BP is elevated (≥140/90 mm Hg).
- Cardiac examination reveals left ventricular hypertrophy.
- Optic fundus should be examined in all patients for hypertensive retinopathy changes. In malignant hypertension, there is papilledema.

Complications of Hypertension

Hypertension is associated with a number of serious adverse effects.

Cardiovascular Complications

- Coronary artery disease (angina, myocardial infarction)
- Heart failure

- Left ventricular hypertrophy and sudden cardiac death
- Premature atherosclerosis of blood vessels.

Central Nervous System Complications

- Transient ischemic attacks
- Stroke: Hypertension is the most common and most important risk factor for stroke.
- Intracerebral hemorrhage
- Subarachnoid hemorrhage
- Hypertensive encephalopathy: This is characterized by very high blood pressure, papilledema, blurring of vision, headache, altered sensorium and focal neurological deficits.

Renal Complications

- Proteinuria
- Chronic renal failure: Hypertension is a risk factor for end-stage renal disease.

Ophthalmic complications: Hypertensive retinopathy.

Malignant hypertension: This is characterized by very high blood pressure with papilledema and end organ damage.

Investigations

Routine Tests

- Urea, creatinine and electrolytes (to assess renal function)
- Urine examination for protein and blood
- Lipid profile
- Blood glucose (to rule out diabetes)
- ECG usually shows evidence of left ventricular hypertrophy.
- Chest X-ray usually shows cardiomegaly

Additional Tests (Done only if Required)

- Renal artery Doppler may be indicated, if renovascular hypertension is suspected.
- 24-hour urinary cortisol and VMA is indicated, if there is clinical suspicion of Cushing's and pheochromocytoma.
- T_3, T_4 and TSH, if hypo- or hyperthyroidism is suspected.

- Growth hormone levels and skull X-ray, if acromegaly is suspected
- Ultrasound abdomen, if polycystic kidney or other renal problems are suspected.
- Ambulatory blood pressure monitoring is used to monitor blood pressure throughout the day. For this, an automatic BP measuring device is worn by the patient throughout the day. It is useful to confirm the diagnosis of hypertension in patients with 'white-coat' hypertension. These devices can also be used to monitor the response of patients to drug treatment and, in particular, can be used to determine the adequacy of 24-hour control with once-daily medication.

Treatment

General Measures

- *Weight reduction:* BMI should be $<25 \text{ kg/m}^2$.
- *Diet:* Low fat, low sodium diet (<6 g sodium chloride per day). Fruit and vegetable consumption should be increased.
- *Habits:* Alcohol consumption should be cut down and smoking should be stopped.
- *Exercise:* Regular exercise, preferably aerobic type for at least 30 minutes per day.
- *Relaxation techniques:* Yoga, meditation.

Antihypertensive Agents

- Antihypertensive drugs should be started, if blood pressure is 150/90 mm Hg or higher in patients 60 years and older, or 140/90 mm Hg or higher in patients younger than 60 years.
- Initial antihypertensive treatment should include a thiazide diuretic or calcium channel blocker or ACE inhibitor or ARB or beta-blocker. There are reports that beta-blockers increase the risk of stroke. Hence, other antihypertensive agents should be preferred over beta-blockers.
- Initially treatment should be initiated with one drug. This drug is increased to maximum tolerated dose gradually till BP is in the desirable range.

- If BP is not controlled within one month with a single drug, addition of a second drug should be considered. Most patients will require a combination of antihypertensive drugs to achieve the recommended targets.
- An easy way to remember the anthypertensive drugs is the pnemonic 'ABCD' (A=ACE inhibitor or angiotension receptor blocker, B=beta-blocker, C=calcium channel blocker, D=diuretics).

Q. What is secondary hypertension? List the causes of secondary hypertension.

In secondary hypertension, a definite reason for hypertension can be found.

Causes of Secondary Hypertension

• *Renal causes*	Renal artery stenosis, glomerulonephritis, polycystic kidney disease, acute and chronic renal failure
• *Endocrine causes*	Pheochromocytoma, hypothyroidism, hyperthyroidism, Cushing's syndrome, Conn's syndrome, acromegaly, hyperparathyroidism, congenital adrenal hyperplasia
• *Drugs*	Oral contraceptives, steroids, NSAIDs, sympathomimetics (phenylephrine, phenylpropanolamine)
• *Miscellaneous*	Coarctation of aorta, obstructive sleep apnea, pre-eclampsia and eclampsia

Q. Hypertensive emergency (malignant hypertension) and hypertensive urgency.

Hypertensive Emergeny

- *Hypertensive emergency* is acute, severe elevation in blood pressure associated with target organ damage. Patients with hypertensive emergency usually present with a blood pressure of more than 180/120 mm Hg.

- Target-organ damage includes hypertensive encephalopathy, pre-eclampsia and eclampsia, acute left ventricular failure, myocardial ischemia, aortic dissection, and renal failure. The characteristic vascular lesion is fibrinoid necrosis of arterioles which causes the clinical manifestations of end-organ damage.
- Investigations to be done include ECG, urinalysis, serum urea and creatinine, and CT head for patients with neurologic symptoms or signs.
- Hypertensive emergency requires ICU admission and lowering of blood pressure by intravenous medications. Sodium nitroprusside infusion is the drug of choice for hypertensive emergencies. Clevidipine is a new, ultra-short-acting (within 1 to 2 minutes), 3rd-generation calcium channel blocker that reduces peripheral resistance without affecting venous vascular tone and cardiac filling pressures. Blood pressure should be lowered gradually over many hours to a target of 170/110 mm Hg. In the next 48 hours, BP can be lowered to normal value. Oral drugs can be added and parenteral therapy slowly tapered off.

Hypertensive Urgency

- *Hypertensive urgency* is acute, severe elevation in blood pressure without evidence of target organ damage. Thus, the main difference between hypertensive emergency and urgency is the presence (hypertensive emergency) or absence (hypertensive urgency) of target organ damage and not the absolute value of blood pressure.
- Hypertensive urgency can be managed by oral drugs. For immediate reduction of BP in hypertensive urgency, labetalol and clonidine are useful.

Q. Discuss the etiology (risk factors) of ischemic heart disease (IHD).

- IHD is a life-threatening disease.
- Atherosclerosis is responsible for almost all cases of IHD. Most risk factors act by

promoting atherosclerosis of the coronary arteries.

Risk Factors for IHD

- **Dyslipidemia:** Elevated LDL-cholesterol, low HDL-cholesterol, and hypertriglyceridemia are associated with increased risk of IHD.
- **Hypertension:** This is a well-established risk factor for IHD.
- **Diabetes mellitus:** Insulin resistance, hyperinsulinemia, and elevated blood glucose are associated with atherosclerotic cardiovascular disease and IHD.
- **Obesity:** Obesity is associated with a number of risk factors for atherosclerosis, such as hypertension, insulin resistance and glucose intolerance, hypertriglyceridemia, and reduced HDL-cholesterol.
- **Metabolic syndrome:** Patients with the constellation of abdominal obesity, hypertension, diabetes, and dyslipidemia are considered to have the metabolic syndrome (syndrome X). Metabolic syndrome is associated with higher risk of coronary artery disease.
- **Sedentary lifestyle:** This leads to obesity, impaired glucose tolerance and is a risk factor for IHD.
- **Smoking:** Cigarette smoking is an important and reversible risk factor. The incidence of an MI is increased sixfold in women and threefold in men who smoke at least 20 cigarettes per day compared to subjects who never smoked.
- **Aging:** As the age advances, atherosclerosis of vessels also increases. Most of the IHD cases occur after 40 years of age. Aging is an independent risk factor for IHD.
- **Family history:** Family history is a significant independent risk factor for IHD, particularly among younger individuals with a family history of premature disease.
- **Diet factors:** A diet rich in calories, saturated fat, and cholesterol is a risk factor for IHD.

Q. Define angina. Describe the etiology, pathogenesis, clinical features, investigations, and management of angina.

Definition

- Angina pectoris may be defined as a discomfort in the chest and/or adjacent area associated with myocardial ischemia.
- It is a common presenting symptom among patients with coronary artery disease (CAD).

Types

- *Stable angina* is usually reproducible and is consistent over time. It is precipitated by effort, and relieved by rest. Stable angina is caused by fixed stenosis in coronary arteries.
- *Unstable angina* is diagnosed when a patient has new-onset angina or angina occurring at rest.
- *Prinzmetal's angina* is due to coronary vasospasm occurring at rest.

Etiology

- Angina is due to transient decrease in blood supply to myocardium.
- It is due to coronary artery (which supply heart) stenosis. In the absence of collateral circulation, stenoses of more than 75% of the cross-sectional area (corresponding to >50% lumen diameter by angiography) result in stable angina. Chest pain can occur at rest due to severe stenosis or thrombus formation or due to vasospasm as in Prinzmetal's angina.
- Stenosis is most commonly due to atherosclerosis.

Clinical Manifestations

History

- Angina means tightening, not pain. Thus, the discomfort of angina is often described as 'pressing', 'squeezing', and 'constricting'.

- Angina usually builds up within 30 seconds and disappears in 5 to 15 minutes. Pain is usually brought on by exertion. The discomfort is most commonly mid-sternal and radiates to the neck, left shoulder, and left arm.
- The clenching of the fist over the sternum while describing the pain (Levine's sign) is classic.
- Pain may be associated with sweating, palpitations, dizziness and dyspnea.
- There may be history of other comorbid conditions like diabetes and hypertension. Smoking history may be positive.

Physical Examination

- *General examination:* May show signs of generalized atherosclerosis like tendon xanthoma, xanthelasmas, thickening of Achilles tendon, locomotor brachialis and corneal arcus. Signs of peripheral vascular disease such as absent peripheral pusles may be noted. Heart rate and BP may be elevated. Excessive sweating may be noted.
- *Systemic examination:* It can be completely normal. 3rd and 4th heart sounds; mitral regurgitation murmur (due to ischemic papillary muscle dysfunction) may be heard during ischemia. Paradoxical splitting of S_2 (from transient left ventricular dysfunction or left bundle-branch block) may be noted. Bilateral basal crepitations may be heard during ischemia due to transient left ventricular dysfunction. Pain is promptly relieved by nitroglycerin. Other systems are usually normal.

Investigations

Resting ECG: This is usually normal between attacks. During an attack, ST depression and T wave inversions in the leads corresponding to ischemic areas may be seen.

Exercise ECG (stress test): Since the resting ECG can be normal in between the attacks, exercise testing can be useful to confirm the diagnosis of angina. Patient is asked to walk on a treadmill and ECG is recorded continuously. Patient may experience chest discomfort during exercise and if ECG shows ST segment depression of >1 mm, it suggests myocardial ischemia.

Cardiac scintigraphy: Myocardial perfusion scans at rest and after stress (i.e. exercise or dobutamine), is a sensitive indicator of ischaemia and useful in deciding if a stenosis seen at angiography is giving rise to ischaemia.

Echocardiography: Ischemic or infarcted ventricular wall does not move properly. This is called regional wall motion abnormally (RWMA) and reflect ischemia or previous infarction.

Coronary angiography (CAG): When all the above tests do not provide an answer to chest pain, CAG can be useful. It can delineate the exact coronary anatomy and areas of stenosis.

Treatment of Angina

General Management

Patients should be reassured. Comorbid conditions such as anemia, hyperthyroidism, diabetes, hypertension, and hypercholesterolemia should be treated. Smoking should be stopped; regular exercise and low fat diet should be encouraged.

Medical Treatment

Glyceryl trinitrate (GTN): Used sublingually, either as a tablet or as a spray, gives prompt relief. If relief is not obtained within 2 or 3 min after nitroglycerin, a second or third dose may be given at 5 min intervals. Oral long-acting preparations of nitrates can be used for daily therapy.

Long-acting nitrates (e.g. isosorbide dinitrate and mononitrate): These are helpful for long-term prophylactic therapy. They reduce venous return and hence intracardiac diastolic pressures, reduce afterload and dilate coronary arteries.

Antiplatelet agents: Aspirin inhibits cyclo-oxygenase activity and inhibits platelet aggregation. It reduces the risk of coronary events in patients with coronary artery disease. All patients with angina should be given aspirin (75–325 mg daily) unless contraindicated. Clopidogrel (300 mg loading and 75 mg daily) is another antiplatelet agent which is as effective as aspirin.

Beta-blockers: Beta-blockers reduce myocardial oxygen demand by decreasing heart rate and the force of ventricular contraction. All patients with angina should be given beta-blockers unless there are contraindications (asthma, heart blocks, COPD). Cardioselective beta-blockers like atenolol, metoprolol, carvedilol, and nebivolol are used commonly.

Angiotensin-converting enzyme (ACE) inhibitors: Clinical trials have shown that ACE inhibitors reduce major adverse events (death, myocardial infarction, and stroke), angina, and the need for revascularization in patients with CAD.

Calcium-channel blockers: These drugs block calcium flux into the cell. They relax coronary arteries, cause peripheral vasodilatation and reduce the force of left ventricular contraction, thereby reducing myocardial oxygen demand. Examples are diltiazem and verapamil.

Nicorandil: This is a potassium-channel activator with a nitrate component. It has both arterial and venous vasodilating properties. It can be used when there are contraindications to other drugs or can be added, if angina is not responding to above drugs.

Ranolazine: This is a cardioselective anti-ischemic agent, indicated for chronic angina unresponsive to other antianginal treatments. Unlike beta-blockers or calcium channel blockers, it does not reduce blood pressure or heart rate.

Coronary Angioplasty

Percutaneous transluminal coronary angioplasty (PTCA) is the technique of dilating coronary stenosis bypassing and inflating a balloon inside the stenosis. The balloon is threaded into the site of stenosis by a thin catheter inserted through radial or femoral artery. A stent can be placed at the site of stenosis to prevent restenosis.

Coronary Artery Bypass Grafting (CABG)

CABG is indicated when patients remain symptomatic despite optimal medical therapy and whose disease is not suitable for PTCA. CABG dramatically improves angina in about 90% of cases. It is also indicated for patients with severe three-vessel disease (significant stenoses in all three main coronary vessels), and in those with left main stem artery disease. CABG provides improved survival in such situations. Usually the left or right internal mammary artery is used in CABG. Long saphenous vein can also be used but is used less commonly now because of higher risk of atheromatous occlusion.

Q. What are acute coronary syndromes?

Acute coronary syndromes (ACS) include:
- o Unstable angina
- o Non-ST-elevation myocardial infarction (NSTEMI)
- o ST-elevation myocardial infarction (STEMI)

Q. Define unstable angina. Describe the etiology, clinical features, investigations, and management of unstable angina.

Q. Non-ST-elevation myocardial infarction (NSTEMI).

Definition

- Unstable angina is defined as angina with at least one of three features: (1) It occurs at rest (or with minimal exertion), (2) it is severe and of new onset (i.e. within the prior 4 to 6 weeks), and/or (3) it occurs with a crescendo pattern (i.e. previously diagnosed angina that has become distinctly more frequent, longer in duration, or more severe in nature).

- Non-ST-elevation myocardial infarction (NSTEMI) is unstable angina with evidence of myocardial necrosis as evidenced by elevated cardiac biomarkers (CK-MB and troponins). Hence, unstable angina + elevated CKMB/tropnin is NSTEMI. In NSTEMI, there will not be any ST elevation on ECG.
- Since the pathogenesis, clinical features and management of both unstable angina and NSTEMI are same, both are described together here.

Etiology

Unstable angina/NSTEMI is caused by rupture or erosion of the atherosclerotic plaque with formation of partially occlusive thrombus. Progressive atherosclerosis is another cause. Sometimes it is caused by coronary spasm (Prinzmetal's angina) or increase in myocardial oxygen demand superimposed on pre-existing CAD.

Clinical Features

- Patients with unstable angina/NSTEMI present with substernal chest pain. Characteristics of chest pain are same as those of stable angina but more severe. Pain usually radiates to the neck, left shoulder, and left arm.
- Examination may be normal or may show diaphoresis, pale cool skin, sinus tachycardia, third and/or fourth heart sound, bilateral basal crepitations, and sometimes hypotension.

Investigations

- *ECG:* Usually shows ST-segment depression, and/or T-wave inversion in the leads corresponding to ischemic area.
- *Cardiac enzymes:* CK-MB and troponins may be elevated.
- Other investigations are same as stable angina.

Treatment

- Patients with unstable angina/NSTEMI should be admitted to ICU and placed on bed rest. High flow oxygen should be started for all patients. Continuous ECG monitoring should be done to detect ST-segment deviation and any arrhythmias. Medical management involves administration of anti-platelet and antithrombotic treatment.
- *Antiplatelet agents:* Aspirin, clopidogrel. They prevent thrombus formation and improve coronary blood flow. They should be given lifelong.
- *Antithrombotic therapy:* Heparin should be given intravenously. Alternatively low molecular weight heparins such as dalteparin or enoxaparin can be used subcutaneously.
- *Other drugs and further treatment for unstable angina is same as stable angina.*

Q. Describe the etiology, pathogenesis, clinical features, diagnosis and management of acute myocardial infarction.

- Myocardial infarction (MI) (also known as heart attack) is the irreversible necrosis of heart muscle secondary to prolonged ischemia. This is usually caused by atherosclerotic plaque rupture with thrombus formation in a coronary vessel, resulting in an acute reduction of blood supply to a portion of the myocardium.
- Myocardial injury is reflected by elevated cardiac enzymes troponin-I, troponin-T, and CK-MB. Two patterns of MI can be recognized based on ECG findings.
  o *Non ST segment elevation MI (NSTEMI):* This isunstable angina accompanied by elevated markers of myocardial injury, such as troponins and CK-MB, but no ST segment elevation in ECG.
  o *ST segment elevation MI (STEMI):* When myocardial injury is accompanied by both enzyme and ST segment elevation it is referred to as *ST segment elevation MI (STEMI).*

- It is important to differentiate between non-ST segment elevation MI and ST segment elevation MI because early recanalization therapy improves the outcome in STEMI but not in NSTEMI. NSTEMI has been described along with unstable angina. The following description is about STEMI.

Etiology

- Atherosclerosis of coronary arteries is responsible for most cases of myocardial infarction. Approximately 90% of myocardial infarctions result from an acute thrombus that obstructs an atherosclerotic coronary artery.
- Non-atherosclerotic causes of myocardial infarction include: Coronary occlusion secondary to vasculitis, ventricular hypertrophy, coronary artery emboli, congenital coronary anomalies, coronary vasospasm, and drug use (e.g. cocaine, ephedrine).

Pathogenesis

- Rupture or erosion of an atherosclerotic plaque in the coronary artery induces local thrombus formation which occludes coronary artery leading to myocardial infarction. Initially subendocardium is affected because this is the least supplied area. With continued ischemia, the infarct zone extends to the entire myocardium, producing a transmural myocardial infarction. Areas of myocardium which are ischemic but not yet undergone infarction can be salvaged by early reperfusion therapy.
- Microscopy shows coagulative necrosis of myocardial fibers that is ultimately followed by myocardial fibrosis.

Clinical Features

- In up to one-half of cases, a precipitating factor appears to be present before MI, such as vigorous physical exercise, emotional stress, or a medical or surgical illness.
- Patients usually present with chest pain, located in the substernal region which frequently radiates to the neck, left shoulder, and left arm. Chest pain of MI is more severe than angina and lasts for more than 20 minutes.
- Examination may reveal diaphoresis, pale cool skin, tachycardia, a third and/or fourth heart sound, bilateral basal crepitations (due to pulmonary edema), and sometimes hypotension.

Investigations

Electrocardiogram (ECG): ECG shows ST elevation MI. ECG changes are seen in leads which correspond to the infarcted region of myocardium.

Biochemical markers: CK–MB, troponin-I, and troponin-T levels are elevated whenever there is myocardial injury.

Echocardiogram: Hypokinesia or akinesia of ventricular wall may be present due to ischemia or infarction.

Coronary angiography (CAG): It can identify the site of block and allow percutaneous coronary intervention.

Radionuclide imaging: Myocardial perfusion imaging with Thallium-201 or technetium-99m-sestamibi can show uptake defects (cold spots) due to infarction.

Other investigations: Full blood count, renal function tests, serum electrolytes, glucose, and lipid profile should be done for all patients.

Management of Myocardial Infarction

Immediate Measures

- Note that time is muscle and treatment should be initiated as early as possible. More delay means more myocardial damage.
- *Oxygen* should be given.
- *Aspirin 300 mg oral and clopidogrel 300 mg oral loading dose should be given and continued at lower doses thereafter. These antiplatelet agents will prevent further*

increase in thrombus and prevent future occurrence of thrombosis.

- *Sublingual glyceryl trinitrate* 0.4 mg. Repeat at 5 min intervals up to 3 doses. This relieves chest pain and improves coronary circulation.
- *Intravenous heparin* is given for all patients unless there is a contraindication. This will prevent further increase in thrombus.
- *Injection morphine 2 to 5 mg,* intravenously, improves chest pain and controls anxiety.
- *Intravenous beta-blocker.* For example, metoprolol, 5 mg every 2 to 5 min for a total of three doses. Beta-blockers decrease heart rate and sympathetic overactivity and hence reduce myocardial oxygen demand.

Reperfusion Therapy

- Coronary reperfusion can be established by two ways: (1) Percutaneous coronary intervention (PCI), and (2) thrombolytic therapy.
- PCI is the treatment of choice, if facilities for PCI are available. If there are no facilities for PCI, patient is treated with fibrinolytic therapy. Currently available fibrinolytic agents include streptokinase, tissue plasminogen activator (tPA), reteplase and tenecteplase. Fibrinolytic agents break the thrombus and reestablish coronary blood flow. The major risk of thrombolytic therapy is bleeding. Intracerebral hemorrhage is the most serious complication. *Percutaneous coronary intervention (PCI)* includes angioplasty and/or stenting.

Coronary Artery Bypass Grafting (CABG)

CABG is indicated for patients with left main stem or triple vessel disease with impaired left ventricular function.

Complications of Myocardial Infarction

- Heart failure
- Myocardial rupture and aneurysmal dilatation
- Ventricular septal defect (VSD)
- Mitral regurgitation
- Cardiac arrhythmias
- Acute pericarditis

Post-MI Drug Therapy

- Extensive clinical trials have shown that many drugs taken indefinitely by MI patients reduce the incidence of recurrent MI and cardiovascular death. Therefore, all MI patients should be taking the following medications lifelong unless there are contraindications.
- **Aspirin and clopidogrel:** They should be given to all patients lifelong. Aspirin is given at a dose of 75–150 mg/day and clopidogrel at 75 mg/day. They inhibit platelet aggregation and prevent thrombus formation thereby reducing the risk of recurrent MI.
- **Beta-blockers:** For example, metoprolol, carvedilol, atenolol. They decrease heart rate and reduce myocardial oxygen demand and should be given to all patients with MI unless there is a contraindication (like asthma or severe LV dysfunction).
- **Oral nitrates:** For example, isosorbide, dinitrate or mononitrate. They dilate the coronary arteries, reduce preload and afterload. They improve the symptoms of angina and heart failure and should be considered for all patients.
- **ACE inhibitors:** For example, enalapril, ramipril, lisinopril, and perindopril. They reduce peripheral resistance (afterload), prevent adverse myocardial remodeling after acute MI and reduce heart failure and death.
- **Statins:** For example, atorvastatin, rosuvastatin, etc. In addition to cholesterol lowering effect, statins also help in plaque stabilization and regression of atherosclerosis.
- **Control of comorbid conditions:** Like diabetes and hypertension help in reducing recurrent MI.

Q. What is infective endocarditis? Discuss the etiology, types, pathogenesis, clinical features, and management of infective endocarditis.

Q. Infective endocarditis prophylaxis.

Q. Duke criteria.

- Infective endocarditis (IE) is the infection of the endocardial surface of the heart.

- It may involve heart valve (native or prosthetic), the lining of a cardiac chamber or blood vessel, a congenital anomaly (e.g. septal defect), or an intracardiac device.

- The causative organism is usually a bacterium, but may be a rickettsia, chlamydia or fungus.

- It is characterized pathologically by the presence of vegetation, which is a mass of platelets, fibrin, microorganisms, and inflammatory cells.

Types

- Endocarditis may be classified according to the temporal evolution of disease as acute and subacute endocarditis.

- *Acute endocarditis* is a serious illness with high-grade fever. It rapidly damages cardiac structures, hematogenously seeds extracardiac sites, and, if untreated, may result in death within weeks.

- *Subacute endocarditis* follows an indolent course, causes structural cardiac damage only slowly if at all, and rarely causes metastatic infection.

Etiology

Acute endocarditis	Subacute endocarditis
• Staphylococcus	• Streptococcus viridans
• Pseudomonas	• Enterococcus fecalis
	• HACEK group

- The causative organism can be bacteria, rickettsia, chlamydia or fungus.

- However, most cases of infective endocarditis are caused by a small number of bacterial species. These include *Streptococcus viridans*, staphylococci, and HACEK organisms (*Haemophilus, Actinobacillus, Cardiobacterium, Eikenella*, and *Kingella*)

originating respectively from oral cavity, skin, and upper respiratory tract. *Streptococcus bovis* originates from GIT, and enterococci from the genitourinary tract.

Pathogenesis

- Organisms that cause endocarditis usually enter the bloodstream from mucosal surfaces, skin, or sites of focal infection.

- Normal endocardium is resistant to infection and to thrombus formation. Endocardial injury (e.g. at the site of impact of high-velocity jets or on the low-pressure side of a cardiac structural lesion, mitral regurgitation, aortic stenosis, aortic regurgitation, ventricular septal defects, and complex congenital heart disease) predisposes to infection or to development of platelet-fibrin thrombus.

- Microorganisms adhere to thrombi but more virulent bacteria (e.g. *S. aureus*) can adhere directly to intact endothelium or exposed subendothelial tissue. If the organisms cannot be removed by defence mechanism, the organisms proliferate and induce a procoagulant state at the site by eliciting tissue factor from adherent monocytes.

- Tissue factor leads to fibrin deposition, and along with platelet aggregation and microorganisms, forms an infected mass called vegetation. Organisms deep in vegetations are relatively resistant to killing by antimicrobial agents. Proliferating surface organisms are shed into the bloodstream continuously some of which are cleared by the reticuloendothelial system and others are distributed to all parts of the body.

- Release of cytokines by inflammatory cells causes constitutional symptoms like fever, malaise.

- Damage to intracardiac structures leads to valvular incompetence and other manifestations.

- Embolization of vegetation fragments leads to infection or infarction of remote tissues.

Clinical Manifestations

The clinical presentation can vary from acute to subacute presentation. Usually the causative microorganism is responsible for the temporal course of endocarditis.

Systemic Manifestations

- In patients with subacute endocarditis, fever is typically low-grade and rarely exceeds 103°F. In acute endocarditis, fever is usually between 103 and 104°F.
- Drenching night sweats, arthralgias, myalgias, and weight loss may accompany fever.

Cardiac Manifestations

- Regurgitant murmurs may occur due to destroyed or distorted valve and its supporting structures. Stenotic murmurs can occur due to large vegetations.
- Valve ring abscess may occur due to local extension of the infection from the valve ring. Valve ring abscesses can cause persistent fever and heart block due to destroyed conduction pathways in the area of the atrioventricular node and bundle of His.
- Myocardial infarction may result from coronary artery embolization.
- Diffuse myocarditis can occur and is probably due to immune complex vasculitis.
- Congestive cardiac failure develops in 30 to 40% of patients due to valvular dysfunction and occasionally due to endocarditis-associated myocarditis or an intracardiac fistula.

Embolic Manifestations

Embolic events result in infarction of numerous organs, such as the lung in right-sided endocarditis or the brain, spleen, or kidneys in left-sided endocarditis. Following are the manifestations of embolic events.

- Cutaneous embolism—produces Janeway lesions. These are hemorrhagic, nonpainful macules most commonly found on the palms and soles.
- Nails—splinter hemorrhages. These are nonblanching, linear, brownish-red lesions in the nail beds.
- Peripheral arteries—claudication, absent pulses and gangrene.
- CNS—seizures, stroke, loss of vision.
- Kidneys—loin pain, hematuria and renal failure
- Lungs—pulmonary infarction, hemoptysis, pleurisy and pleural effusion.
- Septic emboli—suppurative complications such as abscesses, septic infarcts, and infected mycotic aneurysms.

Immunologic Phenomena

- Glomerulonephritis, sterile meningitis, and polyarthritis.
- Mucocutaneous petechiae.
- Roth's spots—circular retinal hemorrhages with central white spot.
- Osler's nodes—painful tender nodules in the pulps of fingers.
- Hepatosplenomegaly may develop with prolonged illness.

Diagnosis

The Duke Criteria (Table 4.4)

Duke criteria are based on clinical, laboratory, and echocardiographic findings. It is highly sensitive and specific for the diagnosis of infective endocarditis. Presence of two major criteria, or one major and three minor criteria, or five minor criteria are required to make a diagnosis of definite endocarditis. If one major and one minor criteria or three minor criteria are present, then it is called possible infective endocarditis.

Blood Cultures

- Isolation of the causative microorganism from blood cultures is important not only for diagnosis but also for treatment. In the absence of prior antibiotic therapy, a total of three blood culture sets, ideally with the first separated from the last by at least 1 hour, should be sent from different venipuncture sites over 24 hours.

Table 4.4: Duke criteria

Major criteria

1. Blood cultures positive

- Typical organism from two cultures (viridans streptococci, *Streptococcus bovis*, HACEK group, *Staphylococcus aureus*), OR
- Blood cultures persistently positive for one of these organisms, from cultures drawn more than 12 hours apart, OR
- Single positive blood culture for *Coxiella brunetii* or IgG antibody titer greater than 1:800

2. Evidence of endocardial involvement

- Positive echocardiographic findings of vegetations
- New valvular regurgitation

Minor criteria

1. **Fever ≥38.0°C (≥100.4°F)**
2. **Immunologic phenomena:** Glomerulonephritis, Osler's nodes, Roth's spots, rheumatoid factor
3. **Vascular phenomena:** Major arterial emboli, septic pulmonary infarcts, mycotic aneurysm, intracranial hemorrhage, conjunctival hemorrhages, Janeway lesions
4. **Echocardiogram results consistent with IE but not meeting major echocardiographic criteria**
5. **Predisposition:** Predisposing heart condition or injection drug use
6. **Microbiological evidence (positive blood culture but not meeting major criterion)**

   Pnemonic to remember above criteria is *"BE FIVE PM"*. B = *Blood culture positivity, E = Endocardial involvement by ECHO; FIVE PM indicates first letter of each minor criteria.*

- Antibiotics should be started immediately in acute endocarditis and in those with hemodynamic instability after the initial three sets of blood cultures are obtained.

ECG

ECG should be done for all to serve as a baseline and to detect any complications like conduction abnormalities, MI, and pericarditis.

Echocardiography

Echocardiography can identify the presence and size of vegetations, detect intracardiac complications, and assess cardiac function. Echocardiograpy should be done for all patients with a clinical diagnosis of endocarditis.

Other Tests

- *Serologic tests* are useful for organisms, which are difficult to culture such as *Brucella, Bartonella, Legionella,* and *Coxiella burnetii.*
- *Culture, microscopic examination, and PCR tests* can also be done on vegetations to identify the causative organism.
- Complete blood count may show anemia and increased WBC count.
- *Urine examination* may show microscopic hematuria (due to renal emboli or focal glomerulonephritis) or macroscopic hematuria (due to renal infarction).
- *Urea and creatinine* may be elevated due to glomerulonephritis.
- *Chest X-ray* may show emboli, cardiac enlargement, and other abnormalities.
- *ESR, CRP, circulating immune complex titer, and rheumatoid factor* concentration are commonly increased in endocarditis.
- *Cardiac catheterization* is useful to assess coronary artery patency in older individuals who are to undergo surgery for endocarditis because CABG also can be done in the same sitting.

Treatment

Antimicrobial Therapy

- In patients with acute endocarditis and hemodynamic instability, empirical antibiotic therapy should be started as soon as possible after drawing blood for cultures. Empirical therapy should be targeted at the most likely pathogens in that particular clinical setting. Antibiotics should be given intravenously for 4 to 6 weeks.

- In most patients, effective antibiotic therapy results in subjective improvement and resolution of fever within 5 to 7 days. Blood cultures should be done daily, and whenever there is fever and 4 to 6 weeks after therapy to document cure.

Antibiotic regimens for infective endocarditis	
Organism	Antibiotic
Viridans streptococci and *Strep. bovis*	Benzyl penicillin and gentamicin
Enterococci	Ampicillin and gentamicin
Staphylococci	Benzyl penicillin

Surgery

Indications for surgery

- Prosthetic valve dysfunction.
- Badly damaged valve (requires replacement).
- Large vegetations (>10 mm) on echocardiography.
- Emergency surgery is required for new onset acute aortic regurgitation and mitral valve and sinus of Valsalva abscess ruptured into right heart.

Complications of Infective Endocarditis

- *Heart failure:* This is the most frequent major complication of IE.
- *Embolization:* The brain and the spleen are the most common sites of embolization.

- *Mycotic aneurysms:* These occur due to septic embolization to the arterial vasa-vasorum, with subsequent spread of infection and weakening of the vessel wall. They occur most frequently in the intracranial arteries and have a particular predilection for the middle cerebral artery and its branches. Mycotic aneurysms are extremely dangerous, because they can rupture and produce sudden intracranial hemorrhage.

- *Periannular extension of infection:* Leads to abscess formation, perforation, fistula development, and hemodynamic deterioration. Persistent fever and bacteremia despite antibiotic therapy, heart failure, or new conduction block should raise suspicion for this complication.

- *Renal dysfunction:* It is a common complication of IE and is often multifactorial due to immune complex deposition, drug-induced nephrotoxicity, and hemodynamic perturbations.

Q. Infective endocarditis prophylaxis.

- Since bacteremia is the first step in the causation of infective endocarditis, prevention of bacteremia can prevent the occurrence of infective endocarditis. Bacteremia is prevented by the administration of antibiotics prior to any procedure known to produce bacteremia. However, not all cardiac lesions are prone for infection. Hence, prophylaxis is recommended only for specific lesions.

- The revised guidelines have narrowed the procedures for which antibiotic prophylaxis is recommended. Antibiotic prophylaxis is no longer recommended for GI/genitourinary tract procedures (including diagnostic esophagogastroduodenoscopy or colonoscopy).

Cardiac Conditions Requiring Antibiotic Prophylaxis (Latest Guidelines)

- Prosthetic cardiac valve.
- Previous infective endocarditis.

- Congenital heart disease
- Cardiac transplantation recipients with cardiac valvular disease
- Rheumatic heart disease with valvular lesions and other acquired valvular diseases have moderate risk of developing infective endocarditis. Prophylaxis is not strongly recommended.

Procedures Requiring Infective Endocarditis Prophylaxis

- *Dental:* All dental procedures that involve manipulation of gingival tissue or the periapical region of teeth or perforation of the oral mucosa. The following procedures and events do not need antibiotic prophylaxis: Routine anesthetic injections through noninfected tissue, taking dental radiographs, placement of removable prosthodontic or orthodontic appliances, adjustment of orthodontic appliances, placement of orthodontic brackets, shedding of deciduous teeth, and bleeding from trauma to the lips or oral mucosa.
- *Respiratory tract:* Invasive procedures of the respiratory tract that involve incision or biopsy of the respiratory mucosa, such as tonsillectomy or adenoidectomy. Routine prophylaxis for bronchoscopy is not recommended unless the procedure involves incision of the respiratory tract mucosa.
- *Infected skin or musculoskeletal:* Surgical procedures that involve infected skin, skin structure, or musculoskeletal tissue.

Antibiotic Regimen for IE Prophylaxis

Table 4.5 describes antibiotic regimens for infective endocarditis prophylaxis.

Q. Janeway leisons.

Q. Osler's nodes.

Q. Roth's spots.

- *Janeway lesions* are due to septic emboli to skin seen in infective endocarditis. They are macular, blanching, nonpainful, erythematous lesions seen on the palms and soles.
- *Osler's nodes* are painful, violaceous nodules found in the pulp of fingers and toes. They are due to immune complex deposition in the skin.
- *Roth spots* are exudative, edematous, oval hemorrhagic lesions with a white centre, seen on retina in infective endocarditis. They are due to emboli occluding small retinal vessels.

Q. Define arrhythmia. Classify different types of arrhythmias.

- An abnormality of the cardiac rhythm is called a cardiac arrhythmia.
- Arrhythmias may cause sudden death, syncope, heart failure, dizziness, and palpitations or can be asymptomatic. They can be either transient or sustained.
- An arrhythmia with a rate of <60 per min is called bradyarrhythmia.
- An arrhythmia with a rate of >100 per min is called tachyarrhythmia.
- Tachyarrhythmias are more symptomatic than bradyarrhythmias. Tachyarrhythmias can be further divided as supraventricular (arise from the atrium or the atrioven-

Table 4.5: Antibiotic regimens for IE prophylaxis	
Situation	*Agent and dose (single dose 30–60 min before procedure)*
Able to take oral medication	Amoxicillin 2 g
Unable to take oral medication	Ampicillin 2 g IM or IV *or* ceftriaxone 1 g IM or IV
Allergic to penicillins or ampicillin	Cephalexin 2 g or other first- or second-generation cephalosporin *or* clindamycin 600 mg

tricular junction) and ventricular (arise from the ventricles).

- Atrial fibrillation (AF) is a supraventricular tachyarrhythmia characterized by uncoordinated atrial activation with consequent deterioration of mechanical atrial function.
- AF is the most common arrhythmia in adults. It can be paroxysmal, persistent, or chronic. Paroxysmal AF refers to episodes that terminate spontaneously. Persistent AF refers to episode sustained for more than seven days, or AF that terminates only with cardioversion. Chronic or continuous AF is the one that is unresponsive to cardioversion.

Etiology

- Emotional stress or following surgery, exercise, excessive caffeine use, smoking, and acute alcoholic intoxication
- Rheumatic heart disease (mitral valve disease such as mitral stenosis or mitral regurgitation)
- Hypertension
- Heart failure
- Hyperthyroidism
- Idiopathic (lone atrial fibrillation)

Pathophysiology

- During AF, the atria have disorganized, rapid, irregular electrical activity (300–600 per minute). The ventricular response is also irregular and variable (irregularly irregular).
- There is no coordinated mechanical contraction of atria giving rise to turbulence and stasis of blood in the atria leading to clot formation. With subsequent resumption of atrial contraction, clot can go into left ventricle and then into systemic circulation causing embolism.

- Excessive ventricular rate does not allow proper filling of ventricles, which leads to reduced cardiac output, pulmonary congestion, or angina pectoris.

Clinical Features

- Atrial fibrillation can be asymptomatic and detected incidentally in some patients.
- Patients may complain of anxiety, palpitations, fatigue and dyspnea. Patients may also present with stroke due to systemic embolism.
- Irregularly irregular pulse which is usally 100 to 150 per minute.
- Varying volume of pulse.
- Apex pulse deficit.
- Variable intensity S_1.

Complications

- Syncope
- Thromboembolism
- Cardiac failure
- Angina
- Hypotension
- Pulmonary edema

Investigations

- ECG shows varying RR intervals. P waves are absent.
- Echocardioagram can detect underlying condition such as mitral steonsis and atrial dilatation and clot formation.
- Other tests include complete blood count (to identify anemia), thyroid function tests (to identify hyperthyroidism), and serum electrolytes (to identify electrolyte imbalance).

Management

- Goals of treatment:
  - Control of ventricular rate
  - Restoration of sinus rhythm, if feasible
  - Prevention of embolic complications
  - Correction of underlying cause.
- If hemodynamically unstable (as evidenced by hypotension, hypoxia, pulmonary

edema, angina), electrical cardioversion (DC shock with 100 to 200 joules) is the treatment of choice.

- If hemodynamically stable, further treatment depends on whether the AF onset is of less than 48 hours or more than 48 hours. If onset of AF is less than 48 hours, then cardioversion can be attempted because the risk of a clot developing in the atria within 48 hours of AF is nil.
- On the other hand, if AF onset is more than 48 hours back, cardiovesrion is risky, because clot formation can occur in the atria, which can be dislodged by cardioversion. For these patients, slowing of ventricular rate should be the initial goal. Ventricular rate control is achieved by intravenous β-blockers (esmolol, metoprolol) and/or calcium channel blockers (*verapamil* or *diltiazem*). Digoxin is an alternative. Once rate control is achieved with above drugs, conversion to sinus rhythm may be attempted by DC shock or antiarrhythmic drugs (amiodarone, flecainide, or ibutilide). Before attempting DC shock for atrial fibrillation of >48 hours old, make sure that there is no clot in the atria, otherwise they will embolize to systemic circulation. Transesophageal echo is the best way to rule out clot. If clot is present, patient should be anticoagulated for at least 3 weeks prior to cardioversion.
- If there is a precipitating factor such as alcohol intoxication, fever, thyrotoxicosis, etc., it should be treated.
- Most of the recent guidelines favor rate control rather than rhythm control in atrial fibrillation, i.e. no need to convert the AF into sinus rhythm, only the ventricular rate needs to be controlled.
- Chronic anticoagulation is required for these patients to prevent clot formation. Warfarin should be used to maintain INR between 2 and 3.
- Patients with poor rate control despite optimal medical therapy should be considered for AV node ablation and pacemaker implantation (*'ablate and pace' strategy*)

Q. Paroxysmal supraventricular tachycardia (PSVT).

PSVT is paroxysmal and recurrent and often seen in young patients with no structural heart disease. Heart rate is usually 140–220 per minute with 1:1 atrioventricular conduction.

Etiology

PSVT is triggered by a reentry mechanism. This may be induced by premature atrial or ventricular ectopic beats. Other triggers include anxiety, hyperthyroidism and stimulants, including caffeine, drugs, and alcohol.

Mechanism

- The most common mechanism for paroxysmal supraventricular tachycardia is reentry, which may be initiated or terminated by a fortuitously timed atrial or ventricular ectopic rhythm.
- The reentry circuit most commonly involves dual pathways (a slow and a fast pathway) within the AV node (known as AV nodal reentrant tachycardia (AVNRT)).

Clinical Features

- It is usually seen in young people. The first presentation is common between ages 12 and 30.
- Attacks may occur spontaneously or may be precipitated by exertion, excess coffee, tea and alcohol.
- Most common symptom of PSVT is rapid regular palpitations, usually with abrupt onset, which can occur spontaneously or precipitated by factors described above. Palpitations are usually terminated by Valsalva maneuvers.
- Other symptoms may include anxiety, dizziness, dyspea, neck pulsation, chest pain, and weakness.
- Very fast heart rate may compromise cardiac output and cause hypotension and congestive heart failure.

- Polyuria may occur because of release of atrial natriuretic peptide in response to increased atrial pressures during the tachycardia.

ECG

- Rate is usually 140–220 per minute.
- P waves are not visible and are buried within the QRS complex.
- QRS complexes are narrow and occur at regular intervals.

Management

- Patients with hemodynamic instability (e.g. hypotension, pulmonary edema) require emergency cardioversion.
- If the patient is hemodynamically stable, vagal maneuvers (right carotid massage, Valsalva maneuver, and facial immersion in cold water) can be tried. Of these, Valsalva maneuver is the best and often easier for the patient to perform.
- If these maneuvers are not successful, intravenous adenosine (6 mg IV fast bolus) should be tried. If required, a second and third dose of 12 mg can be repeated in 1–2 minutes. Adenosine causes complete heart block for a fraction of a second and terminates SVT.
- An alternative treatment is verapamil 5–10 mg IV over 5–10 minutes, IV diltiazem, or beta-blockers (esmolol, propranolol, metoprolol).
- Radiofrequency catheter ablation of accessory pathway can cure SVT.

Q. Ventricular tachycardia (VT).

- VT is a rhythm which originates below the bundle of His at a rate greater than 100 beats per minute. Since it does not conduct through the normal conducting system, it is a wide-complex rhythm.
- It can be monomorphic (uniform QRS complexes) or polymorphic (QRS morphology varies).

- Sustained VT persists for 30 seconds or more. Sustained polymorphic VT is usually unstable and often degenerates into ventricular fibrillation. Sustained monomorphic VT can also degenerate into ventricular fibrillation but usually stable for long periods.
- Torsades de pointes (TdP) is a polymorphic VT with varying axes. It has a characteristic morphology (twisting around an axis) and is associated with prolonged QT interval.

Causes

- Ischemic heart disease
- Dilated cardiomyopathy
- Hypertrophic cardiomyopathy
- MVP
- Myocarditis
- Hypokalemia or hypomagnesemia
- Drugs which prolong QT interval
- Acid–base disturbance.

Clinical Features

- Pulse rate is usually between 120 and 220 per min.
- Sustained VT often results in presyncope (dizziness), syncope, hypotension and cardiac arrest.

Investigations

- *ECG:* Shows a rapid ventricular rhythm with broad QRS complexes.
- *Serum electrolytes:* Calcium, magnesium, sodium, potassium. Hypokalemia, hypomagnesemia, and hypocalcemia may predispose patients to either monomorphic VT or torsades de pointes
- *Drug levels:* For example, digoxin, toxicology screens.
- *Serum cardiac troponin I or T levels and CK-MB:* To evaluate for myocardial ischemia or infarction.
- *Electrophysiologic study:* It is required in patients at high risk for sudden death as a result of significant underlying structural heart disease.

Treatment

- If the patient is hemodynamically unstable (hypotension, pulmonary edema, angina), emergency DC cardioversion is required.
- If hemodynamically stable, intravenous amiodarone or lidocaine can be used to terminate VT. DC cardioversion is necessary, if medical therapy is unsuccessful.
- After resuscitation from VT, the cause of VT should be looked into and treated.

Q. Torsades de pointes.

Torsades de pointes refers to ventricular tachycardia (VT) characterized by polymorphic QRS complexes that change in amplitude and cycle length, giving the appearance of oscillations around the baseline.

Causes

It arises when ventricular repolarization (QT interval) is prolonged. The causes of torsades de pointes thus include causes of long QT syndrome which are as follows.

- *Electrolyte disturbances*: Hypokalemia, hypocalcemia and hypomagnesemia.
- *Drugs:* Phenothiazines, tricyclic antidepressants, quinidine, disopyramide, sotalol, amiodarone, macrolide antibiotics, fluoroquinolones and organophosphates.
- *Miscellaneous:* Bradycardia, acute myocardial infarction.

Clinical Features

- Torsades de pointes causes palpitations and syncope but usually terminates spontaneously.
- It can degenerate to ventricular fibrillation and cause sudden death.

Treatment

Acute Management

- Magnesium sulfate is the drug of choice for torsades de pointes. Magnesium is given at 1–2 g IV and can be repeated in 5–15 minutes.
- Any underlying precipitating factor should be addressed, i.e. correcting any electrolyte imbalances, and stopping drugs causing prolonged QT interval.
- Temporary transvenous pacing: Based on the fact that the QT interval shortens with a faster heart rate, pacing can be effective in terminating torsade.

Long-Term Management

- For congenital long QT syndrome, beta-blockers which shorten QT interval are useful.
- Implantable cardioverter defibrillators (ICD) are useful for patients with recurrent episodes in spite of using beta-blockers.

Q. Ventricular fibrillation (VF).

This is an arrhythmia characterized by disorganized electrical activity with no mechanical contraction and hence no cardiac output.

Causes

VF occurs due to ischemic heart disease, cardiac failure, electrolyte imbalances, Brugada syndrome, etc. Ventricular ectopics during the vulnerable period of ventricular repolarization (R-on-T phenomenon) may initiate VF.

Clinical Features

- The patient is pulseless and rapidly becomes unconscious, and respiration ceases.
- ECG shows shapeless, rapid oscillations without any organized complexes.

Treatment

- VF usually ends in death within minutes unless prompt corrective measures are instituted. The rate of survival in out-of-hospital cardiac arrest has increased with expansion of community-based emergency rescue systems, use of automatic external defibrillators (AEDs), and increasing numbers of laypersons trained in cardiopulmonary resuscitation (CPR).

- VF rarely reverses spontaneously and requires immediate electrical defibrillation. Basic and advanced cardiac life support is needed.
- If ventricular fibrillation occurs after acute myocardial infarction, it usually does not require any prophylactic therapy. However, if the VF has occurred spontaneously without any cause, such patients are at high risk of sudden death and require implantable cardioverter defibrillators (ICDs) to prevent further attacks.

Q. Discuss the etiology, classification, and general clinical features of congenital heart diseases.

- Congenital heart disease affects about 1% of live births.
- Males are affected more commonly except atrial septal defect (ASD) and persistent ductus arteriosus (PDA) which affect females commonly.
- Because of improved medical and surgical management, more children with congenital heart disease are surviving into adolescence and adulthood.

Etiology

Congenital heart diseases are due to abnormal development of a normal structure, or failure of a normal structure to develop fully. Such maldevelopments are due to multifactorial genetic and environmental causes. The recognized risk factors include:

- *Maternal infections:* For example, rubella infection.
- *Drugs:* Alcohol abuse, phenytoin and radiation.
- *Genetic abnormalities:* For example, familial form of atrial septal defect and congenital heart block.
- *Chromosomal abnormalities:* For example, septal defects and tetralogy of Fallot are

associated with Down's syndrome (trisomy 21) or coarctation of the aorta in Turner's syndrome (45, XO).

Classification of Congenital Heart Diseases

Cyanotic congenital heart diseases
- Fallot's tetralogy
- Transposition of the great vessels
- Severe Ebstein's anomaly
- Severe pulmonary stenosis
- Tricuspid atresia

Acyanotic congenital heart diseases
- Atrial septal defect (ASD)
- Ventricular septal defect (VSD)
- Patent ductus arteriosus (PDA)
- Coarctation of the aorta
- Aortic stenosis
- Pulmonary stenosis

General Clinical Features of Congenital Heart Diseases

Congenital heart disease (CHD) should be recognized as early as possible, since early treatment has better outcome. Some general clinical features of congenital heart diseases are as follows:

- In as many as 80% of infants with critical disease, congestive heart failure is the presenting symptom. Difficulty in feeding is common and is often associated with tachypnea, sweating and subcostal retraction. Suspicion of CHD should be raised, if feeding takes more than 30 minutes. On examination, signs of congestive heart failure include an S_3 gallop and crepitations in the lungs.
- *Central cyanosis* occurs in cyanotic congenital heart diseases because of right-to-left shunting of blood or because of mixing of systemic and pulmonary blood flow.
- *Pulmonary hypertension* can happen in left-to-right shunts. Blood from left side of the heart under high pressure enters right side and then into pulmonary artery. This leads to pulmonary hypertension. Pressure in the

pulmonary arterial system can exceed that on left side of the heart which can cause reversal of blood flow from right side to left side. This reversal of blood flow is referred to as *Eisenmenger's syndrome.*

- *Clubbing of the fingers* occurs due to prolonged cyanosis in cyanotic congenital heart diseases.
- *Paradoxical embolism* of thrombus can occur from systemic veins to systemic arterial system when there is a communication between the right and left heart. This can lead to an increased risk of cerebrovascular accidents and abscesses.
- *Growth retardation* is common in children with cyanotic heart disease.
- *Syncope* is common when severe right or left ventricular outflow tract obstruction is present. Exertional syncope may occur in Fallot's tetralogy. Exercise increases pulmonary vascular resistance and decreases systemic vascular resistance. Thus, the right-to-left shunt increases and cerebral oxygenation falls.
- *Squatting* posture is often adopted by children with Fallot's tetralogy. It results in decreased venous return and an increase in the peripheral vascular resistance. This leads to decreased pressure in the right side of heart and increased pressure in left side of the heart which results in reduced right-to-left shunt and improved cerebral oxygenation.
- *Endocarditis* can occur at the sites of shunts and damaged valves.

Genetic Counselling

- A woman with congenital heart disease needs close follow-up during pregnancy. Pregnancy is usually safe, except if pulmonary hypertension is present when the prognosis for both mother and fetus is poor.
- Fetal ultrasound screening during pregnancy is necessary to r/o any heart malformations since patients with congenital heart disease are more likely to have a baby with congenital heart disease.

Q. Ventricular septal defect (VSD).

- VSD is the most common congenital heart disease (1 in 500 live births). It may occur as an isolated anomaly or in association with other anomalies.
- Membranous VSD is the most common type. VSD can close spontaneously or lead to congestive cardiac failure and death in infancy.

Pathophysiology

As left ventricular pressure is higher than right ventricular pressure, blood moves from left to right leading to increased blood flow through pulmonary vasculature. In the long run, this increased flow leads to pulmonary HTN and increased right ventricular pressure so much that right ventricular pressure may be equal to or more than left ventricular pressure (Eisenmenger complex). As a result, the shunt is reduced or reversed (becoming right-to-left) and central cyanosis may develop.

Clinical Features

- *Small VSDs* are asymptomatic and 90% of them close spontaneously by 10 years of age.
- *Moderate and large VSD* leads to pulmonary HTN (Eisenmenger syndrome), which causes exertional dyspnea, chest pain, syncope, and hemoptysis.
- When there is reversal of shunt (right-to-left shunt), central cyanosis, clubbing, and polycythemia develop.
- CVS examination reveals cardiac enlargement and a prominent apex beat. There is often a palpable systolic thrill at the lower left sternal edge. A loud pansystolic murmur is heard in the same area.

Complications

- Congestive cardiac failure
- Pulmonary hypertension
- Eisenmenger's syndrome
- Infective endocarditis
- Right ventricular outflow tract obstruction.

Investigations

- *Chest X-ray* may show features of increased pulmonary flow and pulmonary HTN such as prominent pulmonary artery, 'pruned' pulmonary arteries, and right ventricular hypertrophy.
- *ECG* shows features of both left and right ventricular hypertrophy.
- 2-D echocardiography and color Doppler can confirm the presence, size and location of the VSD, and abnormal blood flow.

Treatment

- Surgery is not recommended for patients with small shunts and normal pulmonary arterial pressures.
- Surgical correction is indicated for moderate to large VSD before the development of severe pulmonary HTN. If severe pulmonary HTN has developed already, it will not reverse or may progress even after surgery.

Q. Atrial septal defect (ASD).

ASD is a defect in interatrial septum. It is common in females.

Types of ASD

There are three main types of ASD—*sinus venosus type*, *ostium secundum* and *ostium primum*.

Pathophysiology

- ASD allows shunting of blood from high pressure left atrium to low pressure right atrium. Hence, there is increase in right ventricular inflow, right ventricular output, and pulmonary blood flow.
- Increased pulmonary blood flow gives rise to increased pulmonary vascular resistance and pulmonary HTN. This usually happens above the age of 30 years.
- Severe pulmonary HTN may lead to increased right atrial pressure, which can be more than left atrium and lead to right-to-left shunting with central cyanosis.

Ultimately, heart failure may develop due to overloading of both ventricles.

- Because of increased blood flow into right side, right atrium and right ventricles dilate and there may be atrial arrhythmias, especially atrial fibrillation.

Clinical Features

Symptoms

- Children with ASD are asymptomatic, but as they reach 3rd decade, they may develop pulmonary HTN as explained above.
- Dyspnea and weakness occur due to pulmonary HTN.
- Recurrent respiratory infections are common due to increased blood flow through pulmonary vasulature and congestion.
- Palpitations may be experienced due to atrial arrhythmias (atrial fibrillation).

Signs

- Precordium is hyperdynamic.
- Signs of pulmonary HTN such as right ventricular heave, prominent pulmonary artery pulsations may be noted.
- On auscultation, the second heart sound is widely split and fixed in relation to respiration. A mid-diastolic rumbling murmur is heard at the fourth intercostal space and along the left sternal border due to increased flow across the tricuspid valve. An ejection systolic murmur may be heard over pulmonary area due to increased blood flow across pulmonary valve.
- Right heart failure may develop and lead to raised JVP and peripheral edema.
- Development of Eisenmenger's syndrome leads to central cyanosis and digital clubbing.

Complications

- Congestive cardiac failure
- Pulmonary hypertension
- Eisenmenger's syndrome
- Infective endocarditis

- Atrial fibrillation
- Paradoxical embolism

Investigations

- *Chest X-ray* shows prominent pulmonary artery and pulmonary vascular congestion. It may also show right atrial and right ventricular enlargement.
- *ECG* mays how right bundle branch block and right axis deviation due to right ventricular hypertrophy and dilatation.
- *Echocardiogram* may show right ventricular hypertrophy, dilated pulmonary artery, and abnormal motion of the interventricular septum. It may also show ASD. Abnormal shunt and blood flow can be assessed by color Doppler.
- *Cardiac catheterization* can confirm the presence of ASD but usually Echo is enough for confirmation. However, it is especially useful when associated coronary artery disease is present as both coronary arteries and ASD can be assessed in the same sitting. Cardiac catheterization shows increased oxygen content of right atrial blood due to blood flow from left atrium.

Treatment

- Surgical closure should be done between 3 and 6 years of age or as soon as possible in significant ASD (i.e. pulmonary flow more than 50% increased compared with systemic flow).
- Angiographic closure is now possible by using a transcatheter device.

Q. Patent ductus arteriosus (PDA).

- The ductus arteriosus is a vessel, which connects the pulmonary artery to the descending aorta distal to the subclavian artery.
- In fetal life, the ductus arteriosus is normally open and diverts blood away from the unexpanded and hence high resistance pulmonary circulation into the systemic circulation, where the blood is re-oxygenated as it passes through the placenta.
- The duct normally closes at birth, due to high oxygen in the lungs and the reduced pulmonary vascular resistance. After closure, a fibrous band is left behind (ligamentum arteriosum).
- If the duct is defective (e.g. less elastic tissue), it will not close. Prenatal hypoxemia and high-altitude environments may impair closure of ductus.
- PDA is more common in females and is sometimes associated with maternal rubella. Premature babies can have PDA which is normal and will close later.

Pathophysiology (Fig. 4.1)

- Since pressure in the aorta is more than pulmonary artery, blood flows from aorta to pulmonary artery throughout the cardiac cycle. This leads to increased flow through the pulmonary vasculature leading to pulmonary HTN.
- Left heart also gets overloaded due to increased pulmonary venous return which may result in left heart failure.
- If pulmonary HTN is very severe, it may lead to reversal of flow from pulmonary artery to aorta (Eisenmenger's physiology).
- One-third of patients with PDA die of heart failure, pulmonary hypertension or endocarditis by the age of 40; two-thirds by the age of 60.

Clinical Features

- Patients may remain asympomatic until later in life when heart failure or infective endocarditis develops.
- High volume peripheral pulses ('bounding') may be noted due to increased venous return to left heart and hence increased stroke volume.
- Auscultation reveals a characteristic continuous 'machinery' murmur heard at the first or second left intercostal space.
- Signs of pulmonary HTN such as loud P2, parasternal heave and prominent epigatsric pulsations may be present.

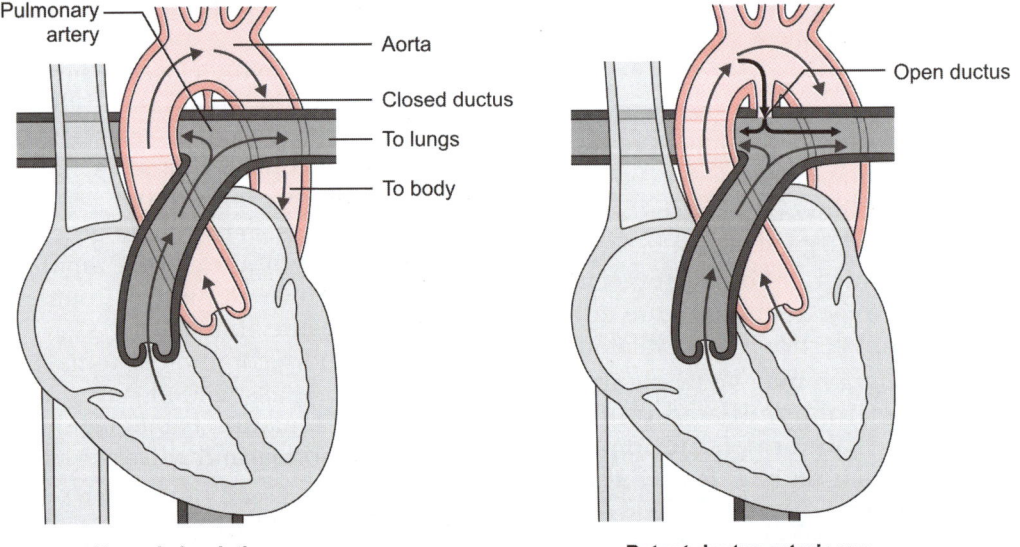

Pulmonary artery	Aorta
	Closed ductus
	To lungs
	To body

Open ductus

Normal circulation   **Patent ductus arteriosus**

Fig. 4.1: Patent ductus arteriosus

- In patients with reversal of shunt (Eisenmenger's physiology), venous blood from pulmonary artery enters descending aorta and leads to differential cyanosis, i.e. cyanois in the lower limbs and sparing of upper limbs especially the right arm.

Complications
- Congestive cardiac failure
- Pulmonary hypertension
- Eisenmenger's syndrome
- Infective endocarditis
- Paradoxical embolism

Investigations
- *Chest X-ray* may show prominent aorta and pulmonary arterial system. It may also show dilated left atrium and ventricle.
- *ECG* shows left ventricular hypertrophy.
- *Echocardiogram* shows dilated left atrium and left ventricle. Color Doppler can visualize PDA and direction of blood flow.

Treatment
Premature infants with PDA are treated medically with indomethacin. Indomethacin closes PDA by inhibiting prostaglandin production which maintains patency.
- In other cases, PDA can be closed surgically or via transcatheter methods.

Q. Fallot's tetralogy (TOF)

Fallot's tetralogy is the most common cyanotic congenital heart disease. It is characterized by 4 features—pulmonary stenosis, VSD, overriding aorta, and right ventricular hypertrophy.

Pathophysiology
Since the right ventricular pressure is more than left ventricle due to pulmonary stenosis, blood is shunted from right to left through the ventricular septal defect, which leads to central cyanosis. Squatting episodes increase systemic arterial rsistance and hence reduce the shunt from right-to-left ventricle.

Clinical Features
- Children are usually asymptomatic at birth.
- Children with Fallot's tetralogy may present with dyspnea and fatigue.

- Growth is usually retarded.
- Exercise leads to drop in systemic vascular resistance and increases the shunting of blood from right-to-left ventricle leading to increased cyanosis and syncope (cyanotic or Fallot's spells). Cyanotic spells occur during crying, feeding, exercise and fever. Sudden death can occur during such spells.
- Squatting is common because it increases peripheral vascular resistance and decreases shunt.
- Polycythemia and clubbing occur due to chronic hypoxemia which may result in thrombotic strokes.
- A parasternal heave is common due to RVH.

Investigations

- *Chest X-ray* shows 'boot-shaped heart'. This shape results from hypertrophied right ventricle coupled with small left ventricle with upturned apex. Pulmonary vascularity is reduced.
- *ECG* shows right ventricular hypertrophy and right-axis deviation. Right bundle branch block may also be present.
- *Echocardiogram* can readily identify overriding aorta and VSD.
- *Cardiac catheterization* is done for patients in whom operative treatment is contemplated or in whom the integrity of the coronary circulation needs to be verified.

Complications

- Intravascular thrombosis and thrombotic stroke can occur.
- Brain abscess can occur because organisms entering right ventricle by venous return can enter systemic circulation through VSD and reach brain.
- Infective endocarditis
- Higher incidence of pulmonary tuberculosis

Treatment

- Complete surgical repair consists of patch closure of the VSD and relief of pulmonary stenosis.

- Occasionally, a palliative procedure—an anastomosis between subclavian artery and pulmonary artery (Blalock-Taussig shunt)—is performed on very young or premature infants.
- Antibiotic prophylaxis for endocarditis is needed.

Q. Define heart failure. Describe the etiology, classification, clinical features, investigations and management of heart failure (congestive cardiac failure).

Q. Precipitating causes of heart failure.

Definition

- Heart failure (HF) is defined as a complex clinical syndrome that can result from any structural or functional cardiac disorder that impairs the ability of the ventricle to fill with or eject blood.
- It is a common health problem especially in industrialized countries.

Etiology of Heart Failure

There are many causes of heart failure. However five causes account for most of the cases of heart failure. These are ischemic heart disease (responsible for 70% of cases), cardiomyopathies, congenital, valvular, and hypertensive heart diseases. Following are the causes of heart failure.

Precipitating Causes of Heart Failure

Precipitating causes make the previously compromised heart fail. These include:
- *Infection:* Any infection may precipitate HF. Fever, tachycardia, hypoxemia, and the increased metabolic demands due to infection may place additional burden on a compromised heart and lead to heart falure.
- *Arrhythmias:* Tachyarrhythmias reduce the time available for ventricular filling, and cause ischemic myocardial dysfunction in patients with ischemic heart disease.

- *Physical, dietary, fluid, environmental, and emotional excesses:* Sudden increase in sodium intake, physical overexertion, excessive environmental heat or humidity, and emotional crises all may precipitate HF.
- *Discontinuation of drugs:* Such as antihypertensives, diuretics, etc. given for heart failure may precipitate heart failure.
- *Ingestion of drugs* such as NSAIDs can precipitate heart failure.
- *Myocardial Infarction:* A new infarction on a previously compromised heart may precipitate heart falure.
- *Pulmonary embolism* may result in right heart falure.
- *Anemia:* In the presence of anemia, the oxygen needs of the metabolizing tissues can be met only by an increase in the cardiac output. An already compromised heart may not be able to tolerate such an increased demand and may fail.
- *Thyrotoxicosis and pregnancy:* Thyrotoxicosis and pregnancy are high cardiac output states which place increased demand on heart.
- *Uncontrolled hypertension:* Uncontrolled BP either due to renal problems or discontinuation of antihypertensives may result in cardiac decompensation.
- *Myocarditis:* Rheumatic, viral, and other forms of myocarditis may precipitate HF in patients with or without pre-existing heart disease.
- *Infective endocarditis:* Valvular damage, anemia, fever, and myocarditis which may occur in infective endocarditis may precipitate HF.

Types

HF can be classified in many ways. It can be acute or chronic, left-sided or right-sided, high-output or low-output, forward or backward, and systolic or diastolic failure.

Acute Versus Chronic Failure

In acute failure, there is sudden reduction in cardiac output which leads to hypotension without peripheral edema, whereas in chronic heart failure, blood pressure is well maintained but there is peripheral edema. Causes of acute heart failure are massive myocardial infarction and valve rupture. Causes of chronic heart failure are valvular heart disease, dilated cardiomyopathy, and systemic hypertension.

Left-sided Versus Right-sided Failure

- In left ventricular failure, there is pulmonary congestion resulting in dyspnea and orthopnea.
- In right-sided failure, systemic congestion leads to raised jugular venous pressure, congestive hepatomegaly, ascites, and lower limb edema.
- Failure of both left and right ventricles is called congestive cardiac failure (CCF) and is seen in long-standing valvular heart disease (aortic and mitral valves), myocarditis, cardiomyopathies, and hypertension.

High-output Versus Low-output Failure

- Examples of high-output failure are severe anemia, hyperthyroidism, beriberi, arteriovenous fistulae, pregnancy, and Paget's disease. Here the cardiac output is more than normal.
- Examples of low-output failure are ischemic heart disease, hypertension, dilated cardiomyopathy, and valvular and pericardial disease. Here the cardiac output is reduced.

Systolic Versus Diastolic Failure

- In systolic heart failure, heart is not able to pump the blood into arterial system. It happens mainly due to myocardial dysfunction. Examples are myocardial infarction, cardiomyopathy, etc.
- Diastolic failure is due to inability of the ventricle to relax and receive blood, which leads to elevation of ventricular diastolic pressure. Examples are left ventricular hypertrophy, constrictive pericarditis, restrictive cardiomyopathy, etc.

Pathophysiology

- In the normal ventricle, stroke volume increases over a wide range of end-diastolic volumes (the Frank-Starling effect). In the failing heart with depressed contractility, there is relatively little increment in systolic function with further increases in left ventricular volume. Systolic dysfunction causes pulmonary congestion (left heart failure) or systemic congestion (right heart failure), or both pulmonary and systemic congestion (CCF), effort intolerance, and organ dysfunction.

- The reduction in cardiac output leads to activation of compensatory mechanisms, viz. increased sympathetic activity, stimulation of the renin–angiotensin–aldosterone system (RAAS) and secretion of antidiuretic hormone (ADH). This neurohumoral activation causes tachycardia, peripheral vasoconstriction, sodium and water retention. The result of these compensatory mechanisms is increase in blood pressure (for tissue perfusion) and blood volume (enhancing preload, stroke volume, and cardiac output by the Frank-Starling mechanism). These compensatory mechanisms help to normalize the hemodynamic disturbances to some extent, but increase the myocardial oxygen and energy requirements. In the long run, these compensatory responses perpetuate myocardial damage and worsen heart failure.

- Other compensatory mechanisms are activation of vasodilatory molecules, such as atrial and brain natriuretic peptides (ANP and BNP), prostaglandins (PGE_2 and PGI_2), and nitric oxide (NO), that offset the excessive peripheral vascular vasoconstriction. ANP and BNP cause natriuresis, vasodilation and inhibition of angiotensin II, aldosterone and ADH secretion, thereby reversing some of the harmful effects.

Clinical Features

Symptoms

Dyspnea

- *Exertional dyspnea* is seen in early heart failure. As heart failure advances, dyspnea occurs with progressively less strenuous activity and ultimately it is present even at rest.

- *Orthopnea* is dyspnea in lying down position and is a later manifestation than exertional dyspnea. Orthopnea is due to redistribution of fluid from the abdomen and lower extremities into the chest in lying position, which increases the pulmonary capillary pressure, combined with elevation of the diaphragm.

- *Paroxysmal nocturnal dyspnea (PND)* is sudden onset dyspnoea and cough occurring usually 1 to 3 hours after the patient retires. Symptoms usually resolve over 10 to 30 minutes after the patient arises, often gasping for fresh air from an open window. PND happens due to accumulation of excessive blood in the lungs during sleep causing pulmonary edema, depression of the respiratory center and decreased sympathetic activity during sleep. The patient gets up suddenly feeling excessively breathless and choked and longs for fresh air. He may bring out pink frothy sputum.

- *Acute pulmonary edema* results from transudation of fluid into the alveolar spaces because of acute rise in capillary hydrostatic pressures due to sudden decrease in cardiac function. Patient may present with cough or progressive dyspnea. Wheezing is common due to bronchospasm. If acute pulmonary edema is not treated earlier, patient may begin coughing up pink (or blood-tinged), frothy fluid and become cyanotic and acidotic. Some patients may present with Cheyne-Stokes respiration (periodic respiration or cyclic respiration) which is characterized by periods of apnea, hypoventilation and hyperventilation.

Fatigue: This is due to reduced perfusion of skeletal muscles.

Cerebral symptoms: Are due to reduced cerebral perfusion and include altered mental status, confusion, lack of concentration, memory impairement, headache, anxiety and insomnia.

Abdominal symptoms: Like nausea, anorexia, and pain abdomen are due to congested gastric mucosa, liver and portal venous system.

Oliguria, nocturia: Reduced renal perfusion during day causes sodium and water retention and oliguria. Renal perfusion increases at night due to shift of fluid from the extravascular to the intravascular compartment, resulting in increased excretion of sodium and water and nocturia.

NYHA classification of heart failure: The New York Heart Association (NYHA) classification system is the simplest and most widely used method to gauge symptom severity. The classification system is a well-established predictor of mortality and can be used at diagnosis and to monitor treatment response.

Functional capacity	Description
I	No limitations of physical activity No heart failure symptoms (fatigue, palpitation, dyspnea)
II	Mild limitation of physical activity Heart failure symptoms with significant exertion; comfortable at rest or with mild activity
III	Marked limitation of physical activity Heart failure symptoms with mild exertion; only comfortable at rest
IV	Discomfort with any activity Heart failure symptoms occur at rest

Physical Signs

Vital signs
- Pulse is fast and of low volume. Pulsus alternans may be seen in LVF.
- BP is low in severe heart failure.
- Respiratory rate may be high due to pulmonary edema.

General examination
- Patient is dyspneic and orthopneic. Peripheries are cold and may be cyanosed. JVP is usually elevated with positive abdominojugular reflux. Pitting pedal edema may be present. Sacral edema is seen in bedridden patients. In chronic, severe heart failure, weight loss may occur.

CVS: Cardiac enlargement (apex beat shifted down and out) may be seen. Third and fourth heart sounds are often audible. Pansystolic murmur may be heard due to incompetence of mitral and tricuspid valve due to dilatation of ventricles.

RS: Tachypnea may be present due to pulmonary edema. Bilateral fine basal crepitations and ronchi may be heard due to pulmonary edema. Sometimes signs of pleural effusion may be present.

Abdomen: Liver may be enlarged and tender due to congestion. Ascites may be present.

NS: Confusion, memory disturbances may be seen.

Investigations

- *Chest X-ray:* The presence of cardiomegaly is a strong indicator of heart failure. Pulmonary edema may be seen as bilateral batwing hilar haziness, generalized haze (due to interstitial edema), and Kerley's B lines (due to prominent interlobular lymphatics) at the lung base. Bilateral pleural effusion may be seen which is usually more on right side.
- *Electrocardiogram (ECG):* It can show cardiac rhythm, identify ischemia, prior or recent MI, and detect evidence of left ventricular hypertrophy.
- *Echocardiogrphy:* Transthoracic echo can confirm the presence of heart failure and also quantify it.
- *Natriuretic peptide measurements:* Elevated serum levels ANP (atrial natriuretic peptide) and BNP (brain natriuretic peptide) are seen in heart failure.
- *Radionuclide studies:* Provide non-invasive and accurate measurement of wall motion abnormalities, ventricular volume and ejection fraction.
- *Cardiac catheterization:* In heart failure, there is increased end-diastolic ventricular

pressure, reduced cardiac output and reduced ventricular ejection fraction. Coronary angiogram can identify the extent of coronary artery disease.

Treatment of Heart Failure

The ideal approach would be to treat both the underlying and precipitating causes. Correction of underlying cause (e.g. surgical correction of valvular defects) may dramatically improve heart failure. Correction of underlying cause may not always be possible (e.g. old myocardial infarction). Precipitating causes like infections, severe anemia, hyperthyroidism, etc. should be looked for and corrected.

Control of Excessive Fluid

- *Low salt diet and fluid restriction:* Can help in decreasing many of the clinical manifestations of heart failure.
- *Diuretics:* These agents reduce ECF volume expansion and reduce edema. Many agents are available and almost all are effective in controlling fluid retention. These agents include frusemide, torsemide, thiazides, spironolactone, amiloride, etc.

Prevention of Deterioration of Myocardial Function

- Chronic activation of the renin–angiotensin–aldosterone system (RAAS) and of the adrenergic nervous systems in HF causes ventricular remodeling, further deterioration of cardiac function and/or potentially fatal arrhythmias. Drugs that block these two systems are useful in the management of HF and decrease long-term mortality.
- *Angiotensin-converting enzyme (ACE) inhibitors:* ACE inhibitors slow the maladaptive remodeling of ventricles, and reduce the afterload by causing vasodilatation. ACE inhibitors has been shown to prevent or retard the development of HF in patients with left ventricular dysfunction without HF, enhance exercise tolerance, and reduce long-term mortality and rate of readmission to hospitals. ACE inhibitor should be given indefinitely to patients with heart failure. Examples of ACE inhibitors are captopril, enalapril, lisinopril, ramipril, perindopril, etc.

- *Angiotensin receptor blockers (ARB):* These agents have similar effects as ACE inhibitors. They are used when patients cannot tolerate ACE inhibitors due to cough, angioneurotic edema, and leucopenia. Examples of ARBs are losartan, telmisartan, olmesartan, etc.
- *Aldosterone antagonist:* The activation of the RAAS in HF increases the levels of angiotensin II and aldosterone. Aldosterone causes Na^+ retention (hence fluid retention), sympathetic activation, myocardial, vascular, and perivascular fibrosis, and vasoconstriction. Spironolactone is an antagonist of aldosterone and when given to heart failure patients on long-term basis reduces mortality and sudden death. Eplerenone is a new, more selective aldosterone inhibitor that can be used instead of spironolactone.
- *Beta-adrenoceptor blockers:* Beta-blockers have been shown to improve the symptoms of HF, and to reduce long-term mortality, sudden death, and rehospitalization for HF. They should be given only for patients with moderately severe HF (classes II and III). They should not be given for patients with class IV heart failure, hypotension (systolic pressure <90 mm Hg).
- *Vasodilators:* Direct vasodilators are helpful in patients with severe heart failure who have systemic vasoconstriction despite ACE inhibitor therapy. Decrease in peripheral resistance enhances cardiac output by decreasing afterload. Sodium nitroprusside, nitroglycerin, hydralazine and nesiritide are vasodilators, which have to be given by continous IV infusion. Hydralazine and isosorbide dinitrate are useful for chronic oral administration.

Enhancement of Myocardial Contractility

- *Cardiac glycosides (digitalis and digoxin):* Cardiac glycosides enhance myocardial contractility and hence improve symptoms of heart failure.

- *Sympathomimetic amines:* These are dopamine and dobutamine which act on β-adrenergic receptors and improve myocardial contractility. They have to be given by constant intravenous infusion and can be given for several days.
- *Phosphodiesterase inhibitors:* Examples are amrinone and milrinone. Both these drugs exert positive inotropic and vasodilator actions by inhibiting phosphodiesterase III.

Circulatory Assist Devices/Cardiac Transplantation

When patients do not respond to all the above measures, have class IV heart failure, and are unlikely to survive one year, they should be considered for assisted circulation and/or cardiac transplantation.

Non-Pharmacological Measures

- *Rest:* Rest reduces the demand on the heart. Adequate rest reduces venous pressure and pulmonary congestion. Absolute bed rest is not required even for patients with severe HF.

- *Diet:* The diet should provide adequate calories to maintain ideal weight. Obese patients should have a low-calorie diet. Oils and fats should be cut down. Sodium intake should not exceed 6 g of salt per day. Potassium-rich foods are advised for those receiving diuretics.

Hematology

Q. Define anemia.

Q. Write the causes and classification of anemia.

- Anemia is defined as a reduction in the number of circulating RBCs.
- Anemia can be classified based on the underlying cause or morphology of RBCs.

Classification of Anemia

I. Based on underlying cause

Decreased RBC production
- Iron, vitamin B_{12}, or folate deficiency
- Bone marrow disorders (e.g. aplastic anemia, myelodysplasia, tumor infiltration)
- Bone marrow suppression (e.g. drugs, chemotherapy, irradiation).
- Anemia of chronic disease/inflammation

Increased RBC destruction
- Hemolytic anemias (e.g. hereditary sphero-cytosis, sickle cell disease, thalassemia major, autoimmune hemolytic anemia)

Blood loss
- Trauma, hematemesis, hemoptysis, bleeding ulcer or carcinoma

II. Based on the morphology of RBC

Microcytic anemia (MCV below 80 fL)
- Iron deficiency
- Anemia of chronic disease
- Thalassemia

Macrocytic anemia (MCV above 100 fL)
- Vitamin B_{12} and folate deficiency

Normocytic anemia (MCV normal, i.e. between 80 and100 fL)
- Acute blood loss

Q. Enumerate the causes of microcytic anemia. Discuss the etiology, clinical features, investigations and management of iron deficiency anemia.

Q. Pica.

Q. Plummer-Vinson syndrome (Paterson-Kelly syndrome).

Q. Oral iron therapy.

Q. Parenteral iron therapy.

Causes of Microcytic Anemia (MCV Below 80 fL)

- Iron deficiency
- Anemia of chronic disease
- Sideroblastic anemia
- Thalassemias

IRON DEFICIENCY ANEMIA

- Iron deficiency is the most common cause of microcytic anemia. Other than hemoglobin, iron is also a part of many enzymes in the body which are vital for tissue respiration and organ function.
- Iron is the commonest deficiency disease all over the world. It is widely prevalent in India and is more common in pregnant women.

Causes of Iron Deficiency

Decreased iron intake or absorption
- Inadequate diet
- Malabsorption (celiac sprue, Crohn's disease, post-gastrectomy)
- Acute or chronic inflammation

Increased demand for iron
- Rapid growth in infancy or adolescence
- Pregnancy

Increased iron loss
- Blood loss (blood donation, trauma, peptic ulcer, GI malignancy, hookworm infestation)

Clinical Features

Symptoms

- Insidious onset of weakness, dyspnea, and easy fatigability.
- Palpitations, tinnitus and headache due to hyperdynamic circulation.
- Dysphagia due to formation of mucosal webs at the pharyngo-oesophageal junction (also called Plummer-Vinson syndrome).
- Menstrual disturbances can occur (amenorrhea or menorrhagia).
- Pica is seen in some people. *Pica* is the persistent eating of substances such as dirt or paint that have no nutritional value. Pica is relieved by iron therapy.

Signs

- Glossitis (inflammation of tongue) and angular stomatitis may be present.

Papillary atrophy of the tongue makes it appear smooth and pale (bald tongue).
- Flattening and concavity of the nails are called platynychia and koilonychia respectively, and is a feature of iron deficiency.
- Mild hepatosplenomegaly may be present.
- The triad of dysphagia due to esophageal webs, koilonychia and splenomegaly in a patient with iron deficiency anemia is known as the *Plummer-Vinson* or *Patterson-Kelly syndrome*. Webs and dysphagia do not respond to iron therapy. Dysphagia is treated by passage of bougei and dilatation. These webs are premalignant.

Investigations

Investigations are required to confirm iron deficiency and to determine its cause.

- *Complete blood picture:* RBC count, hemoglobin, hematocrit, MCV, MCH and MCHC are all decreased in iron deficiency anemia.
- *Peripheral blood smear:* Shows microcytic hypochromic RBCs. There may be other morphological abnormalities such as poikilocytosis and presence of target cells.
- *Serum iron and ferritin* are decreased, and TIBC is increased.
- *Bone marrow:* Shows micronormoblasts. Iron stores are absent or markedly reduced.
- *Investigations to identify the cause of iron deficiency:* Stool for occult blood and helminthiasis, upper GI scopy to rule out peptic ulcer or malignancy, etc. depending on the clinical presentation.

Treatment

Treatment involves replacement of iron and correction of the cause of iron deficiency. Iron can be given orally or parenterally.

Oral Iron Therapy

- Oral Iron therapy is safer and cheaper than parenteral, and is preferred.

- Iron is best given as a single dose at bedtime.
- There are many iron salts available such as ferrous fumarate, ferrous sulfate and ferrous gluconate. There is no significant difference in the absorption of these salts. Oral iron is better tolerated, if given after food, but may be absorbed less efficiently.
- Hemoglobin level will normalize in about 6 weeks of iron therapy. However, iron therapy has to be continued for a total of 6 months to ensure repletion of the body iron stores.
- Adverse effects of oral iron include nausea, vomiting, epigastric discomfort, constipation or diarrhea. They are dose-related, and can be reduced by gradually increasing the dose and giving it after meals.

Parenteral Iron Therapy

- *Indications:* It is indicated in patients who cannot tolerate oral iron and in pregnant women who present with severe anemia very late in pregnancy. Patients with gastrointestinal diseases such as peptic ulcer and ulcerative colitis are likely to be aggravated by oral iron and need parenteral iron.
- *Parenteral preparations:* There are many parenteral iron preparations available. These are iron dextran (can be given either IM or IV), ferric gluconate complex and iron sucrose (only for IV use). Injection should be given after a test dose because there is a small risk of anaphylaxis.
- *Side effects:* Both local and systemic side effects can occur following use of iron dextran. Local reactions include pain, muscle necrosis, and phlebitis in adjacent vessels. Anaphylactic reactions also can occur with all the preparations but less with ferric gluconate complex and iron sucrose than iron dextran.

Treatment of Cause of Iron Deficiency

- For example, treatment of hookworm infestation, piles, peptic ulcer disease and any other bleeding lesions.

Q. Enumerate the causes of macrocytic anemia. Discuss the etiology, clinical features, diagnosis and management of vitamin B_{12} (cyanocobalamin) deficiency.

RBCs with MCV more than 100 fL (femtoliters) are called macrocytes (megaloblasts).

Causes of Macrocytic Anemia

- Vitamin B_{12} deficiency
- Folic acid deficiency
- Drugs: 6-mercaptopurine, azathioprine, 5-fluorouracil, hydroxyurea, acyclovir, zidovudine

Vitamin B_{12}

- Vitamin B_{12} is found in animal proteins and dairy products. Vegetables contain practically no vitamin B_{12}. Vegetarians get their vitamin B_{12} by dairy products.
- Normal recommended dietary allowance for vitamin B_{12} is 2 µg/day. Total body stores of vitamin B_{12} is 2 to 5 mg, half of which is in the liver. These stores are enough for approximately 3 years, and hence, it takes approximately 3 years to develop manifestations of vitamin B_{12} deficiency after absorption of dietary vitamin B_{12} ceases.
- Dietary vitamin B_{12} is liberated in the stomach in the presence of acid and pepsin in the stomach and binds to gastric-derived intrinsic factor (IF). IF is a glycoprotein with very high affinity for vitamin B_{12}. The IF vitamin B_{12} complex is absorbed in the ileum. In the plasma, vitamin B_{12} is bound to a protein called transcobalamin.

Physiological Role of Vitamin B_{12} (Fig. 5.1)

- Vitamin B_{12} is very important for nucleic acid synthesis in every cell. Actively growing and dividing cells, which synthesise DNA rapidly (e.g. mucosal cells and hemopoietic cells), are likely to be particularly affected by vitamin B_{12} deficiency. It is also important for the normal integrity of nervous system.

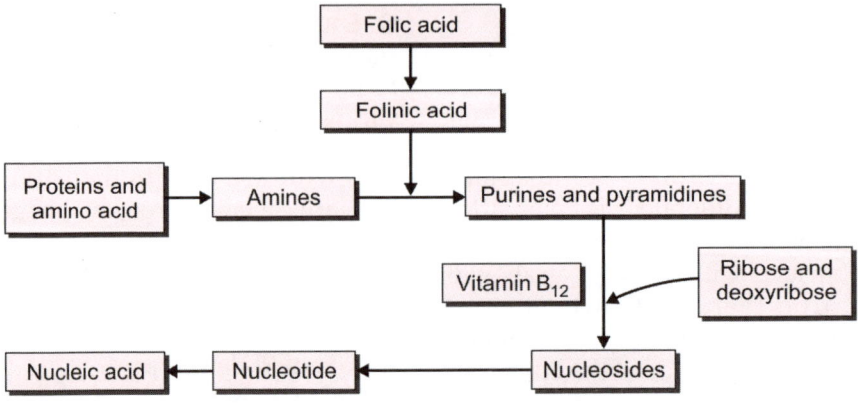

Fig. 5.1: Role of vitamin B_{12} and folic acid in the synthesis of nucleic acid.

- Thymine (a purine) is important for DNA synthesis. Synthesis of thymine requires tetrahydrofolate (THF). Vitamin B_{12} is required for conversion of methyl THF to THF. Thus lack of vitamin B_{12} causes impaired DNA synthesis and cell division. RNA synthesis continues, resulting in a large cell with a large nucleus. All cell lines have dyspoiesis, in which cytoplasmic maturity is greater than nuclear maturity; this dyspoiesis produces megaloblasts in the marrow before they appear in the peripheral blood. Dyspoiesis results in intramedullary cell death (intramedullary hemolysis), making erythropoiesis ineffective and causing indirect hyperbilirubinemia and hyperuricemia. Because dyspoiesis affects all cell lines, pancytopenia develops in advanced stages of vitamin B_{12} deficiency. Hypersegmentation of neutrophils is common, the mechanism of which is unknown.

Etiology of Vitamin B_{12} Deficiency

Inadequate intake
- Strict vegetarians

Intrinsic factor deficiency
- Pernicious anemia
- Gastrectomy
- Atrophic gastritis

Decreased absorption
- Malabsorption syndromes
- Ileal resection or bypass

- Crohn's disease
- Blind loops
- Fish tapeworm infestation
- Pancreatitis

Agents that block absorption
- Neomycin
- Biguanides (e.g. metformin)
- Proton pump inhibitors (e.g. omeprazole)

Clinical Features
- Symptoms related to anemia such as easy fatigability, weakness, dyspnea, and effort intolerance.
- Hyperdynamic circulation due to anemia may lead to palpitations, tinnitus and headache.
- Vitamin B_{12} deficiency causes atrophic glossitis and neurologic symptoms.
- Vitamin B_{12} deficiency causes peripheral neuropathy (with paresthesias, ataxia, loss of vibration and position sense). In severe deficiency, subacute combined degeneration (SCD) of the spinal cord may develop. In SCD, there is degeneration of posterior columns and corticospinal tract. Manifestations of SCD are paresthesias, ataxia, loss of vibration and position sense due to posterior column involvement and weakness, spasticity, clonus, and paraplegia due to corticospinal tract involvement.
- Other neurologic symptoms of vitamin B_{12} deficiency include memory loss, irritability, and dementia.

Investigations

Complete blood count
- Hemoglobin level is low.
- Mean corpuscular volume (MCV) is over 100 fL (normal 80–100).
- Mean corpuscular hemoglobin (MCH) and mean corpuscular hemoglobin concentration (MCHC) are usually normal.

Peripheral smear: It shows macrocytes. Hypersegmented neutrophils are common. When the anemia is severe, there may be leukopenia and thrombocytopenia (pancytopenia).

Bone marrow
- Bone marrow is hypercellular with increased myeloid: erythroid ratio.
- Megakaryocytes are decreased with basophilic agranular cytoplasm and hypersegmented nucleus.

Vitamin B_{12} and folic acid levels: The normal vitamin B_{12} level is 300 to 900 pg/mL; values <200 pg/mL indicate clinically significant deficiency.

Other tests
- Schilling test can be done to diagnose the cause of vitamin B_{12} deficiency.
- Upper GI scopy is useful in cases of pernicious anemia.
- Jejunal biopsy is useful in malabsorption disorders.

Treatment

General Management

This is similar to other cases of anemia. For severe symptomatic anemia (Hb <7 g/dL), packed red cell transfusion is given. Before transfusion, it is necessary to collect samples for vitamin B_{12} and folic acid estimation.

Vitamin B_{12} Replacement
- Vitamin B_{12} should be replaced by parenteral route since malabsorption is the cause most of the time. 1000 µg should be given intramuscularly per week for 8 weeks, followed by 1000 µg every month for the rest of the patient's life.
- Oral replacement therapy with 2 mg vitamin B_{12} per day is also effective, if malabsorption is not the cause of deficiency.
- Any underlying cause of vitamin B_{12} deficiency should be treated (e.g. antibiotics for intestinal bacterial overgrowth, deworming for tapeworm infestation).

Q. Pernicious anemia.

- Pernicious anemia is due to vitamin B_{12} deficiency caused by the absence of intrinsic factor, due to either atrophy of the gastric mucosa or autoimmune destruction of parietal cells. The disease was given its common name because it was fatal (pernicious) prior to the discovery of treatment.
- It is common in whites, and rare in Asians. Females are affected more often than males. It is a disease of the elderly, the average patient presenting near age 60; it is rare under age 30.

Pathogenesis
- Intrinsic factor is important for the absorption of vitamin B_{12}. Intrinsic factor deficiency causes less absorption of vitamin B_{12} and its deficiency. Gastric atrophy also results in hypochlorhydria and malabsorption of vitamin B_{12}.
- Pernicious anemia may be associated with other autoimmune diseases such as thyroid disorders, Addison's disease, hypoparathyroidism, diabetes mellitus, and rheumatoid arthritis.
- 90% of patients have parietal cell antibody in serum and 50% have antibody to intrinsic factor which inhibits binding of vitamin B_{12} to intrinsic factor.

Clinical Features

Clinical features are similar to vitamin B_{12} deficiency anemia.

Investigations
- In addition to tests done for vitamin B_{12} deficiency, antibodies to parietal cell and antibodies to intrinsic factor may be demonstrated in serum and gastric juice.

- *Histamine or pentagastrin test:* Acid secretion does not increase even after injection of histamine or pentagastrin.
- *Barium meal examination:* Shows atrophic mucosal pattern of stomach.
- *Upper GI scopy and mucosal biopsy:* They show atrophic gastritis.

Treatment

Treatment is similar to vitamin B_{12} deficiency anemia.

Q. What are the causes of blood loss anemia? How do you manage it?

Causes of Blood Loss Anemia

Acute blood loss
- Trauma
- Hematemesis
- Hemoptysis
- Rupture of ectopic pregnancy

Chronic blood loss
- Slowly bleeding peptic ulcer
- GI malignancy
- Hookworm infestation

Clinical Features

- Anemia due to acute blood loss is symptomatic, if severe. Loss of up to 20% of the blood volume can be asymptomatic. Blood loss more than this can cause anxiety, hypotension, syncope, tachycardia, breathlessness, and shock. Hemoglobin level immediately after the bleed may be normal as it takes some time for hemodilution to occur.
- Chronic blood loss as happens in hookworm infestation, peptic ulcer, etc. can produce severe anemia which can be asymptomatic. Symptoms will not appear until severe anemia develops.

Treatment

- In acute blood loss, volume replacement either by blood transfusion, or IV fluids is very important.

- In chronic blood loss anemia, if the patient is severely anemic, packed RBC should be transfused.
- Underlying cause of blood loss should be treated in both acute and chronic blood losses.

Q. Anemia of chronic disease.

The anemia of chronic disease (ACD), also termed the anemia of chronic inflammation, is associated with many chronic diseases (infectious, inflammatory, neoplastic disease, severe trauma, heart disease, diabetes mellitus, etc.). Though ACD occurs in chronic diseases, it can begin acutely during virtually any infection or inflammation.

Pathophysiology

Three pathophysiologic mechanisms have been identified in ACD: (1) Shortened RBC survival, (2) Impaired erythropoiesis due to decreases in both erythropoietin (EPO) production and marrow responsiveness to EPO, and (3) impaired intracellular iron metabolism.

Clinical Features

Most patients have mild anemia that produces no symptoms. Signs and symptoms of underlying disease may be present.

Investigations

- The anemia is normocytic-normochromic and rarely microcytic-hypochromic.
- Reticulocyte count, leukocyte count and platelet counts are normal.
- The serum iron concentration and transferrin level (also measured as total iron binding capacity, TIBC) are both low and the percent saturation of transferrin is usually normal, which should distinguish ACD from iron deficiency anemia, in which transferrin saturation is low.

Treatment

- Correction of the underlying disorder.
- Iron supplements.
- Administration of recombinant human erythropoietin, if anemia is severe.

Q. Discuss the classification, clinical features, diagnosis and management of hemolytic anemias.

- Anemia resulting from increased red cells destruction is called hemolytic anemia. Hemolysis can be defined as a shortening of RBC survival to less than 100 days (normal 120 days).
- Normal marrow has tremendous capacity to compensate for hemolysis, hence anemia occurs only when compensation is not adequate.
- Hemolysis may be an extravascular or an intravascular phenomenon. Autoimmune hemolytic anemia (AIHA) and hereditary spherocytosis are examples of extravascular hemolysis because the red blood cells are destroyed in the spleen and other reticuloendothelial tissues. Others are due to intravascular hemolysis.

Classification of Hemolytic Anemias

Hereditary
- Hereditary spherocytosis, G6PD-deficiency, thalassemias, sickle cell anemia

Acquired
- Paroxysmal nocturnal hemoglobinuria (PNH), autoimmune hemolytic anemia, incompatible blood transfusion, prosthetic heart valves, drugs (dapsone, primaquine), malaria.

Clinical Features

History

- Patient may complain of fatigue and other symptoms of anemia.
- Mild jaundice (lemon yellow).
- History of passing red-brown urine (due to hemoglobinuria).
- Left hypochondrial pain due to splenomegaly.
- Right hypochondrial pain due to cholelithiasis. Pigment stones occur due to increased production of bilirubin from hemolysis.
- Family history may be present.
- Drug history may be positive.
- Symptoms of any underlying disease responsible for hemolysis.

Physical Findings

- Anemia
- Mild jaundice
- Splenomegaly
- Hemolytic facies due to marrow hyperplasia in skull bones and other bones
- Ankle ulcers (seen in sickle cell anemia)
- Signs of any underlying disease responsible for hemolysis

Investigations

Evidence of increased RBC destruction
- Indirect hyperbilirubinemia.
- Increased urobilinogen excretion in urine.
- Decreased plasma haptoglobin and hemopexin.
- Increased plasma lactate dehydrogenase (LDH).
- Shortened RBC survival as demonstrated by chromium-51 labeled RBCs.

Evidence of increased RBC production
- Increased reticulocyte count (reticulocytosis).
- Finding premature RBCs in peripheral smear (macrocytes, polychromasia, nucleated RBCs).
- Erytroid hyperplasia of bone marrow.

Additional findings in intravascular hemolysis
- Hemoglobinuria
- Hemosiderinuria

Tests to diagnose underlying cause of hemolysis

- Peripheral blood smear examination.
- Coombs test (to detect antibodies causing hemolysis).
- Hemoglobin electrophoresis (for thalassemias).
- Osmotic fragility, sucrose lysis and hams test (for RBC membrane defects).
- Measurement of enzyme activity (for G6PD deficiency).
- Other tests are done depending on the suspected underlying cause.

Treatment

Supportive Therapy

- Blood transfusion for severe anemia
- Replacement of vitamins due to increased erythropoiesis (iron, folic acid)
- Treatment of infections
- Treatment of ankle ulcers
- Splenectomy in selected cases

Specific Therapy

This depends on the underlying cause—steroids for immune hemolytic anemia, splenectomy in sickle cell anemia and hereditary spherocytosis, withdrawal of offending drug, etc.

Q. Discuss the etiology, clinical features, diagnosis and management of autoimmune hemolytic anemia (AIHA).

- Hemolysis secondary to antibodies against red cell antigens is called immune hemolysis.
- In autoimmune hemolytic anemia, antibodies are directed against person's own RBCs.

Etiology of Immune Hemolytic Anemias

- Idiopathic
- Chronic lymphocytic leukemia (CLL)
- Hodgkin's lymphoma
- Systemic lupus erythematosus
- Drugs
- Viral infections

Clinical Features

- Onset is insidious.
- *Symptoms of anemia*—fatigue, palpitations.
- *Symptoms of hemolysis*—mild jaundice, dark urine
- Presence of pallor
- Splenomegaly

Investigations

- Features of hemolysis
- Positive Coombs test

Treatment

- *Blood transfusions*—for significant anemia.
- *Corticosteroids:* Any significant hemolysis is treated with 60 mg of prednisolone daily for 3 to 4 weeks and then tapered; many need maintenance therapy. Parenteral methyl prednisolone is often used in acutely ill patients.
- *Splenectomy:* Patients who do not respond to steroids and/or require large maintenance dosage are candidates for splenectomy.
- *Immunosuppressive drugs* like azathioprine or cyclophosphamide are used, if significant hemolysis continues despite splenectomy. Intravenous gammaglobulin, danazol, cyclosporine and antithymocyte globulin are used in occasional refractory cases.
- *Folic acid supplements* should be given to all patients with hemolysis because of increased requirements due to increased erythropoiesis.
- *Treatment of underlying cause.*

Q. Define aplastic anemia. Discuss the etiology, classification, clinical features, investigations and management of aplastic anemia.

- Aplastic anemia is defined as pancytopenia with an empty (hypoplastic or aplastic) bone marrow.
- Pancytopenia means decrease in the number of all three blood cells, i.e. RBCs, WBCs, and platelets.

Etiology and Classification of Aplastic Anemia

- Idiopathic (no identifiable cause)
- Cytotoxic drugs (anticancer drugs)
- Exposure to radiation
- Toxic chemicals (benzene, lindane, glue vapors)
- Viral infections (parvovirus B19, HIV infection, Epstein-Barr virus)
- Immune disorders (SLE)
- Fanconi's anemia
- Diamond-Blackfan anemia

Pathogenesis

In idiopathic cases, there is no identifiable cause but in all such cases there is a stem cell defect (diminished numbers, impaired maturation, proliferation and differentiation). In all other cases, there is damage to bone marrow which may be dose-related or idiosyncratic reaction to radiation, drugs, chemicals or infectious agents.

Clinical Features

- The onset is insidious and symptoms and signs are due to anemia, leukopenia and thrombocytopenia (pancytopenia).
- Anemia causes easy fatigability, exertional dyspnea and pallor.
- Leucopenia causes recurrent infections (pneumonia, urinary tract infections, fungal infections, septicemia).
- Thrombocytopenia causes bleeding manifestations (mucosal hemorrhages, menorrhagia, and petechiae).
- Remember that splenomegaly and lymphadenopathy *are not features* of aplastic anemia.

Investigations

- Hemoglobin is low.
- There is pancytopenia.
- Reticulocyte count is low in relation to the degree of anemia.
- ESR is elevated.

- Peripheral blood smear shows pancytopenia and normochromic-normocytic RBCs. No abnormal cells are seen in peripheral blood.
- Bone marrow examination shows profoundly hypocellular marrow with a decrease in all cell elements. The marrow space is composed mostly of fat cells and marrow stroma.

Prognosis

Prognosis depends upon two factors—disease severity and patient age. Severe aplastic anemia is associated with reduced survival rate and there is a strong inverse relation between patient age and 5-year survival.

Treatment

Supportive Therapy

- Involves treatment of infection, correction of anemia with blood transfusion, correction of thrombocytopenia by platelet transfusion.
- Antifibrinolytic agents such as tranexamic acid or epsilon-amino caproic acid (EACA) are also useful to control bleeding in severe cases.
- Blood and platelet transfusions should be used sparingly in patients who are candidates for hematopoietic stem cell transplantation to avoid sensitization.

Definitive Therapy

- *Bone marrow transplantation* is curative in aplastic anemia. This is the treatment of choice in patients below 45 years, if an HLA-matched donor is available.
- *Immunosuppressive regimens* are recommended for those above 45 years. They are not curative, but improve survival. A combination of anti-thymocyte globulin, cyclosporine, and corticosteroids with or without granulocyte-colony stimulating factor (G-CSF) can be used for immunosuppression.

- Treatment of the underlying cause or agent.

- The sickle cell anemia is characterized by the presence of hemoglobin S (HbS) caused by a mutation in the β-globin gene that changes the 6th amino acid from glutamic acid to valine (glutamic acid goes).
- If both genes encoding for beta chain are abnormal, it is called *sickle cell disease*. It is more severe and is inherited as autosomal recessive manner.
- If only one gene is abnormal, and other gene is normal, it is called *sickle cell trait*. These patients have mild disease and can be asymptomatic.

Pathophysiology

- RBCs containing HbS turn into sickle-shaped cells on deoxygenation. Other factors leading to sickling are fever, sluggish blood flow, and acidosis. Sickling happens due to polymerization of HbS which distorts the shape of RBC.
- Sickling of RBCs leads to hemolysis causing anemia. Sickled RBCs cannot negotiate through small blood vessels leading to vascular occlusion and consequent ische-mic damage to organs.
- Presence of high amount of HbF (fetal hemoglobin) may decrease the symptoms of sickle cell disease because HbF interferes with polymerization of HbS.

Clinical Manifestations

- Clinical manifestations include anemia (due to hemolysis), pain (due to vascular occlusion causing ischemia), infections (due to damage to spleen), and damage to organ systems.
- Growth retardation and psychosocial problems are common.
- Splenic infarcts result in frequent life-threatening episodes of septicemia. Many types of crisis such as painful crisis, splenic sequestration crisis and aplastic crisis can occur which are life-threatening unless treated promptly.
- Vaso-occlusion can cause organ damage (particularly heart and kidney in adults and brain in children).

Painful Crisis (Sickle Cell Crisis)

- Vascular occlusion can lead to ischemic pain in many areas of the body. Pain is the commonest cause of debility in HbS disease. Acute episode of severe pain is called painful crisis or sickle cell crisis. Acute pain is the first symptom of disease in many patients and is the most frequent symptom after the age of two years.
- Pain may be precipitated by events such as weather conditions (e.g. high wind speed/low humidity), dehydration, infection, stress, menses, alcohol consumption, and nocturnal hypoxemia. However, the majority of painful episodes have no identifiable cause.
- Pain can affect any area of the body, but common in the back, chest, extremities, and abdomen. Dactylitis (acute pain in the hands and/or feet) is common in children.
- Pain can vary from mild to excruciating. Pain may be accompanied by systemic symptoms such as fever, tachypnea, hypertension, nausea, and vomiting.
- Painful episodes last for two to seven days.
- Frequent pain may lead to psychosocial problems, depression and interfere with daily life.

Splenic Sequestration Crisis

- Vaso-occlusion can occur within the spleen and RBCs can get trapped in the spleen. Most of the circulating red cell mass is sequestrated in the spleen and the spleen rapidly enlarges (within hours). There is marked fall in hemoglobin concentration. There is a risk of hypovolemic shock.

- The patients who are susceptible to this syndrome are those whose spleens have not yet undergone fibrosis. Splenic sequestration crisis is associated with a 10 to 15% mortality rate, occurring before transfusions can be given.
- Sequestration can be recurrent in survivors and hence, splenectomy is recommended after the first attack. Milder cases can be managed with transfusion and careful observation.

Aplastic Crisis

- In aplastic crisis, there is transient arrest of erythropoiesis, leading to sudden decrease in hemoglobin. Bone marrow shows decrease in red cell precursors.
- Most cases of aplastic crisis are precipitated by infections such as parvovirus B19.
- Affected patients require blood transfusion. Patients usually recover within a few days.

Infections

- Sickle cell patients are prone to a variety of infections. Absent splenic function (autosplenectomy due to splenic infarcts) leads to infections with the encapsulated organisms, e.g. *Streptococcus pneumoniae* and *H. influenzae*. Pneumococcal infections can result in death within hours.
- Urinary tract infections (due to *E. coli*) and osteomyelitis are also common. *Salmonella typhimurium* is another common infecting organism.

Investigations

- *Features of hemolysis:* Mild to moderate anemia, reticulocytosis, unconjugated hyperbilirubinemia, elevated serum LDH and low serum haptoglobin.
- *Peripheral blood smear* reveals sickled RBCs, polychromasia indicative of reticulocytosis, and Howell-Jolly bodies reflecting hyposplenia.

- *Sickle test:* Sickling of RBCs occurs when mixed with a solution of sodium metabisulphite.
- *Hemoglobin electrophoresis* allows the definitive diagnosis of sickle cell disease. Most of the hemoglobin is HbS.
- *Genetic analysis* can show the specific mutation.

Management

General Measures

- Avoidance of dehydration, cold weather and hypoxia
- Psychosocial support
- Dietary advice (adequate calorie intake, folic acid, vitamin C, vitamin E and zinc)

Specific Measures

- *Infections:* Infections can be prevented by prophylactic penicillin and immunizations. Pneumococcal and *H. influenzae* vaccination should be given to all patients with sickle cell anemia. Hepatitis B vaccination is also necessary. Febrile episodes should be investigated appropriately and treated with early antibiotic therapy.
- *Pain management:* Pain should be controlled by aggressive use of analgesics. Most of the time opioid analgesics such as morphine, fentanyl or tramadol are required.
- *Blood transfusions:* Transfusions can be used to correct anemia and also in emergencies such as splenic sequestration syndrome.
- *Hydroxyurea:* Hydroxyurea induces the synthesis of fetal hemoglobin. High levels of fetal hemoglobin (HbF) decrease the severity of crisis and prolong survival in sickle cell patients.
- *Bone marrow transplantation* offers the only chance of cure at present.

Prognosis

Patients now survive up to 6th or 7th decade. Common causes of death include organ failure (predominantly renal) and sickle cell crisis. A high level of fetal hemoglobin(HbF) predicts prolonged survival.

Q. What are thalassemias? Classify thalassemias.

- Thalassemias are a group of inherited anemias characterized by reduced or absent production of one or more globin chains of hemoglobin.
- Thalassemia is common in the Mediterranean region especially amongst Italians and Greeks. The thalassemia belt extends to India and south East Asia. In India, it is found in Punjab, Gujarat, Maharashtra, Karnataka, Bengal and Assam. It is relatively less common in the southern states. On an average, 3% of Indians carry the thalassemia gene (chiefly beta thalassemia). The highest incidence is found in Lohanas and Sindhis.

Classification

Thalassemias are named according to globin chain deficiency, e.g. in beta thalassemia, there is deficiency of beta chain, and in alpha thalassemia, there is deficiency of alpha chain.

Beta thalassemias
- *Beta thalassemia major* (Cooley's anemia) (patient is homozygous, i.e. both genes defective).
- *Beta thalassemia minor* (also known as thalassemia trait, patient is heterozygous, i.e. one gene defective, other gene normal).

Alpha thalassemias
- Loss of one or more of alpha globin genes

Q. Discuss the etiology, pathogenesis, clinical features, investigations and management of thalassemia major (Cooley's anemia).

Etiology

Beta thalassemias usually arise from point mutations in the gene which encodes beta globin chain of hemoglobin. The 'beta gene' cluster is located on the short arm of chromosome 11.

Pathophysiology

- Impaired synthesis of globin chain decreases the production of hemoglobin causing hypochromia and microcytosis. There is accumulation of unaffected alpha globin chains since their production proceeds at a normal rate.
- In the presence of reduced beta chains, the excess alpha chains are unstable and precipitate, leading to damage of red blood cell membranes. This leads to hemolysis causing anemia.
- Ongoing hemolysis stimulates bone marrow to produce more RBCs leading to bone marrow hyperplasia. Marked expansion of the bone marrow may cause severe bony deformities, osteopenia, and pathologic fractures.

Clinical Features (Table 5.1)

- Symptoms start late in the first year of life when fetal hemoglobin levels decline.
- Pallor, irritability, growth retardation, hepatosplenomegaly and jaundice develop due to severe hemolytic anemia.
- Anemia and hemolysis stimulate erythropoiesis leading to extensive marrow expansion leading to characteristic chipmunk facies (frontal bossing and prominent cheeckbones).
- 80% of untreated children die within the first five years of life as a result of severe anemia, high output heart failure, and infections.

Investigations

- Signs of hemolysis such as anemia, increased indirect (unconjugated) bilirubin, increased LDH and reduced haptoglobin levels.
- HbA is markedly reduced and HbF is raised.
- Peripheral smear shows hypochromia, microcytosis, anisopoikilocytosis, tear drop cells and target cells. Nucleated red cells are abundant but reticulocyte count is low due to ineffective erythropoiesis.

Table 5.1: Differences between β thalassemia major and minor

Features	Thalassemia major	Thalassemia minor
• Symptoms	Symptomatic	Asymptomatic
• Genes resposnsible for globin chain synthesis	Both defective	One is normal, one is defective
• Anemia	Severe	Mild
• Peripheral smear	Severe hypochromasia, microcytosis	Mild hypochromasia and microcytosis
• Hb electrophoresis	HbF elevated, HbA reduced/absent	HbA2 elevated
• Parents	Both having thalassemia minor	One parent having thalassemia minor

- Bone marrow shows marked hyper-cellularity.
- The osmotic fragility test is significantly reduced.
- Skull X-ray shows widened diploic space and hair-on-end appearance. Compression fractures of the vertebrae and marked osteoporosis are common.

Management

- Beta thalassemia major requires regular blood transfusions to maintain hemoglobin at >10 g/dL. Correction of anemia leads to normal growth and development.
- Repeated blood transfusions lead to iron overload. Hence, iron chelation therapy should be given (desferrioxamine infusion subcutaneously 5 days a week or oral iron chelator deferiprone).
- Folic acid supplements should be given to all patients because of increased require-ments due to increased red cell turnover.
- Splenectomy for gross symptomatic splenomegaly or hypersplenism.
- Allogeneic bone marrow transplantation is the treatment of choice for β-thalassemia major and can cure it.
- Genetic counseling and prenatal diagnosis should be offered to affected parents.
- Thalassemia minor requires no treatment except genetic counseling, avoidance of inappropriate iron therapy and close monitoring during pregnancy.

Q. Etiology of leukemias.

- **Idiopathic (**majority of cases are idiopathic)
- **Ionizing radiation (**atomic bombing, X-ray exposure, radiotherapy)
- **Viruses** [Human T cell lymphotropic virus type I (HTLV-I), HTLV-II, Epstein-Barr virus]
- **Immune deficiency states** (e.g. HIV and hypogammaglobulinemia)
- **Genetics factors**
- **Chemicals and drugs (**benzene, tobacco, cyclophosphamide, melphalan, etc.)
- **Chromosomal abnormalities**

Q. Classification of leukemias.

Acute leukemias
- Lymphoid (lymphoblastic)
- Myeloid (myeloblastic)

Chronic leukemias
- Lymphoid (lymphocytic)
- Myeloid (myelocytic)

Q. Define acute leukemia. Discuss the etiology, clinical features, investigations and management of acute leukemia.

- Acute leukemia is defined as a malignant clonal proliferation of lymphoid or myeloid precursor cells which replace the bone marrow and ultimately spill over to the peripheral blood and infiltrate lymph nodes, spleen, liver or other organs.

- Normally hematopoietic stem cells proliferate and differentiate into various cellular components of blood. In acute leukemia, an early hematopoietic precursor fails to differentiate and instead continues to proliferate in an uncontrolled fashion. As a result, immature myeloid (in AML) or lymphoid cells (in ALL), called *blasts*, rapidly accumulate and replace the bone marrow which in turn results in decreased production of normal red cells, white cells, and platelets. Eventually leukemic blasts will pour out into the blood and also infiltrate lymph nodes, spleen, and other vital organs. Acute leukemia is rapidly fatal and most patients die within months of diagnosis. However, in many patients, it can be controlled or cured with appropriate therapy.

Incidence

ALL (acute lymphoblastic leukemia) is more common in children and AML (acute myeloid leukemia) is more common in adults.

Etiology

- **Idiopathic (**majority of cases are idiopathic)

- **Ionizing radiation (**atomic bombing, X-ray exposure, radiotherapy)

- **Viruses** [Human T cell lymphotropic virus type I (HTLV-I), HTLV-II, Epstein-Barr virus]

- **Immune deficiency states** (e.g. HIV and hypogammaglobulinemia)

- **Genetics factors**

- **Chemicals and drugs (**benzene, tobacco, cyclophosphamide, melphalan, etc.)
- **Chromosomal abnormalities**

Clinical Features

- Two things happen in leukemia which causes all the signs and symptoms. One is leukemic blasts fill the bone marrow and interfere with its function. Another is leukemic blasts infiltrate normal organs and lead to their dysfunction.

- Decreased bone marrow function leads to deficiency of all three cell lines causing anemia, thrombocytopenia, and granulocytopenia. Anemia is present at diagnosis in most patients and causes fatigue, pallor, and headache and in severe cases angina or heart failure. Thrombocytopenia causes bleeding manifestations in the form of petechiae, ecchymoses, bleeding gums, epistaxis, or hemorrhage. Granulocytopenia results in increased incidence of infections.

- Infiltration of normal organs by leukemic blasts lead to enlargement of lymph nodes, liver, and spleen. Bone pain may be present and is due to leukemic infiltration of the periosteum or expansion of the medullary cavity. Leukemic cells sometimes infiltrate the skin and result in a raised, nonpruritic rash, a condition termed *leukemia cutis*. Leukemic cells may infiltrate the leptomeninges and cause leukemic meningitis.

- Certain clinical manifestations are unique to specific subtypes of leukemia. For example, DIC (disseminated intravascular coagulation) is common in promyelocytic leukemia (AML-M3) due to release of tissue thromboplastins by dying leukemic cells.

Differences between AML and ALL

Table 5.2 describes differences between AML and ALL.

Laboratory Findings

- Presence of anemia and thrombocytopenia.

Table 5.2: Differences between AML and ALL

	AML	ALL
• Cell linage	Myeloid precursors	Lymphoid precursors
• Auer rods	Present	Absent
• Age group affected	Commonly adults	Commonly children
• Common genetic abnormalities	t(8;21), t(15;17), and inv(16)(p13;q22).	t(9;22) and t(4;11).
• Nuclear enzyme, terminal deoxynucleotidyl transferase (Tdt) in leukemic blasts	Rarely present	Present in more than 90%
• Lymphadenopathy	Uncommon	Common
• Hepatosplenomegaly	Uncommon	Common
• CNS involvement	Uncommon	Common
• Cytochemical staining (myeloperoxidase, sudan black B)	Positive	Negative

- Total leukocyte count is markedly raised (often as high as 100,000/mm^3). However, normal neutrophil count is low (granulocytopenia).
- Peripheral blood smear shows circulating blasts. However, blasts may not always be seen in peripheral smear (aleukemic leukemia).
- Bone marrow is usually hypercellular with the presence of blasts. More than 20% blasts are required to make a diagnosis of acute leukemia.
- Serum LDH, uric acid and alkaline phosphatase levels are elevated due to rapid cell turnover.
- The Auer rod, an eosinophilic needle-like inclusion in the cytoplasm, is pathognomonic of AML.
- ALL is diagnosed when there is no morphologic or histochemical evidence of myeloid or monocytic lineage. The diagnosis of ALL is confirmed by demonstrating surface markers of primitive lymphoid cells, by flow cytometry and monoclonal antibodies.
- Cytogenetic studies reveal many chromosome abnormalities which can also predict the prognosis in acute leukemias.

Treatment

Chemotherapy is the mainstay of therapy for acute leukemias. The aim of chemotherapy is to induce remission and maintain it. The type of initial chemotherapy depends on the subtype of leukemia.

AML: AML is treated with a combination of daunorubicin, cytarabine and etoposide. After remission induction, further therapy with curative intent includes standard chemotherapy and autologous or allogeneic bone marrow transplantation. If the leukemia recurs after initial chemotherapy, the prognosis is worse.

ALL: ALL is treated with combination chemotherapy, including daunorubicin, vincristine, prednisone, and asparaginase. As with AML, patients may be treated with either chemotherapy or high-dose chemotherapy plus bone marrow transplantation.

Chronic myeloid leukemia (CML) is a myeloproliferative disorder characterized by overproduction of myeloid cells.

Pathophysiology

- CML is characterized by a specific chromosomal abnormality called the Philadelphia chromosome (Fig. 5.2) which occurs due to reciprocal translocation between chromosomes 9 and 22. The abnormal chromosome 22 is known as Philadelphia chromosome.
- The oncogene *c-ABL*, normally situated in the long arm of chromosome 9, gets translocated to chromosome 22, where a specific gene called *BCR* (breakpoint cluster region) is situated. Both *ABL* and *BCR* form a fusion gene, *ABL/BCR*, which is important in the pathogenesis of CML. The fusion gene BCR/ABL produces a protein possessing tyrosine kinase activity. This leads to tumor cell proliferation.

Natural Course

- The disease has three stages: (1) Chronic stable phase, (2) accelerated phase, and (3) blast crisis.
- The chronic phase is characterized by a large increase in peripheral blood leukocytes. These leucocytes have almost normal maturity. Most patients are in stable phase at presentation. This phase may last for months to years.
- In accelerated phase, neutrophil differentiation becomes progressively impaired and leukocyte counts are more difficult to control. There is worsening anemia, thrombocytopenia, worsening splenomegaly, and increasing marrow or blood blasts.
- In blast crisis, myeloid or lymphoid blasts fail to differentiate and large number of blasts are found in peripheral blood. Blasts in blood or marrow increase to >20%. Blast crisis carries very poor prognosis.

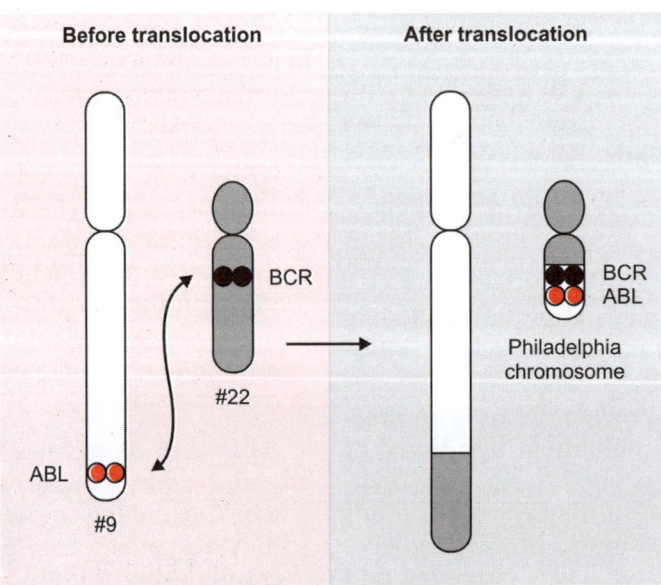

Fig 5.2: Philadelphia chromosome.

Clinical Features

- CML has an annual incidence of 1 to 2 cases per 100,000 with a slight male predominance. CML is a disorder of middle age (median age is 50 years).
- Patients usually present with fat, weight loss, night sweats, and low-grade fever.
- Bleeding episodes are common due to platelet dysfunction.
- Abdominal fullness, early satiety, left upper quadrant pain, and discomfort may be complained of due to massive splenomegaly.
- Acute gouty arthritis may be present due to overproduction of uric acid.
- Examination reveals pallor, massive splenomegaly, and sternal tenderness due to bone marrow hyperplasia. Hepatomegaly may also be present.

Laboratory Findings

- Anemia
- High WBC count (usually above 1 lakh/µL.
- Normal or low or elevated platelet count.
- Basophil and eosinophil count is almost always increased.
- Peripheral blood smear shows presence of myelocytes and metamyelocytes which are immature WBCs. RBC morphology is normal.
- Bone marrow aspiration and biopsy in patients with CML in chronic phase shows myeloid hyperplasia. There is increase in the myeloid-to-erythroid ratio in the bone marrow as well as a marked increase in the number of megakaryocytes and the number of immature forms. Blast crisis is diagnosed when blasts are more than 20% in the bone marrow.
- The diagnosis of CML is established by demonstration of the Philadelphia chromosome or the BCR-ABL fusion gene. BCR-ABL can be detected in the peripheral blood by polymerase chain reaction (PCR) test, which has now supplanted cytogenetics.

Treatment

Tyrosine Kinase Inhibitors (Imatinib Mesylate, Dasatinib)

The treatment of CML has been revolutionized by the introduction of tyrosine kinase inhibitors, such as imatinib mesylate, which inhibit the tyrosine kinase activity of the *BCR/ABL* oncogene. Imatinib inhibits proliferation and induces apoptosis of cells positive for *BCR/ABL*. Tyrosine kinase inhibitors are the first-line drugs for chronic and accelerated phase of CML. Imatinib is well tolerated and controls the disease in 98% of chronic phase patients with positive Philadelphia chromosome. In chronic phase of CML, the dose of imatinib is 400 mg orally daily. Blood counts normalize and splenomegaly regresses within 3 months. Philadelphia chromosome becomes negative within 6 months (maximum 12 months). However, tyrosine kinase inhibitors do not cure CML. It controls the disease as long as it is given.

Omacetaxine

- Omacetaxine is a new drug introduced for the treatment of CML. It is a protein translation inhibitor that is indicated when there is resistance and/or intolerance to *hydroxyurea*
- These agents suppress the bone marrow and reduce the leukocyte count. Conventional treatment of CML in chronic phase has been single agent therapy with busulphan or hydroxyurea. However, due to the availability of newer agents such as imatinib, these agents are being used less commonly now.
- Hydroxyurea is preferred over busulphan. It is given orally daily. Blood counts should be monitored and the dose is adjusted as per the counts.

Interferon Therapy

Alpha IFN inhibits the late progenitors which may be the major phase of CML clonal expansion. Patients in chronic phase respond better. Reduction of 'BCR-ABL' oncogene expression has been reported after therapy with IFN. However, due to the availability of newer agents such as imatinib, interferon alpha is now used only for refractory cases in combination with other agents.

Bone Marrow Transplantation

If the patients do not respond to imatinib, this is the 2nd choice of therapy. The best results (80% cure rate) are obtained in patients under 40 years of age, if transplanted within 1 year after diagnosis. Bone marrow should be obtained from HLA matched siblings.

Course and Prognosis

In the past, median survival was 3 to 4 years. However, after the introduction of imatinib mesylate, 4-year survival and remission is 80%.

Q. Blast crisis in CML.

- Blast crisis represents transformation of CML into an acute leukemia (myeloblastic or lymphoblastic). A variety of mutations have been associated with progression to blast crisis. Mutations of the BCR-ABL tyrosine kinase domain have been observed in up to 80% of patients.
- Blast crisis can develop from days to decades after diagnosis of CML.
- Clinical features include fever, hemorrhage, generalized lymphadenopathy, abrupt increase in spleen size, bone pain and sternal tenderness.
- Peripheral smear or bone marrow shows more than 20% blasts.

Treatment of Blast Crisis

Blast crisis can be treated with acute myeloid leukemia (AML) induction chemotherapy regimens (daunorubicin, cytarabine and etoposide) in combination with a tyrosine kinase inhibitor; some patients can be treated with a tyrosine kinase inhibitor such as imatinib alone. Stem cell transplantation can also be considered at this phase.

Q. Define lymphomas.

Q. Discuss the classification, clinical features, clinical staging, investigations and management of Hodgkin's lymphoma.

Lymphomas are malignant transformations of lymphoid cells. They are divided into two major types: non-Hodgkin's lymphoma (NHL) and Hodgkin's lymphoma (HL). NHL is the most common type of lymphoma.

HODGKIN'S LYMPHOMA

Hodgkin's lymphoma is named after the British physician who first described it. The cancer cells in Hodgkin's lympoma are known as Reed-Sternberg cells (named after the physicians who discovered them) which are derived from B lymphocytes.

Etiology

- Exact cause is unknown, but genetic susceptibility; occupation such as woodworking; history of treatment with phenytoin, radiation therapy, chemotherapy; infection with Epstein-Barr virus, *Mycobacterium tuberculosis*, herpesvirus type 6, and HIV play a role.
- Immunosuppressed state (e.g. post-transplant patients taking immunosuppressants, congenital immunodeficiency disorders) also increases the risk of developing Hodgkin's lymphoma.

Pathological Classification

- Pathologically, Hodgkin's lymphoma is divided into four subtypes:

Type	Prognosis
Lymphocytic predominant	Very good
Mixed cellularity	Good
Nodular sclerosis	Fair
Lymphocyte depleted	Poor

- Nodular sclerosis is the most common type and lymphocyte depleted is the least common type.

Clinical Features

- Hodgkin's lymphoma has bimodal age distribution, with one peak in the 20s and a second over age 50 years.

- More common in males.

- The majority of patients present with overt disease, most often as an asymptomatic enlarged lymph node or a mass on chest X-ray.

- Lymphadenopathy is most often found in neck. Other sites of lymph node involvement are cervical, supraclavicular, axillary, inguinal, mediastinal and intra-abdominal nodes. Involved lymph nodes are painless and non-tender with a rubbery consistency.

- Constitutional symptoms such as fever, drenching night sweats, and weight loss are designated as symptomatic 'B' disease. Fever is usually of low grade and irregular. Rarely, a cyclic pattern of high fever for 1 to 2 weeks alternating with afebrile periods of similar duration is present at diagnosis. This fever pattern is called *Pel-Ebstein fever* and is virtually diagnostic of Hodgkin's lymphoma.

- Compression of various structures by tumor masses can produce many signs and symptoms. These are: Jaundice due to bile duct obstruction, leg swelling due to lymphatic obstruction in the pelvis or groin, dyspnea due to tracheobronchial compression, paraplegia due to compression of the spinal cord, Horner syndrome due to compression of cervical sympathetic chain by enlarged lymph nodes, hoarseness of voice due to compression of recurrent laryngeal nerves, radicular pain due to compression of nerve roots, superior vena cava obstruction due to compression by enlarged mediastinal lymph nodes, etc.

- Hepatosplenomegaly may be present.

- An unusual symptom of Hodgkin's disease is pain in an involved lymph node following alcohol ingestion.

- Patients may have a variety of nonspecific symptoms reflecting organ involvement or paraneoplastic syndromes.

Staging of Hodgkin's Lymphoma

- Based on the extent of the disease, it can be staged as follows (Ann Arbor staging):

Stage I: One lymph node region involved
Stage II: Involvement of two or more lymph node areas on one side of the diaphragm
Stage III: Lymph node regions involved on both sides of the diaphragm
Stage IV: Extranodal involvement (bone marrow, lungs, liver)

- In addition, patients are designated as stage A, if they lack constitutional symptoms and stage B, if they have constitutional symptoms (weight loss, fever, or night sweats).

Investigations

- *Complete blood count* shows normocytic normochromic anemia, normal WBC count and elevated ESR. Lymphopenia, if present is a bad prognostic factor.

- *Alkaline phosphatase (ALP)* may be elevated due to liver or bone involvement.

- *LDH levels* may be raised and indicate bad prognosis.

- *Liver function tests* may be abnormal due to hepatic infiltration. An obstructive pattern may be caused by enlarged nodes at the porta hepatis.

- *Chest X-ray* can show mediastinal widening due to involvement of mediastinum and lymph nodes.

- *CT scan of the thorax, abdomen, and pelvis* is used to establish the extent of disease.

- *Whole-body positron emission tomography scan (PET scan)* is more sensitive imaging technique than CT scan to find out the extent and staging of disease. PET scan can differentiate malignant from non-malignant lesions.

- *Lymph node biopsy* can establish the diagnosis of lymphoma. Presence of Reed-Sternberg cells is characterictic of Hodgkin's lymphoma.
- *Bone marrow biopsy* is required sometimes, if infiltration to bone marrow is suspected.

Treatment

Radiotherapy

Radiotherapy is used as initial treatment only for patients with low-risk stage IA and IIA disease. Radiotherapy is also indicated for lesions causing serious pressure problems.

Chemotherapy

- Limited chemotherapy can be given for some patients treated with radiotherapy.
- Most patients with Hodgkin's disease are best treated with combination chemotherapy using adriamycin, bleomycin, vincristine, and dacarbazine (ABVD). Another regimen includes: Cyclophsophamide, oncovin, procarbazine, and prednisolone (COPP).

Autologous stem cell transplantation: Should be considered for patients who relapse after initial chemotherapy.

Q. Reed-Sternberg cells.

- These are the histologic hallmark of Hodgkin's lymphoma (HL). The presence of these cells differentiates Hodgkin's from non-Hodgkin's lymphoma.
- These are large malignant lymphoid cells of B cell origin with paired, mirror imaged nuclei (binucleate) with large nucleoli. There is a characteristic clear area around the nucleoli giving an 'owl's eyes' appearance to the nuclei (Fig. 5.3).
- They are often only present in small numbers but are surrounded by large numbers of reactive normal T cells, plasma cells and eosinophils.

Q. Disuss the classification, clinical features, clinical staging, investigations and management of non-Hodgkin's lymphoma (NHL).

The non-Hodgkin's lymphomas (NHL) are a heterogeneous group of cancers of lympho-

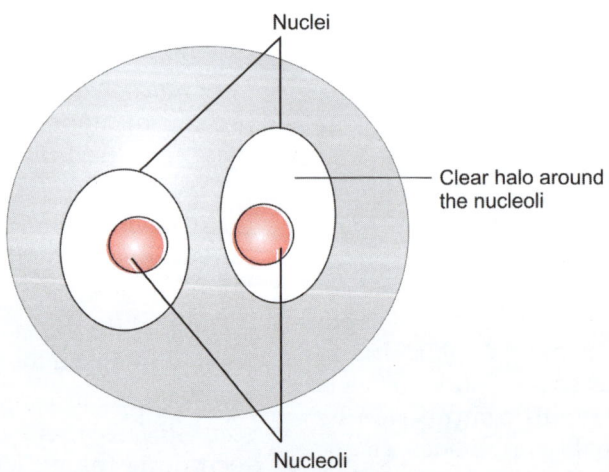

Nuclei

Clear halo around the nucleoli

Nucleoli

Fig. 5.3: Reed-Sternberg cells

cytes. NHL is more common than Hodgkin's lymphoma.

Classification

WHO Classification of the Non-Hodgkin's Lymphomas

Precursor B lymphomas
Mature B lymphomas
Precursor T lymphomas
Mature T lymphomas

Etiology

The exact etiology is unknown in most of the cases. Many risk factors have been identified which are as follows.

Immune deficiency states
- AIDS
- Ataxia telangiectasia
- Immunosuppressive therapy

Occupational and environmental exposure
- Organic solvents
- Hair dyes
- Ultraviolet rays

Infectious agents
- EBV
- HTLV-1
- HHV-8
- Hepatitis C
- *H. pylori* (gastric lymphoma)

Pathology

- Most (80 to 85%) NHL arise from B cells; the remainder arise from T cells or natural killer cells. Either precursor or mature cells may be involved.
- In most cases of non-Hodgkin's lymphoma, activation of proto-oncogenes is the major abnormality. In some cases, there may be deletion of tumor suppressor genes.

Clinical Features

- NHL is more common in men than women.
- Its incidence increases with age and is higher in whites than in other ethnic groups. Median age is 65–70 years.

- Clinical presentation can be indolent to aggressive. Patients with indolent lymphomas usually present with painless enlargement in one or more of the lymph nodes, particularly in the neck, axilla, or inguinal areas. Lymph nodes in the thorax, abdomen and pelvis can be involved. Even the indolent lymphomas are usually disseminated at the time of diagnosis, and bone marrow involvement is common.
- Patients with intermediate and high-grade lymphomas may have constitutional symptoms such as fever, night sweats, or weight loss (B-symptoms). Patients with Burkitt's lymphoma may complain of abdominal pain or fullness due to frequent involvement of nodes in the abdomen.
- NHL can involve any organ in the body, and there may be clinical features relating to that organ dysfunction. Examples are neurological symptoms with CNS lymphoma, breathlessness with MALT lymphomas in the lung, epigastric pain and vomiting with gastric MALT or diffuse large B cell lymphomas, bowel obstruction with small bowel lymphomas, testicular masses with testicular lymphoma, and skin lesions with cutaneous lymphomas. SVC obstruction can occur due to mediastinal lymphadenopathy. Bone marrow involvement leads to bone marrow failure manifesting as recurrent infections, bleeding, and anemia.
- Examination reveals lymphadenopathy which is rubbery and non-tender. Hepatosplenomegaly may be present.

Investigations

- Anemia is usually present.
- ESR is raised.
- Serum LDH is usually elevated.
- Chest X-ray may show a mediastinal mass due to lymph node enlargement.
- CT scan of the chest, abdomen, and pelvis, blood tests, bone marrow biopsy, and PET scan.
- Peripheral smear is usually normal.
- Bone marrow aspiration and biopsy.

- CSF cytology, if CNS involvement is suspected.
- Lymph node or tissue biopsy to confirm the diagnosis.
- Immunophenotyping of surface antigens to distinguish T and B cell tumors. This may be done on blood, marrow or nodal material.
- Genetic studies will help to find the molecular abnormality.

Treatment

Treatment depends on whether the behavior of many of these neoplasms is indolent or aggressive, localized or disseminated and the patient condition. Some lymphomas can be managed initially with observation, whereas other situations such as spinal cord compression require emergency treatment.

Radiotherapy

Local radiotherapy can be used for localized low grade lymphomas either alone or in combination with chemotherapy.

Chemotherapy

Most patients require chemotherapy, either single or combinations of drugs. Common chemotherapy regimens include the combination of rituximab, cyclophosphamide, vincristine, and prednisone (R-CVP); or rituximab, cyclophosphamide, hydroxydaunomycin, oncovin (vincristine), and prednisone (R-CHOP). Combination chemotherapy is especially helpful in intermediate and high grade lymphomas.

Autologous stem cell transplantation: Individuals with very high-risk lymphoma are best treated with stem cell transplantation.

Splenectomy

- Can improve cytopenias
- Palliative therapy for symptomatic splenomegaly.

Q. Enumerate the differences between Hodgkin's and non-Hodgkin's lymphoma.

Table 5.3 describes differences between Hodgkin's and non-Hodgkin's lymphoma.

Table 5.3: Difference between Hodgkin's and non-Hodgkin's lymphoma		
Feature	Hodgkin's lymphoma	Non-Hodgkin's lymphoma
Peak incidence	Bimodal peak, one peak in the 20s and another peak over age 50 years.	65–70 years
Reed-Sternberg cells	Present and pathognomonic	Absent
B-symptoms	More common	Less common
Alcohol-induced pain in involved lymph nodes	Yes	No
Dissemination at presentation	Well localized	Widespread
Origin	B lymphocytes and unifocal	B or T cells and multifocal
Involvement of extralymphatic organs	Late	Early
Involvement of mediastinum	Common	Uncommon
Involvement of bone marrow	Late	Early

Q. Burkitt lymphoma.

- Burkitt lymphoma is a highly aggressive B cell non-Hodgkin's lymphoma (NHL).
- It often presents with extranodal disease and occurs most often in children and immunocompromised hosts.
- Epstein-Barr virus (EBV) has been implicated in the causation of disease.

Pathology

- Most cases are associated with t(8:14), i.e. translocation between chromosomes 8 and 14.
- Burkitt lymphoma is the most rapidly growing human tumor, and pathology reveals a high mitotic rate, a monoclonal proliferation of B cells, and a 'starry-sky' pattern of benign macrophages that have engulfed apoptotic malignant lymphocytes.

Clinical Features

Three clinical forms of Burkitt's lymphoma can be recognized: Endemic, sporadic (non-endemic), and immunodeficiency-associated.

1. The endemic form presents as a jaw or facial bone tumor that spreads to extranodal sites.
2. The nonendemic form has an abdominal presentation, with massive disease and ascites.
3. Immunodeficiency-related cases more often involve lymph nodes.

Investigations

- Histology shows tumor cells, frequent mitotic figures and starry sky appearance.
- Chromosome analysis may show 8/14 translocation.
- Antibodies against EBV may be detected.

Treatment

- Treatment should be initiated within 48 hours of diagnosis.

- Combination chemotherapy CHOP (cyclophosphamide, hydroxydoxorubicin, oncovin, and prednisolone).
- Intrathecal methotrexate for meningeal prophylaxis.

Q. Dicsuss the mechanism of coagulation (hemostasis).

Q. Coagulation cascade.

Normal Hemostasis

- The normal hemostatic process can be divided into primary and secondary components.
- *Primary hemostasis* consists of platelet plug formation at sites of injury. It occurs within seconds of injury and is of prime importance in stopping blood loss from capillaries, small arterioles, and venules. Platelet plug attaches to vessel wall through von Willebrand factor (vWF).
- *Secondary hemostasis* consists of fibrin formation which involves many steps in plasma coagulation system (coagulation cascade). Secondary hemostasis requires several minutes for completion and is important to prevent bleeding in larger vessels and late bleeding occurring hours or days after the injury.
- Actually these two events do not occur separately. They occur simultaneously. As the primary hemostatic plug is being formed, plasma coagulation proteins are activated to initiate secondary hemostasis.

Coagulation Cascade (Fig. 5.4)

Coagulation cascade (secondary hemostasis) involves a number of steps. Each step leads to activation of a molecule which in turn activates next molecule. Coagulation cascade can start by two independent activation pathways—the intrinsic pathway and extrinsic pathway (tissue factor-mediated). Both pathways merge at the point of factor X activation and subsequent steps are same for both.

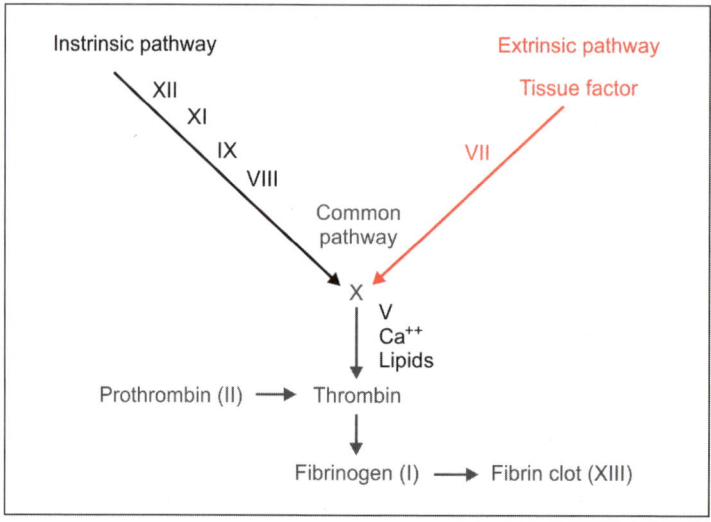

Fig. 5.4: Coagulation cascade

Anticoagulants (Coagulation Inhibitors)

- Just like there are factors which help in coagulation of blood (procoagulants), there are factors which inhibit coagulation. These are called anticoagulants. A fine balance between procoagulant and anticoagulant factors maintains the fluidity of blood.
- The flow of the blood itself inhibits coagulatiuon. Hence, blood clots when it stagnates.
- Antithrombin, proteins C and S are important natural anticoagulant factors that maintain blood fluidity. Reduced levels of antithrombin, proteins C and S, result in a hypercoagulable or prothrombotic state.

Q. Discuss the evaluation of a patient with a bleeding disorder.

Q. Discuss the approach to hemorrhagic disorders.

Q. How will you investigate a case of bleeding disorder?

Q. Differences between bleeding and clotting disorders. (Table 5.4)

- Bleeding results either from a breach of the vessel wall due to a specific insult (e.g. trauma) or from a defect in the hemostatic system.
- Defects in the hemostatic system may be due to a deficiency of one or more of the coagulation factors, thrombocytopenia, or occasionally excessive fibrinolysis (e.g. after fibrinolytic therapy with tPA or streptokinase).
- Detailed history and physical examination are important in finding out the cause of bleeding disorder.

History

The following points should be elicited from the history:

- *Site of bleeds:* Superficial bleeds (skin and mucous membranes), epistaxis, gastrointestinal hemorrhage or menorrhagia indicate a platelet disorder, thrombocytopenia or von Willebrand disease. Deep-seated bleeding such as bleed into muscle, joint or retroperitoneum indicate a coagulation defect. Recurrent bleed at the same site indicates a local structural abnormality.

- *Duration of history:* Onset in childhood may suggest an inherited coagulation disorder such as hemophilia.
- *Precipitating causes:* Bleeding arising spontaneously indicates a more severe defect than bleeding that occurs only after trauma.
- *Surgery or trauma:* Ask about all past surgeries or trauma. Bleeding from a platelet disorder usually occurs immediately after trauma or surgery, and is easily controlled by local measures (such as local pressure). Bleeding due to coagulation defects (e.g. hemophilia) occurs hours or days after injury, and cannot be controlled by local measures.
- *Family history:* A family history of bleeding suggests an inherited hemostatic disorder such as hemophilia.
- *Systemic illnesses:* Enquire about the presence of liver disease, renal failure, paraproteinemia or a connective tissue disease (vasculitis) which can cause bleeding.
- *Drugs:* Many drugs can cause bleeding either by bone marrow suppression or by inhibiting vit-K dependent clotting factors and platelets. Examples are aspirin, clopidogrel, warfarin, etc.

Physical Examination

- Examination should note the presence of any bleeding in the skin and mucous membranes such as petechiae, ecchymoses and hematomas.
- Bleeding into body cavities, the retroperitoneum, or joints is common in coagulation disorders such as hemophilia.
- Joint deformities may be present in coagulation disorders due to recurrent bleeding.
- Hematomas can also compress nerves and lead to neurological deficits. For example, retroperitoneal hematoma can compress femoral nerve. Intracerebral bleed can lead to stroke and altered sensorium. Intracerebral bleed is the leading cause of death in hemostatic disorders.
- Look for evidence of liver disease; splenomegaly may cause thrombocytopenia due to hypersplenism.

Investigations

- Platelet count, bleeding time, clotting time, prothrombin time, fibrinogen level, and clotting factor level, etc.
- Additional tests such as liver function tests to rule out any underlying disorder.

Table 5.4: Differences between primary (bleeding) and secondary (clotting) hemostatic disorders

Features	Primary hemostatic disorder (bleeding disorder, e.g. thrombocytopenia)	Secondary hemostatic disorder (coagulation disorder, e.g. hemophilia)
• Onset of bleeding after trauma	Immediate	Delayed—hours or days
• Age of onset	Late	Childhood
• Sites of bleeding	Superficial: Skin and mucous membranes	Deep: Joints, muscle, retroperitoneum
• Physical findings	Petechiae, ecchymoses	Hematomas, hemarthroses
• Family history	Usually absent	Usually present
• Inheritance	Autosomal dominant	Autosomal or X-linked recessive
• Local measures	Can control bleeding	Cannot control bleeding

Q. Causes of thrombocytopenia.

Q. Define thrombocytopenia. Discuss the causes, clinical features, investigations and management of thrombocytopenia.

Q. Tourniquet test (capillary resistance test; Hess test).

Thrombocytopenia is defined as a platelet count less than 150,000/μL (normal 150,000 to 450,000)

Causes of Thrombocytopenia

- Aplastic anemia
- Marrow infiltration (leukemia, myeloma, carcinoma, myelofibrosis, osteopetrosis)
- Myelodysplasia
- Vitamin B_{12} and folic acid deficiency
- Drugs (anticancer drugs)
- Radiation therapy
- Idiopathic thrombocytopenic purpura (ITP)
- HELLP syndrome (hemolytic anemia, elevated liver function tests, and low platelet count) in pregnant women
- Hypersplenism
- Disseminated intravascular coagulation (DIC)
- Sepsis
- Infections (dengue, malaria, HIV, parvovirus)

Clinical Features

- Bleeding manifestations may not occur until the platelet count falls below 10,000/μL.
- Patients present with bleeding manifestations from cutaneous and mucous membranes.
- Bleeding manifestations include epistaxis, petechiae, purpura, ecchymosis, GI bleed and genitourinary bleeding. Women may present with menorrhagia. Intracranial bleeding can occur in severe thrombocytopenia and cause death.
- *Tourniquet test (Hess test):* A sphygmomanometer cuff is tied around the arm and inflated above diastolic blood pressure but below systolic pressure. Cuff is deflated after 5 minutes. In thrombocytopenia, petechial spots appear in the forearm. More than 20 petechial spots in 3 cm area is considered positive Hess test. It is due to the increased capillary fragility in thrombocytopenia.

Investigations

- Low platelet count
- Prolonged bleeding time
- Anemia may be present due to blood loss.
- *Peripheral smear:* This gives information on morphology of cells, presence or absence of platelet clumping, etc. Peripheral smear can also diagnose diseases such as leukemia.
- *Bone marrow examination:* This may show aplasia, an infiltrative disease, or increased number of megakaryocytes in excessive peripheral destruction (e.g. in ITP).
- *Other tests:* Should be directed at the suspected cause. HIV serology, liver function tests, ultrasound abdomen to look for splenomegaly, etc. are helpful.

Management

- Treat the underlying cause.
- Platelet transfusion is required, if the platelet count is less than 10,000/cumm.

Q. Describe the etiology, clinical features, diagnosis and management of idiopathic (autoimmune) thrombocytopenic purpura (ITP).

- Idiopathic thrombocytopenic purpura (ITP) is an autoimmune disorder due to the presence of an IgG autoantibody against platelets.

Etiology

ITP is due to development of antibodies to one's own platelets, usually triggered by a preceding infection. Any infection can trigger antibody production but common cause is viral infections.

Pathogenesis

Antibody bound platelets are destroyed in the spleen, where splenic macrophages with Fc receptors bind to antibody-coated platelets. Since the spleen is the major site both of antibody production and platelet destruction, splenectomy is highly effective therapy for ITP.

Clinical Features

- ITP is a disease of young. Peak incidence is between ages 20 and 50 years.
- Females are more commonly affected than males.
- Patients present with mucosal or skin bleeding. Common types of bleeding are epistaxis, oral bleeding, menorrhagia, purpura, and petechiae. Intracerebral bleed can be fatal in these patients.
- On examination, patient appears well. Bleeding manifestations such as petechiae and purpura may be noted. In ITP, usually there is no splenomegaly and presence of splenomegaly should make one suspect an alternative diagnosis.

Laboratory Features

- The hallmark of the disease is thrombocytopenia.
- Bleeding time is prolonged due to low platelet count but clotting time is normal.
- Other counts are usually normal except for occasional mild anemia due to bleeding.
- Peripheral smear is normal except reduced platelets.
- Bone marrow is normal except increased number of megakaryocytes.

Treatment

A Few patients may have spontaneous remission, but most will require treatment.

Platelet transfusions: Platelet transfusions are given, if the platelet count is below 10,000/μL because spontaneous bleeding can occur below this level. However, even these exogenous platelets are destroyed and the effect lasts only a few hours. Platelet transfusion should be reserved for cases of life-threatening bleeding in which even fleeting hemostasis may be of benefit.

Steroids: Prednisolone 1–2 mg/kg/day acts by decreasing the affinity of splenic macrophages for antibody-coated platelets. It also reduces the production of antibody and binding of antibody to the platelet surface. Platelet count will usually begin to rise within a week, and responses are almost always seen within 3 weeks. Steroids are continued until the platelet count is normal, and the dose should then be gradually tapered. Dexamethasone can also be used.

Immunoglobulin therapy

- Intravenous immunoglobulin (IVIG), 1 g/day for 3 days, is highly effective in raising the platelet count.
- IVIG works by blocking Fc receptors on macrophages, thereby inhibiting phagocytosis. However, this treatment is expensive, and it should be reserved for bleeding emergencies.

Splenectomy: Splenectomy is indicated, if patients do not respond to other therapies such as steroids or immunoglobulin.

Other therapies: These are tried, if the patient does not respond to above therapies.
  - o Danazol
  - o Immunosuppressive agents (vincristine, azathioprine, cyclosporine, and cyclophosphamide)
  - o Rituximab.
  - o High-dose immunosuppression and autologous stem cell transplantation.

Prognosis

Prognosis is good and most patients will recover with medical line of management. Patients may die due to intracranial hemorrhage.

Q. Discuss the etiology, clinical manifestations, investigations and management of von Willebrand disease.

Q. von Willebrand factor.

von Willebrand disease is the most common congenital bleeding disorder and is transmitted in an autosomal dominant pattern. Rarely it can be acquired also.

Etiology
- von Willebrand disease is due to deficient or defective von Willebrand factor (vWF).
- vWF is important for platelet adhesion to subendothelium. vWF is synthesized by megakaryocytes and endothelial cells.
- vWF also acts as a carrier for factor VIII in the circulation, increasing the half-life of factor VIII. Hence, in von Willebrand's disease, there may be secondarily coagulation disturbance due to decreased levels of factor VIII.

Clinical Features
- von Willebrand disease affects both men and women.
- Most cases are mild.
- Patients present with mucosal bleeding (epistaxis, gingival bleeding, menorrhagia).
- Some patients may come to attention because of excessive bleeding after surgical incisions or tooth extraction. Bleeding tendency is exacerbated by aspirin.

Investigations
- Bleeding time is prolonged in the presence of normal platelet count.
- Defective or absent platelet aggregation.
- Levels of von Willebrand factor in plasma are reduced.
- Ristocetin cofactor test is the most specific and shows decreased biological activity of vWF.

Management
- Since the bleeding is mild, no treatment is necessary except before surgery or dental procedures.

- Desmopressin acetate (DDAVP) can increase the vWF levels by two- to threefold by releasing stored vWF from endothelial cells. It can be given before surgery or dental procedures.
- The antifibrinolytic agent epsilon-aminocaproic acid (EACA) is useful as adjunctive therapy during dental procedures. It is given after DDAVP.

Q. Discuss the etiology, clinical features, investigations and management of Hemophilia A.

Q. Factor VIII (antihemophilic factor).

- Hemophilia A (classic hemophilia) is a hereditary clotting disorder due to deficiency of coagulation factor VIII.
- Hemophilia is an X-linked recessive disease, and hence, males are usually affected. This is because females have two X chromosomes and even if one is affected, other one compensates. However, rarely, female can be affected, if their normal X chromosome is also disproportionately inactivated. One in 10,000 males is born with deficiency or dysfunction of the factor VIII molecule.
- Antenatal diagnosis can be made by chorionic villous sampling or amniocentesis.

Pathogenesis
- Factor VIII (antihemophilic factor) is a large single-chain protein that regulates the activation of factor X by proteases generated in the intrinsic pathway. Hence deficiency of factor VIII leads to defective coagulation and bleeding.
- Factor VIII is synthesized in liver and circulates in the blood. Von Willebrand factor (vWF) acts as a carrier of factor VIII in blood.
- Hemophilia is classified as severe, if factor VIII level is less than 1%; moderate, if level is 1–5%; and mild, if level is greater than 5%.

Clinical Features

- Hemophilia A is the second most common congenital hemostatic disorder after Von-Willebrand's disease. It is a severe clotting disorder.
- Family history of hemophilia is usually positive.
- The bleeding tendency is related to factor VIII levels. Patients with mild hemophilia bleed only after major trauma or surgery, those with moderately severe hemophilia bleed with mild trauma or surgery, and those with severe disease bleed spontaneously.
- Bleeding can occur anywhere but commonly occurs in deep tissues such as joints (knees, ankles, elbows), muscles, and from GIT.
- Bleeding into joints (hemarthroses) is common in hemophilia A and is almost diagnostic of the disorder. Recurrent bleeding into joints leads to joint destruction and joint deformities.

Investigations

- Partial thromboplastin time (PTT) is prolonged.
- Platelet count and PT are normal.
- Bleeding time and fibrinogen levels are also normal.
- Factor VIII levels are reduced.

Treatment

- Treatment of hemophilia A involves infusion of factor VIII concentrates, either recombinant or heat treated.
- For mild hemophiliacs, DDAVP (desmopressin) is enough for minor surgeries. It causes release of stored factor VIII and will raise the factor VIII levels two- to threefold for several hours.
- EACA (epsilon-aminocaproic acid) may be added, if bleeding persists after treating with factor VIII and desmopressin.
- Fresh frozen plasma can be used, if factor VIII concentrate is not available.

- Gene therapy is currently in the developmental phase.
- Avoid the use of aspirin (antiplatelet agent) in these patients.

Prognosis

Prognosis is good now because of the availability of factor VIII concentrates. Intracerebral hemorrhage is the usual cause of death but uncommon.

> **Q. Discuss the etiology, clinical features, investigations and management of Hemophilia B (Christmas disease).**

- Hemophilia B (Christmas disease) is a hereditary clotting disorder due to deficiency of coagulation factor IX. It is sometimes called Christmas disease, named after Stephen Christmas, the first patient described with this disease. Inheritance is same as hemophilia A (X-linked recessive).
- Factor IX deficiency is less common than factor VIII deficiency but is otherwise clinically and genetically identical.

Clinical Features

Same as hemophilia A, but less severe.

Investigations

- Factor IX levels are reduced.
- Other laboratory features are same as factor VIII deficiency.

Treatment

- Transfusion of factor IX concentrates. Recombinant factor IX is available now.
- Fresh frozen plasma can be used in emergencies, if factor IX concentrate is not available.
- DDAVP is not useful in this disorder.
- Aspirin should be avoided.

Prognosis

Prognosis is same as hemophilia A.

Q. Causes of splenomegaly.

Mild splenomegaly
- *Acute infections:* Typhoid, malaria, septicemia, subacute bacterial endocarditis

Moderate splenomegaly
- Leukemia
- Lymphoma
- Polycythemia vera
- Hemolytic anemias
- Cirrhosis of liver

Massive splenomegaly
- Chronic myeloid leukemia (CML)
- Myelofibrosis
- Gaucher's disease
- Chronic lymphocytic leukemia (CLL)
- Hairy cell leukemia
- Kala-azar (visceral leishmaniasis)
- Tropical splenomegaly syndrome
- Thalassemia major

Q. Enumerate the causes of generalized lymphadenopathy.

Lymphadenopathy is classified as localized when it involves only one region and generalized when it involves 2 or more noncontiguous body regions.

Causes of Generalized Lymphadenopathy

- *Infections:* Disseminated tuberculosis, cat-scratch disease, secondary syphilis, HIV, infectious mononucleosis, histoplasmosis, coccidioidomycosis, cryptococcosis, toxoplasmosis
- *Malignancy:* Metastatic carcinoma, lymphoma, leukemia.
- *Connective tissue diseases:* Rheumatoid arthritis, SLE, sarcoidosis
- *Drugs:* Phenytoin

Q. Define neutropenia and agranulocytosis. Describe the etiology, clinical features and management of neutropenia/agranulocytosis (febrile neutropenia).

- Neutropenia is defined as an absolute neutrophil count (ANC) of less than $1500/\mu L$.
- Agranulocytosis refers to ANC less than $500/\mu L$.
- The risk of infection increases whenever there is neutropenia and agranulocytosis.

Etiology

Decreased production
- Anticancer drugs
- Aplastic anemia
- Tumor invasion of bone marrow (myeloma, leukemias, myelofibrosis)
- Nutritional deficiency—vitamin B_{12}, folate (especially alcoholics)
- Infections—tuberculosis, typhoid fever, brucellosis, infectious mononucleosis, parvovirus infection, AIDS

Increased destruction
- Hypersplenism
- Antineutrophil antibodies
- Autoimmune disorders—Felty's syndrome, rheumatoid arthritis, systemic lupus erythematosus

Clinical Features

- Can be asymptomatic.
- Increased risk of recurrent infections and sepsis. Common infective organisms include *Staphylococcus aureus*, gram-negative organisms and fungi.
- Common sites of infection include the oral cavity and mucous membranes, skin, perirectal and genital areas.
- Classic presentation is sore throat and fever.
- Ulcers in the throat and mouth.
- Toxemia and sepsis can lead to death.

Investigations

- Total WBC count is low.
- Neutrophil count is low.
- Peripheral smear shows absence of neutrophil and band forms.

- Bone marrow examination shows myeloid aplasia or hypoplasia or myeloid maturation arrest.
- Blood culture may grow the infective organism.
- Imaging studies such as chest X-ray, X-ray of paranasal sinuses, CT scan of the abdomen, etc. may be done based on history and examination findings to identify the focus of infection.

Treatment

- Treatment depends upon the cause and degree of the neutropenia.
- Patients with bone marrow hypoplasia and/or severe infections should receive aggressive antibacterial therapy for fever, even in the absence of signs of infection. Broad-spectrum antibiotics to coverage both gram-positive and gram-negative bacteria should be used. Patients with an ANC less than $500/\mu L$ and marrow aplasia should always be treated on an inpatient basis with parenteral antibiotics.
- G-CSF (granulocyte colony-stimulating factor) should be given to patients with inadequate response to antibiotics. It increases neutrophil count.

Q. Oral manifestations of hematologic disease.

- Diseases of blood frequently affect soft and hard tissues of mouth with different characteristics.
- Every dentist should be familiar with the wide variety of oral manifestations of the blood diseases to differentiate from other diseases.

Polycythemia

Abnormal increase of erythrocytes is called polycythemia.

Clinical features: Patient will have headache, tinnitus, dyspepsia, and visual disturbance. The skin will be reddened.

Oral manifestations

- Mucous membrane appears dark red.
- Gingiva is congested, enlarged and may have spongy bleeding
- Petechia and ecchymosis are common in mucosa
- Cyanosis can occur.

Iron Deficiency Anemia

This anemia is mainly caused due to inadequate dietary intake of iron, faulty absorption of iron and increased requirement for iron. The Plummer-Vinson syndrome is a form of anemia with iron deficiency, dysphagia, kolinychia and atrophic glossitis.

Oral manifestations

- Pale and bald tongue, the mucous membrane appears pale.
- Cracks or fissure at the corners of mouth (angular stomatitis).

Vitamin B$_{12}$ Deficiency Anemia

Vitamin B$_{12}$ is essential for erythropoiesis. Deficiency leads to megaloblastic anemia. Patient presents with fatigue, pallor and peripheral neuropathy.

Oral manifestations

- The tongue is inflamed and beefy red in colour either entirely or partly. The papilla undergoes atrophy.
- Small shallow ulcers like apthous ulcers can be seen.

Treatment

Vitamin B$_{12}$ injection

Aplastic Anemia

- Anemia is caused by lack of bone marrow activity.
- Reduction of red blood cell count, white blood cell count and platelets causing pancytopenia.

Oral manifestations

- Oral mucosa is pale, and atrophic due to anemia.

- The dorsum of the tongue is smooth, bald and sore.
- Angular stomatitis present.
- Bleeding from gums due to low platelet count.
- Ulcerations may be present.

Thalassemia

This is a hereditary disease—a congenital defect of globin synthesis resulting in defective and unstable hemoglobin.

Clinical features

- Features of hemolytic anemia.
- Splenomegaly and hepatomegaly may develop.

Oral manifestations

- Pale oral mucosa.
- An unusual prominence of the premaxilla, maxillary teeth are irregularly arranged. Intraoral radiograph shows peculiar trabecular pattern of maxilla. Coarsening of trabecula and blurring and disappearance of other resulting 'salt and pepper effect' thickening of diploe of skull. Inner and outer plates become elongated producing bristals like crew cut or hair on end appearance.

Bleeding and Clotting Disorders

Oral manifestations

- Petechiae, ecchymoses
- Spontaneous gingival hemorrhage
- Prolong bleeding following oral surgery
- Gingival enlargement
- Mucosal ulcers

Leukemia

Oral manifestations

- Mucosal bleeding
- Ulceration
- Petechiae
- Gingival enlargement

Renal System

Definition

- Acute kidney injury(AKI) earlier known as acute renal failure refers to rapid decrease in renal function over days to weeks, causing an accumulation of nitrogenous products in the blood (azotemia).
- It is usually reversible.

Causes

Prerenal
- **Decreased perfusion of kidneys:** Heart failure, septic shock, hemorrhage, vomiting, diarrhea.
- **Drugs:** ACE inhibitors, NSAIDs

Intrarenal
- Acute pyelonephritis, acute glomerulonephritis, vasculitis, malignant hypertension

Postrenal
- **Obstruction to urine flow:** Stone, tumor, prostate enlargement, urethral stenosis

Pathogenesis

Glomerular filtration occurs due to pressure gradient from the glomerulus to the Bowman space. Glomerular pressure depends on renal blood flow. Almost all the causes of AKI cause reduction in renal blood flow which is the common pathologic pathway for decreasing glomerular filtration rate (GFR). The etiology of AKI consists of three main mechanisms: Prerenal, renal (intrinsic), and postrenal.

- *Prerenal causes* are the most common cause of acute renal failure. All prerenal causes act through renal hypoperfusion. If hypoperfusion is rapidly reversed, renal parenchymal damage does not occur. If hypoperfusion persists, ischemia can result, causing renal failure.

- *Renal causes* of AKI either damage glomerulus (glomerulonephritis) or tubules (ATN).

- *Postrenal causes* are the least common cause of acute renal failure. It occurs when urinary flow from either kidneys, or a single functioning kidney, is obstructed. This leads to elevated intraluminal pressure in the nephron, causing a decrease in GFR. If the obstruction is relieved, this type of renal failure is reversible.

Clinical Features

- Uremia (increase in blood urea) occurs in renal failure. Uremia can cause nausea, vomiting, malaise, altered sensorium, flapping tremors and seizures.
- Platelet dysfunction can lead to bleeding.

- Decreased or no urine output can occur. Signs and symptoms of fluid overload can occur such as pedal edema, ascites, pleural and pericardial effusions.
- Arrhythmias can occur due to electrolyte imbalance such as hyper- and hypokalemia.
- The lung examination may show crepitations due to volume overload.
- There may be signs and symptoms of underlyng disorder causing renal failure.

Investigations

- Anemia may be present in prerenal AKI due to hemorrhage.
- *Urea and creatinine* are elevated. In prerenal AKI, there is disproportionate elevation of urea in relation to creatinine (usually >20:1).
- *Urine analysis may show presence of* RBCs and WBCs in AKI due to glomerulonephritis. RBC casts indicate glomerular injury or rarely interstitial nephritis.
- *Electrolyte abnormalities* include hyperkalemia, hypocalcemia and hyperphosphatemia.
- *ECG* may reveal changes of hyperkalemia and also any cardiac problems.
- *Anti-streptolysin O titre*: If post-streptococcal glomerulonephritis is suspected.
- *Other serology*: If clinically suspected, e.g. hepatitis B, hepatitis C, leptospirosis, syphilis, Hantavirus.
- If diagnosis is not clear from above investigations, consider ANA, ANCA, complement levels, etc. to rule out connective tissue disorder.
- *Renal ultrasound* is usually required urgently especially renal failure due to obstruction is suspected. *Renal Doppler* can identify patency of renal arteries and veins.
- *Chest X-ray* may show evidence of pulmonary edema.
- *Renal biopsy* is indicated when renal function does not return for a prolonged period and a prognosis is required to develop long-term management.

Management

- Correct the underlying cause of the AKI.
- Treat fluid and electrolyte abnormalities. Loop diuretics such as frusemide or torsemide can be used, if there is fluid overload. On the other hand, fluids should be given if there is hypovolemia causing renal failure. Hyperkalemia should be corrected by antihyperkalemia measures such as salbutamol nebulization, potassium binding resins, etc.
- Correct metabolic acidosis with oral or IV bicarbonate.
- Nephrotoxic drugs such as NSAIDs, aminoglycosides, etc. should be avoided.
- Restriction of water (unless there is hypovolemia), sodium, phosphate, and potassium intake, but provision of adequate protein.
- Hemodialysis is required for the following if conservative measures fail.

Indications for Hemodialysis

- Urea >180 mg/dL and creatinine >8 mg/dL.
- Refractory fluid overload with pulmonary edema.
- Resistant hyperkalemia.
- Severe metabolic acidosis (pH less than 7.1).
- Signs of uremia, such as pericarditis, neuropathy, or altered mental status.

Q. Define chronic kidney disease (CKD). Discuss the causes, clinical features, investigations and management of CKD.

- *Chronic kidney disease (CKD)* (earlier known as chronic renal failure) is defined as either kidney damage or a decreased glomerular filtration rate (GFR) of less than 60 mL/min/1.73 m² for 3 or more months.
- CKD can be divided into following stages.

Stage 1	Kidney damage with normal or increased GFR (>90 mL/min/1.73 m²)
Stage 2	Mild reduction in GFR (60–89 mL/min/1.73 m²)
Stage 3	Moderate reduction in GFR (30–59 mL/min/1.73 m²)

| Stage 4 | Severe reduction in GFR (15-29 mL/min/1.73 m²) |
| Stage 5 | Kidney failure (GFR <15 mL/min/1.73 m² or dialysis) |

- CKD stage 1 and 2 cannot be diagnosed based on GFR alone as GFR can be normal in these stages. Stage 5 CKD is also known as end stage renal disease (ESRD).

Etiology of CKD

- **Primary glomerular diseases:** Focal and segmental glomerulosclerosis (FSGN), membranoproliferative glomerulonephritis (MPGN), IgA nephropathy, membranous nephropathy

- **Secondary glomerular diseases:** Diabetic nephropathy, hypertension, postinfectious glomerulonephritis

- **Tubulointerstitial nephritis**: Drugs, reflux/chronic pyelonephritis

- **Obstructive nephropathies:** Prostate enlargement, kidney stones, tumor

- **Vascular diseases:** Renal artery stenosis

- **Hereditary diseases**: Polycystic kidney disease

Clinical Features

Fluid and Electrolyte Imbalance

- In most patients with stable CKD, there is retention of sodium and water leading to fluid overload. Fluid overload manifests as peripheral edema, acites, pleural and pericardial effusions.

- Hyperkalema is seen in CKD, as potassium excretion is impaired.

Acid–Base Disturbance

Metabolic acidosis is common due to inability to excrete acid load due to less ammonia formation in the kidneys. In severe metabolic acidosis, patient may have deep respiration (Kussmaul's respiration), anorexia, nausea, vomiting, hiccoughs, pruritus, muscular twitching, fits, drowsiness and coma.

Uremia

- Uremia refers to a constellation of signs and symptoms seen in renal failure. Manifestations of the uremic state include anorexia, nausea, vomiting, growth retardation, peripheral neuropathy, altered sensorium, seizures, and coma.

- Bleeding may occur due to abnormal platelet adhesion and aggregation due to uremia.

- Pericarditis and pericardial effusion also occurs in uremia and is an indication for dialysis.

Disturbances in Calcium and Phosphate Metabolism

Renal osteodystropy: Kidney is the site of formation of 1, 25-dihydroxycholecalciferol (active vitamin D). Diminished active vit-D formation in CKD leads to hypocalcemia and hyperphosphatemia (due to phosphate retention). Hypocalcemia and hyperphosphatemia stimulate PTH production. Increased PTH (hyperparathyroidism) stimulates bone turnover and leads to osteitis fibrosa cystica characterized by marrow fibrosis and bone cysts.

Anemia

Anemia is due to reduced renal erythropoietin production. It is normocytic and normochromic.

Hypertension

Hypertension is due to volume expansion and/or activation of the renin–angiotensin system.

Growth Impairment

Growth failure is common in childhood CKD, and is multifactorial. It is due to metabolic acidosis, decreased caloric intake, renal osteodystrophy, and alterations in growth hormone metabolism.

Investigations

- Urea and creatinine are elevated. The level of serum creatinine correlates with the degree of renal impairement.
- *Urine analysis:* It shows fixed specific gravity of around 1.010 (isosthenuria, because of loss of urine concentrating ability of kidneys) and presence of broad casts. WBCs are present in the urine in UTI, papillary necrosis, BPH and renal tuberculosis. RBC casts are seen in glomerulonephritis.
- *Serum electrolytes:* Hyperkalemia, hypocalcemia, and hyperphosphatemia are seen. Bicarbonate levels are reduced.
- Anemia is seen which is usually normocytic normochromic.
- *Ultrasound abdomen:* Usually shows bilateral small sized kidneys. Ultrasound can also rule out obstruction, polycystic kidney disease, etc.
- *Chest X-ray:* May show pulmonary edema and pericardial effusion
- *ECG:* It may show signs of hyperkalemia or cardiac disease.
- *Renal artery Doppler:* If renal artery stenosis is suspected.
- Hepatitis B, C and HIV serology, if dialysis is needed (vaccination against hepatitis B, if no previous infection; isolation of dialysis machine, if positive)
- ANA if connective tissue disease is suspected.
- Renal biopsy to establish the diagnosis in selected cases.

Management

Treatment of Underlying Cause

Identify the underlying cause of renal failure and institute treatment for that. For example, control of diabetes, hypertension, immunosuppression in glomerulonephritis, etc.

Slowing the Progression of CKD

- ACE inhibitors have been shown to slow the progression of CKD in diabetics. ACE inhibitors should be used, where tolerated. Monitor creatinine and potassium after starting on ACE inhibitors as there can be worsening of GFR and hyperkalemia. Angiotensin II receptor antagonists also have similar effect.
- Restriction of dietary protein intake also delays the progression of CKD.

Treatment of the Complications of Renal Failure

- *Anemia:* Recombinant human erythropoietin is effective in correcting the anemia of CKD. Severe anemia should be corrected by blood transfusion.
- *Volume overload:* It should be treated by a combination of dietary sodium restriction and diuretic therapy, usually with a loop diuretic given daily.
- *Hyperkalemia:* It should be treated by low potassium diet, diuretics such as frusemide, and potassium binding agents (Kayexalate 5 grams with each meal). Salbutamol nebulizations are also useful to decrease potassium.
- *Metabolic acidosis:* Sodium bicarbonate (in a daily dose of 0.5 to 1 mEq/kg per day) should be given to maintain serum bicarbonate concentration above 22 mEq/L. Sodium citrate may be used in patients unable to tolerate sodium bicarbonate.
- *Hyperphosphatemia:* This is treated by oral phosphate binders to maintain serum phosphorus levels less than 5 mg/dL.
- *Renal osteodystrophy:* This is treated by calcitriol (1, 25-dihydroxyvitamin D) and control of phosphate levels.
- *Hypertension:* It is controlled by a combination of antihypertensives and diuretics. ACE inhibitors or angiotensin II receptor blocker can be used initially, if creatinine is not high. Other antihypertensives are calcium channel blockers, clonidine, betablockers and alpha-blockers.

Renal Replacement Therapy

- If conservative measures are inadequate, hemodialysis must be planned.

- Renal transplantation can be considered in suitable patients.

Q. Distinguishing acute kidney injury (AKI) from chronic kidney disease (CKD).

Table 6.1 shows distinguishing features of AKI and CKD.

Q. Discuss the etiology, clinical features, investigations and management of nephrotic syndrome.

Nephrotic syndrome is defined as proteinuria of more than 3 g/day due to a glomerular disorder accompanied by hypoalbuminemia and edema.

Etiology

Idiopathic or primary nephrotic syndrome
- Minimal change disease
- Focal segmental glomerulosclerosis (FSGS)
- Membranous nephropathy
- Membranoproliferative glomerulonephritis

Secondary nephrotic syndrome
- Diabetes mellitus
- SLE and other collagen diseases
- Amyloidosis
- Vasculitis (Wegener's granulomatosis, rapidly progressive glomerulonephritis, Goodpasture's syndrome, etc.)
- Infections (post-streptococcal, hepatitis B, hepatitis C, HIV infection, filariasis)
- Drugs (penicillamine, NSAIDs, lithium, street heroin)
- Malignancy (Hodgkin's lymphoma, leukemia)

Pathophysiology

- Nephrotic syndrome is characterized by proteinuria, hypoalbuminemia and peripheral edema.
- Proteinuria occurs because of damage to glomerular capillary endothelial cells, the glomerular basement membrane (GBM), or podocytes, which normally filter serum protein selectively by size and charge.
- Hypoalbuminemia is due to urinary protein loss. Catabolism of filtered albumin by the proximal tubule as well as redistribution of albumin within the body also contribute to hypoalbuminemia.
- Salt and water retention in nephrotic syndrome can be explained by two different mechanisms. In the classic theory, proteinuria leads to hypoalbuminemia, a low

Table 6.1: Distinguishing features of acute kidney injury (AKI) from chronic kidney disease (CKD)

Finding	Comment
Previously documented elevation of serum creatinine	Most reliable evidence of CKD
Small kidneys on ultrasound	Seen in CKD
Normal or enlarged kidneys on ultrasound	Usually favours AKI. Can be seen in some forms of CKD (diabetic nephropathy, polycystic kidney disease, myeloma, rapidly progressive glomerulonephritis, infiltrative diseases amyloidosis, obstruction)
Oliguria, daily increases in serum creatinine and BUN	Favours AKI
Eye-band keratopathy	Favours CKD
Presence of anemia	Favours CKD
Hypocalcemia	Favours CKD

plasma oncotic pressure, and intravascular volume depletion leading to under-perfusion of the kidneys. This stimulates renin–angiotensin system causing incre-ased renal sodium and water retention. Decreased oncotic pressure in the capil-laries also causes fluid leakage and edema.

- Another mechanism may be primary renal sodium retention at a distal nephron site, perhaps due to altered responsiveness to hormones such as atrial natriuretic factor.

Clinical Features

- Nephrotic syndrome occurs at any age but is more prevalent in children, mostly between ages 1½ and 4 years.
- Peripheral edema is the hallmark of the nephrotic syndrome. Initially it is noted in the dependent areas such as the lower extremities, but later becomes generalized. Early morning facial puffiness is seen in most patients even before the development of generalized edema.
- Patients can experience dyspnea due to pulmonary edema and pleural effusion.
- Ascites may be present.
- Patients are more prone to infection due to loss of immunoglobulins and complements in the urine.
- Patients also have hypercoagulable state due to urinary losses of antithrombin III, protein C, and protein S and increased platelet activation. Patients are prone to renal vein thrombosis and other venous thromboemboli.
- Microcytic hypochromic anemia may result from loss of transferrin in the urine.
- Vitamin D deficiency may result from loss of cholecalciferol binding protein.

Investigations

- Urine analysis shows heavy proteinuria. 24-hour urine protein excretion should be measured and it shows nephrotic range proteinuria (>3 g/day). Normal protein excretion is <150 mg/day. Minimal hema-turia may also be present.

- Serum albumin is low (<3 g/dL).
- Urea and creatinine may be elevated, if there is renal failure.
- Total cholesterol and LDL-cholesterol is elevated in most patients. HDL-cholesterol is normal or decreased.
- Blood sugar and glycosylated hemoglobin tests for diabetes.
- Antinuclear antibody (ANA) and ANCA test for collagen vascular disease and vasculitis.
- Serum anticoagulants and complement levels are decreased.
- Hepatitis B and C serology, HIV serology.
- Renal biopsy, if the cause is not clear especially in an adult patient.

Management

Protein loss: The daily total dietary protein intake should replace the daily urinary protein losses so as to avoid negative nitrogen balance. Angiotensin-converting enzyme (ACE) inhibitors and angiotensin receptor blockers reduce the amount of proteinuria.

Edema: This can be managed by dietary salt restriction and diuretics. Commonly used diuretics include thiazide and loop diuretics.

Hyperlipidemia: Dietary modification and exercise should be adviced. HMG-CoA reduc-tase inhibitors (statins) can be used in patients not responding to dietary measures.

Hypercoagulable state: Anticoagulation therapy is given for at least 3–6 months in patients with evidence of thrombosis. Patients with renal vein thrombosis and recurrent thromboemboli require indefinite anticoa-gulation.

Treatment of the Underlying Cause

- Minimal change disease responds to steroids.
- Steroids are beneficial in only 20–30% cases of focal segmental glomerulosclerosis (FSGS). Cyclophosphamide and cyclo-sporine are alternatives.
- Membranous nephropathy responds to alternating monthly corticosteroids and

monthly oral chlorambucil over 6 months. Recent controlled studies using only corticosteroids for 6 months have shown similar beneficial results. Membranous nephropathy with progressive renal failure may benefit from cyclophosphamide plus corticosteroids.

Q. Minimal change disease (nil disease or lipoid nephrosis).

- Minimal change disease accounts for most cases of nephrotic syndrome in children and 10 to 15% of idiopathic nephrotic syndrome in adults.
- Most of the cases are idiopathic but some cases are associated with drugs (NSAIDs, lithium) and hematological malignancies (Hodgkin's disease and leukemias).

Clinical Features

- Patients typically present with periorbital and peripheral edema. Periorbital edema is noted first.
- Malaise, easy fatiguability and weight gain.

Investigations

- Urea and creatinine are normal.
- Urine analysis shows nephrotic range proteinuria and occasionally hematuria. RBC casts are absent. (RBC casts are seen in glomerulonephritis.)
- Serum albumin is low.
- Serologic workup (including antinuclear antibodies and complements) is normal.
- Kidney biopsy is usually not required in children except in atypical cases. However, kidney biopsy is required in adults. Biopsy shows no glomerular abnormalities on light microscopy. The tubules may show lipid droplet accumulation from absorbed lipoproteins (hence also called lipoid nephrosis). Complement and Ig deposits are absent on immunofluorescence. Electron microscopy shows effacement or 'fusion' of the foot processes of epithelial podocytes.

Treatment

- Initial therapy is with steroids, prednisolone 1 to 2 mg/kg body weight per day (maximum of 60 mg/day). When proteinuria disappears, prednisolone is continued at the same dose for 1 month and then on alternate day (at the same daily dose) for 2 months. Thereafter, the alternate day dose is gradually decreased.
- Complete remission occurs in >80% of patients treated with corticosteroids, and treatment is usually continued for 1 to 2 years. Response may be slower in adults.
- Relapses can occur in children and adults. First relapse is treated similarly as the initial episode. Patients who relapse third time or who become steroid dependent may be treated with a 2-month course of an alkylating agent (cyclophosphamide 2 mg/kg/day or chlorambucil). Another alternative is low dose cyclosporine (4 to 6 mg/kg/day for 4 months), but this carries the risk of nephrotoxicity.

Q. Discuss the etiology, clinical features, investigations and management of glomerulonephritis (nephritic syndrome).

Glomerulonephritis literally means 'inflammation of glomeruli'. Here the glomeruli are damaged due to inflammation.

Etiology

Primary glomerular diseases: Diffuse proliferative glomerulonephritis, focal segmental glomerulosclerosis (FSGS), membranous glomerulonephritis, membranoproliferative glomerulonephritis, cresentic glomerulonephritis, IgA nephropathy

Systemic diseases: SLE, Wegener's granulomatosis, polyarteritis, Henoch-Schonlein purpura,

Infections: Post-streptococcal glomerulonephritis, subacute bacterial endocarditis, hepatitis B and C, malaria.

Miscellaneous: Malignancy, eclampsia, serum sickness, drugs (penicillamine), malignant hypertension

Pathogenesis

- Most types of glomerulonephritis are immunologically mediated. Glomerular injury occurs by two main mechanisms, either by deposition of antibody in the glomerular basement membrane or by deposition of immune complexes.
- Immune complexes are formed 'in situ' by antibodies which complex with glomerular antigens, or with other antigens ('planted' antigens, e.g. viral or bacterial ones) that have localized in glomeruli.
- The antibodies and immune complexes trigger injury by complement activation, fibrin deposition, release of cytokines and recruitment of inflammatory cells.

Clinical Features

Patients present with hematuria, hypertension, oliguria and edema. Edema is found first in body parts with low tissue tension, such as the periorbital and scrotal regions.

Investigations

- Urine analysis shows hematuria, moderate proteinuria (usually <2 g/d), RBC casts, and WBCs. Red cell casts are specific for glomerulonephritis.
- Complement levels (C3, C4) are usually decreased.
- ASO titer may be increased in post-streptococcal glomerulonephritis.
- Anti-GBM antibody levels are elevated.
- ANCA, ANA, if connective tissue disease is suspected.
- Hepatitis serologies.
- Renal ultrasound.
- Renal biopsy, if the cause is not clear.

Treatment

- Depending on the nature and severity of disease, treatment may involve high-dose steroids and cytotoxic agents such as cyclophosphamide.
- Plasmapheresis can be used in Goodpasture's disease as a temporary measure until chemotherapy takes effect.
- Underlying disease requires specific treatment.

Q. What are the differences between nephrotic and nephritic syndrome?

Differences between nephrotic and nephritic syndrome are given in Table 6.2.

Table 6.2: Differences between nephrotic and nephritic syndrome		
	Nephrotic syndrome	*Nephritic syndrome*
Proteinuria	Massive (>3 g/day)	Moderate (<2 g/day)
Hematuria	Minimal	Significant
RBC casts in urine	Absent	Present
Hypoalbuminemia	Present	Rarely
Generalized edema	Present	Rarely present in cases of renal failure
Hyperlipidemia/hyperlipiduria	Yes	No
Hypertension	Absent	Present
Urea and creatinine	Usually normal	Often elevated

Q. Discuss the etiology, pathogenesis, clinical features, investigations, complications and management of post-streptococcal glomerulonephritis.

Post-streptococcal glomerulonephritis is acute glomerulonephritis occurring after infection with streptococci.

Etiology

Group A beta hemolytic streptococci are responsible for post-streptococcal glomerulonephritis. Skin and throat infections with this organism are followed by glomerulonephritis.

Pathogenesis

- Post-streptococcal glomerulonephritis is an immune-mediated disease involving streptococcal antigens, circulating immune complexes, and activation of complement in association with cell-mediated injury.
- Many streptococcal antigens have biochemical affinity for glomerular basement membrane and in this location act as target for antibodies.
- The immune response to these antigens leads to acute glomerulonephritis.

Clinical Features

- It occurs in children between the ages of 5 and 15 years, but can occur in adults also.
- It is more common in males.
- Patients present with hematuria, proteinuria, pyuria, red blood cell casts, edema, hypertension, and oliguric renal failure.
- Systemic symptoms of headache, malaise, anorexia, and flank pain (due to swelling of the renal capsule) may be present.
- Subclinical disease is common and is characterized by asymptomatic microscopic hematuria.

Investigations

- Urine analysis shows hematuria, proteinuria, pyuria, and RBC casts. Proteinuria can sometimes be in the nephrotic range.
- Urea and creatinine may be elevated.
- Serum complement levels are low.
- Streptococcal culture may be positive from the infected site (throat or skin).
- ASO titre, anti-DNase or antihyaluronidase antibodies are increased.
- Renal biopsy is rarely required. It shows mesangial and endothelial cell proliferation, glomerular infiltration with polymorphonuclear leukocytes, granular subendothelial immune deposits and subepithelial deposits.

Complications

Pulmonary edema, hypertensive encephalopathy, and permanent renal failure.

Management

- Treatment is mainly supportive.
- The measures are salt restriction, diuretics, antihypertensives and dialysis, if required.
- Antibiotic treatment for streptococcal infection should be given to all patients and their cohabitants. Antibiotic choices are pencillins (ampicillin, amoxicillin) or cephalosporins or macrolides or clindamycin. Oral penicillin V or amoxicillin are the 1st drugs of choice and are given for 10 days.
- Steroids and cytotoxic drugs are of no value.
- Prognosis is good and permanent renal failure is uncommon.

Nutritional Disorders

Q. Balanced diet.

- The modern definition of balanced diet is "a diet that contains the proper proportions of carbohydrates, fats, proteins, vitamins, minerals, and water necessary to maintain good health". Malnutrition results from an unbalanced diet, this can be due to an excess of some dietary components and lack of other components, not just a complete lack of food. Too much of one component can do as much harm to the body as too little. Deficiency diseases occur when there is a lack of a specific nutrient, although some diet-related disorders are a result of eating in excess. An adequate diet provides sufficient energy for the performance of the body to function.

- A healthy person should aim to get *45 to 65% of their calories from carbohydrates, 10 to 35% of their calories from protein and 20 to 35% of their calories from fat.*

- Our body uses carbohydrates as its preferred source of energy. We get most of our carbohydrates from grains, fruits and milk products. Examples of carbohydrate-rich grains are rice, wheat, jowar, millets, oats and barley, starchy vegetables like potatoes, sweet potatoes, corn and squash.

- Healthy fats include butter, ghee, cheese, coconut oil, avocado oil, etc. Unhealthy fats are transfats which are found in margarine, pastries, hydrogenated vegetable oils, etc.

- Coming to proteins, proteins are the main building blocks of our body. Our muscles are mainly made of protein. Sources of protein include grains, vegetables, pulses, eggs and meat. Pulses, eggs and meat are especially rich in proteins.

- Vitamins and minerals are present in most foods. But fruits and vegetables are a rich source of vitamins and antioxidants.

- Good amount of fiber is also important for the body. Fibers are not absorbed from the gastrointestinal tract and hence, they add to the bulk of the stools and prevent constipation. Unpolished cereals, green leafy vegetables are good sources of fiber.

- Water is very important for the body for all its metabolic functions and to eliminate waste products. A healthy adult requires around 2 to 2.5 litres of water per day. About one litre of this requirement comes from the food itself (hidden water). Remaining 1.5 litres should be taken as water and other beverages.

Q. Vitamin A (retinol) deficiency.

- Vitamin A is lipid soluble and is found in three forms—retinols, beta-carotenes, and carotenoids. Retinol, also known as preformed vitamin A, is the most active form and is mostly found in animal sources of food. Beta-carotene, also known as provitamin A, is the plant source of retinol.

- Vitamin A was the first fat-soluble vitamin to be discovered.
- The recommended daily intake of vitamin A is 800 to 1000 μg.

Functions of Vitamin A

- Night vision.
- Differentiation of epithelial cells.
- Normal growth, fetal development, fertility, hematopoiesis and immune function.

Causes of Vitamin A Deficiency

- *Poor intake:* It is endemic in areas such as southern and eastern Asia, where rice, devoid of β-carotene, is the staple food.
- *Malabsorption:* Celiac disease, cystic fibrosis, pancreatic insufficiency, duodenal bypass, chronic diarrhea.

Clinical Features

- Vitamin A deficiency is an important cause of blindness.
- Night blindness is the earliest sign due to an impairment of the dark adaptation process.
- Xerophthalmia (dry eyes) is caused by inadequate function of the lacrimal glands and is characterized by Bitot's spots, corneal xerosis and keratomalacia.
- Bitot's spots: These are glistening white plaques of desquamated thickened conjunctival epithelium, usually triangular in shape and firmly adherent to the conjunctiva.
- Keratomalacia: It is the final consequence of deficiency and leads to corneal ulceration, scarring and irreversible blindness.
- Dermatological abnormalities, such as hyperkeratosis and phrynoderma (follicular hyperkeratosis).
- Impairment of humoral and cell-mediated immunity via direct and indirect effects on the phagocytes and T cells.

Investigations

- Serum retinol level is low.
- A serum RBP (retinol binding protein) is less expensive than a serum retinol study. Level is low in vitamin A deficiency.

Treatment

- For treatment of xerophthalmia, vitamin A is given in three doses. The first dose (2 lakh U) is given immediately on diagnosis, the second on the following day, and the third dose at least two weeks later. If there is vomiting or diarrhea, vitamin A is given by intramuscular injection.
- In countries where vitamin A deficiency is endemic, pregnant women should be advised to eat dark green leafy vegetables and yellow fruits. A single prophylactic oral dose (2 lakh U) is given to pre-school children. Repeated oral administration of these doses to children every 4–6 months is used in some endemic areas.

Q. Vitamin B₁ (thiamine) deficiency.

Q. Beriberi.

Q. Wernicke-Korsakoff syndrome.

Thiamine (vitamin B_1) is found in larger quantities in yeast, legumes, pork, rice, and cereals.

Importance of Thiamine

- Thiamine is required for carbohydrate metabolism. Thiamine pyrophosphate (TPP) is an essential coenzyme in the conversion of pyruvate to acetyl CoA. This is the bridge between glycolysis and the tricarboxylic acid (Krebs) cycle.
- TPP is the coenzyme for transketolase of the pentose phosphate pathway.
- Thiamine is also important for nerve impulse conduction.

Thiamine Deficiency

- Cells cannot metabolize glucose aerobically leading to accumulation of pyruvic and lactic acids, which produce vasodilatation and increased cardiac output. There is also less ATP generation.
- Thiamine deficiency is mainly seen in chronic alcoholics due to poor diet and impaired absorption. Deficiency is also seen in people eating mainly polished rice.

Clinical Features

- *Infantile beriberi* is seen in exclusively breastfed infants of thiaminhe-deficient mothers, and is invariably fatal.
- *Dry beriberi* mainly affects nervous system and is characterized by peripheral neuropathy with wrist and/or foot drop, Wernicke's disease and Korsakoff psychosis. Wernicke's disease is a triad of nystagmus, ophthalmoplegia, and ataxia, along with confusion. Korsakoff's psychosis is impaired short-term memory and confabulation with otherwise grossly normal cognition. These two are almost exclusively seen in alcoholics with thiamine deficiency.
- *Wet beriberi* mainly affects heart and causes congestive cardiac failure with pulmonary and peripheral edema.

Treatment

- Thiamine injection is given for 7 to 14 days IV or IM. Then oral thiamine should be given until full recovery is achieved.
- Korsakoff's psychosis is irreversible and does not respond to thiamine treatment.

Q. Niacin deficiency (pellagra).

- Niacin is an essential component of the coenzymes nicotinamide adenine dinucleotide (NAD) and nicotinamide adenine dinucleotide phosphate (NADP), which are involved in many oxidation-reduction reactions.

- The major food sources of niacin are protein foods, cereals, vegetables, and dairy products. It is also synthesized by the body in small amounts from tryptophan.

Causes of Niacin Deficiency

- Pellagra is now uncommon except in parts of Africa, alcoholics and in patients with anorexia nervosa, or malabsorptive disease.
- Pellagra can occur in Hartnup's disease which is characterized by impaired absorption of tryptophan from which niacin is synthesized.
- It may also be seen in carcinoid syndrome, where tryptophan is utilized for the production of 5-HT rather than the synthesis of niacin.

Deficiency (Pellagra)

- Pellagra (meaning 'raw skin') is characterized by three Ds—**d**ermatitis, **d**iarrhea, and **d**ementia.
- *Dermatitis:* It appears as erythema resembling severe sunburn, symmetrically over the parts of the body exposed to sunlight, particularly the dorsum of hands and feet, and neck are involved (Casal's necklace). Skin lesions are dark, dry, and scaling.
- *Diarrhoea:* It is often associated with glossitis, stomatitis and dysphagia, reflecting the presence of inflammation throughout the gastrointestinal tract.
- *Dementia:* It begins with lethargy, insomnia and irritability, and progresses to confusion, memory loss, hallucinations, and psychosis.

Treatment

- Nicotinamide is given in a dose of 100 mg 8-hourly by mouth or by the parenteral route for 5 days.
- Intake of diet rich in niacin such as meats, milk, peanuts, green leafy vegetables, whole or enriched grains, and brewers' dry yeast.

Q. Vitamin B$_{12}$ deficiency

- Vitamin B$_{12}$ deficiency causes megaloblastic anemia, and neurological degeneration.
- Vitamin B$_{12}$ is required for the integrity of myelin. In severe deficiency, there is demyelination. It may be clinically manifest as peripheral neuropathy or spinal cord degeneration affecting both posterior and lateral columns (subacute combined degeneration of the spinal cord). In addition, there may be cerebral manifestations (resembling dementia) or optic atrophy.
- Treatment is with parenteral hydroxocobalamin.
- Vitamin B$_{12}$ is discussed in detail in hematology chapter.

Q. Vitamin C (ascorbic acid) deficiency; scurvy.

- Vitamin C plays a role in collagen, carnitine, hormone, and amino acid formation. It is essential for wound healing and facilitates recovery from burns. Vitamin C is also an antioxidant, supports immune function, and facilitates the absorption of iron.
- It takes part in the hydroxylation of proline and lysine to hydroxyproline and hydroxylysine which is present in collagen.
- Ascorbic acid is present in fresh fruit and vegetables. It is very easily destroyed by heat. Hence, many traditional cooking methods reduce or eliminate it.

Causes of Deficiency

- Lack of dietary fruit and vegetables >2 months
- Infants fed exclusively on boiled milk
- Severely malnourished individuals
- Drug and alcohol abusers
- Extreme poverty

- Defective formation of collagen impairs wound healing, causes capillary hemorrhage and reduced platelet adhesiveness (normal platelets are rich in ascorbate).

Clinical Features

- Severe deficiency causes scurvy.
- Symptoms develop after weeks to months of vitamin C depletion. Lassitude, weakness, irritability, weight loss, and vague myalgias and arthralgias may develop early.
- Gums become swollen, purple, spongy, friable and bleed easily. Eventually, teeth become loose and avulsed.
- Other features are perifollicular hemorrhages, petechiae and purpura, splinter hemorrhages, hemarthroses, and subperiosteal hemorrhages. Intracerebral hemorrhage can cause death.
- Anemia
- Impaired wound healing

Diagnosis

Diagnosis is based on clinical features. Serum ascorbic acid levels of <0.2 mg/dL (<11 mmol/L) indicate vitamin C deficiency, but this test is not routinely done.

Treatment

- Scurvy is treated with 300–1000 mg of ascorbic acid orally per day.
- Eating raw fruits and vegetables especially citrus fruits.

Q. Fluorosis.

- Excess fluoride consumption (water fluoride content >3 to 5 ppm) can cause fluorosis or hypomineralization of the dental enamel. The mechanism by which excessive fluoride causes fluorosis is not fully understood.
- The earliest signs of fluorosis are chalky-white patches on the surface of the enamel. These patches become stained yellow or brown, producing a characteristic mottled appearance. Severe toxicity weakens the

enamel, pitting its surface and teeth become brittle and easily breakable.

- Other features are sclerosis of the bones, especially of spine, pelvis and limbs. Ligament and tendon calcification also can occur.
- Fluorosis is primarily a cosmetic concern, but it can make the teeth more susceptible to wear and breakage. Fluorosis can be prevented by avoiding excess fluoride consumption (e.g. avoiding swallowing of fluoridated toothpaste or mouthrinses).

Q. Vitamin D deficiency.

- Vitamin D is a fat-soluble vitamin. There are two chemical forms of vitamin D; ergocalciferol (vitamin D_2) and cholecalciferol (vitamin D_3). Ergocalciferol (vitamin D_2) is present in food. Cholecalciferol (Vitamin D_3) is synthesized in the skin on exposure to sunlight from 7-dehydrocholesterol.
- Natural dietary sources of vitamin D include egg yolk, liver, fatty fish, butter and milk.
- Vitamin D is hydroxylated in the liver to 25-hydroxyvitamin D (calcidiol), which is the major circulating form of vitamin D and is the best index of vitamin D levels. Calcidiol is hydroxylated in the kidney to 1, 25-dihydroxyvitamin D (calcitriol), which is the most active form.
- Vitamin D deficiency is present when serum levels of 25-hydroxyvitamin D is less than 20 ng/mL.
- Vitamin D deficiency produces defective mineralization of bone, leading to rickets in children and osteomalacia in adults.
- A minimum intake of 200 IU of vitamin D per day is recommended for adults. For pregnant and lactating women, a minimum of 400 IU per day is recommended.

Actions

- Vitamin D has a variety of actions on calcium, phosphate, and bone metabolism.
- It increases serum calcium and phosphate concentration by increasing intestinal calcium and phosphate absorption, increasing renal calcium reabsorption, and enhancing PTH-mediated bone resorption.

Causes of Vitamin D Deficiency

- Deficient intake
- Inadequate sunlight exposure
- Decreased absorption (small intestine problems, pancreatic insufficiency)
- Loss of vitamin D binding protein (nephrotic syndrome)
- Defective hydroxylation (cirrhosis of liver, renal failure)

Clinical Features of Vitamin D Deficiency

Vitamin D deficiency causes rickets in children and osteomalacia in adults.

Investigations

- Serum vitamin D level will be low. A level of less than 20 ng/mL indicates vitamin D deficiency.
- Serum parathyroid hormone level will be elevated. But PTH measurement is not routinely required.

Treatment of Vitamin D Deficiency

- Initial treatment with 50,000 units of vitamin D_2 or D_3 orally once per week for 6 to 8 weeks, and then 800 to 1000 IU of vitamin D_3 daily thereafter. Vitamin D_3 is better than vitamin D_2 for vitamin D supplementation. Loading dose is not recommended in pregnant women.
- All patients should maintain a daily calcium intake of at least 1000 mg per day.

Q. Rickets.

- Rickets refers to the changes caused by deficient mineralization at the growth plate. It occurs in children. Osteomalacia refers to impaired mineralization of the bone matrix and occurs in adults.
- Hypocalcemic rickets is due to calcium deficiency.

- Hypophosphatemic rickets is due to phosphate deficiency.

Etiology

It is due to vitamin D deficiency.

Clinical Manifestations

Rickets manifests initially at sites of rapid bone growth such as distal forearm, knee, and costochondral junctions (Fig. 7.1).

Skeletal Findings

- Delay in the closure of the fontanelles.
- Parietal and frontal bossing.
- Craniotabes (soft skull bones).
- Enlargement of the costochondral junction visible as beading along the anterolateral aspects of the chest (the 'rachitic rosary').
- Development of Harrison sulcus caused by the muscular pull of the diaphragmatic attachments to the lower ribs.

- Enlargement of the wrist and bowing of the distal radius and ulna.
- Progressive lateral bowing of the femur and tibia.

Extraskeletal Findings

- Decreased muscle tone, seizures, increased sweating and hypoplasia of the dental enamel are seen in hypocalcemic rickets.
- Abscesses of the teeth occur in hypophosphatemic rickets.

Laboratory Findings

- Alkaline phosphatase is markedly increased.
- Serum calcium concentration is low in hypocalcemic rickets.
- Serum concentration of 25-hydroxyvitamin D is low in vitamin D deficiency.
- *Radiographic findings:* The shafts of the long bones are osteopenic, with thin cortex.

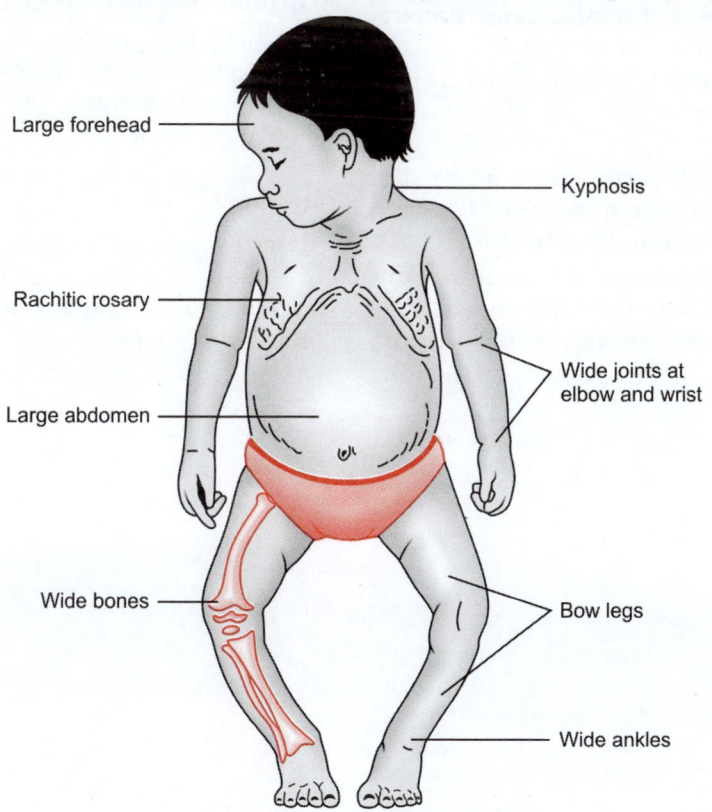

Large forehead

Rachitic rosary

Large abdomen

Wide bones

Kyphosis

Wide joints at elbow and wrist

Bow legs

Wide ankles

Fig. 7.1: Clinical features of rickets

Trabecular pattern is reduced and becomes coarse. Bone deformities are usually present and in severe rickets, pathological fractures and Looser zones may be noted.

Treatment

- Rickets caused by vitamin D deficiency is treated with vitamin D_2 or vitamin D_3 and calcium supplementation daily. After 3–4 months, the dose of vitamin D is reduced to a maintenance level.
- Treatment of hypophosphatemic rickets is with phosphate supplements, combined with vitamin D to promote intestinal calcium and phosphate absorption.

Q. Vitamin K.

- The name 'K' comes from the German/ Danish word koagulations vitamin (clotting vitamin). Vitamin K plays an important role in coagulation by acting as a cofactor for the post-translational carboxylation of coagulation factors II, VII, IX, and X. Without carboxylation, coagulation reactions occur slowly and hemostasis is impaired.
- Vitamin K is primarily supplied by diet (green vegetables like spinach and broccoli) and synthesis by intestinal bacteria.
- Vitamin K is a fat-soluble vitamin. Pancreatic and biliary functions need to be intact for proper vitamin K absorption.

Dietary vitamin K is protein-bound and requires pancreatic enzymes in the small intestine for liberation. Bile salts then solubilize vitamin K into luminal micelles for absorption.
- Deficiency develops because of inadequate diet, use of broad-spectrum antibiotics, liver and pancreatic disorders. A patient not taking orally and is put on broad spectrum antibiotics can develop vitamin K deficiency in as little as 1 week.

Clinical Features

There are no specific clinical features. Bleeding can occur at any site. Vitamin K deficiency is common in the newborn and can manifest as hemorrhagic disease of the newborn. Hence, parenteral vitamin K is given routinely to newborns.

Laboratory Findings

- In mild vitamin K deficiency, only the PT is prolonged.
- In severe vitamin K deficiency, both PT and PTT are prolonged, but PT is more prolonged than aPTT.

Treatment

Vitamin K should be replaced parenterally either subcutaneously or intravenously. A single dose of 15 mg will completely correct laboratory abnormalities in 12–24 hours.

Nervous System

Q. Define coma. How do you examine and manage a case of coma?

Coma is a clinical state in which patient is unresponsive to external stimulation and unarouseable (unarousable unresponsiveness).

Mechanisms of Coma

Consciousness is maintained by an interaction of reticular activating system of brainstem and cerebral cortex. Hence, altered consciousness including coma can be produced by any pathology in the brainstem, reticular formation and cerebral cortex.

Causes of Coma

Diffuse brain dysfunction
- Drug overdose (sedatives, anesthetic agents, alcohol)
- Hypoglycemia
- Hyperglycemia (DKA, HHS)
- Hypoxic/ischemic brain injury
- Uremia
- Hepatic failure
- Respiratory failure
- Electrolyte imbalances (hypercalcemia, hypocalcemia, hyponatremia, hyperntremia)
- Hypothyroidism

- Head injury
- Infections (encephalitis, meningitis, cerebral malaria, sepsis)

Brainstem problems
- Brainstem hemorrhage or infarction

Examination of a Patient with Coma

Immediate Assessment
- Take care of CABs first (circulation, airway, breathing).
- Get a quick short history from those who brought the patient. Many patients with diabetes, epilepsy or hypoadrenalism, carry identification which may give clue about the cause of coma.
- Record depth of coma by using Glasgow Coma Scale.
- Next go for full general and neurological examination.

General Examination
- Many general examination findings may provide clues to the cause of coma.
- *Temperature:* Body temperature is high in infection and hyperpyrexia, and low in hypothermia and hypothyroisism. Pontine hemorrhage also can cause elevated body temperature.
- *Cyanosis:* Coma may be due to respiratory failure or cardiac failure.

- *Jaundice:* Coma may be due to liver failure, sepsis.
- *Petechiae and purpura:* Coma may be due to intracranial bleed due to some bleeding or clotting disorder.
- *Hyperpigmentation:* Coma may be due to Addison's disease.
- *Injection marks:* Coma may be due to drug abuse.
- *Coarse and dry skin:* Coma may be due to hypothyroidism.
- *Breathing:* Look for smell of ketones, alcohol, or ammonia. Arsenic poisoning produces the odor of garlic. OP compound poisoning produces kerosene smell. *Kussmaul (acidotic) respiration* is deep, sighing hyperventilation seen in diabetic ketoacidosis and uremia.

Neurological Examination in Coma

- *Head, neck, and spine:* Note trauma, skull burr-holes and bruits, neck stiffness.
- *Pupils:* Check size and reaction to light. Unilateral dilated pupil indicates compression of the third nerve due to temporal lobe uncus herniation (coning). This happens in raised intracranial pressure on one side (e.g. an extradural hematoma). Bilateral fixed, dilated pupils are seen in brainstem death, and deep coma of any cause. Bilateral pinpoint pupils are seen in pontine lesions (e.g. a pontine hemorrhage) and opioid intoxication.
- *Fundi:* Presence of papilledema suggests raised intracranial tension. Look for retinal hemorrhage.
- *Ocular movements:* Vestibulo-ocular reflexes. Passive head turning produces conjugate ocular deviation away from the direction of rotation (doll's eye reflex). This reflex is absent in deep coma and brainstem lesions. In *caloric stimulation test,* ocular deviation towards the irrigated ear is seen when ice-cold water is irrigated into the external auditory meatus. This is also absent in brainstem death.

- *Abnormalities of conjugate gaze: Lateral deviation* occurs towards a destructive frontal lesion. Rarely, an irritative lesion in one frontal lobe can make the eyes deviate to opposite side. In a pontine lesion, conjugate lateral deviation occurs away from the lesion. *Skew deviation* (one eye deviated up and the other down) indicates a brainstem or cerebellar lesion.
- *Other findings:* Look for any asymmetry in tone, reflexes and plantar responses.

Cardiac Examination

Cardiac diseases such as atrial fibrillation, infective endocarditis, MI, etc. can produce embolic stroke and cause coma.

Abdominal Examination

Look for abnormal bowel sounds, organomegaly, masses, and ascites. Bowel sounds are absent in an acute abdominal condition, as well as with anticholinergic poisoning. Increased bowel sounds occur in organophosphorus compound poisoning. Hepatomegaly is seen in hepatoma or metastatic disease which indirectly suggests brain metastases as the cause of coma. Look for evidence of cirrhosis such as ascites and splenomegaly which suggests hepatic encephalopathy as the cause of coma.

Respiratory System Examination

Look for evidence of COPD, pneumonia or any other lung disease which can produce respiratory failure and coma.

Investigations

- Tests should be chosen according to the clues available from history and examination.
- Routine biochemistry (urea, creatinine, electrolytes, glucose, calcium, liver function tests)
- Metabolic and endocrine studies (TSH, serum cortisol)

- Blood cultures, malaria test to rule out cerebral malaria and sepsis.
- Drugs screen (e.g. diazepam, narcotics, etc.).
- Urine examination for ketone bodies.
- Arterial blood gas analysis (hypoxia and hypercarbia can cause coma).
- *Imaging:* CT or MRI brain should be done to rule out any intracranial pathology.
- *CSF examination:* This is helpful to rule out meningitis and subarachnoid hemorrhage.
- *Electroencephalography:* EEG is of some value in the diagnosis of metabolic coma, encephalitis and ongoing non-convulsive seizures.

Management

- The underlying cause of coma should be treated. For example, correction of blood glucose in hypoglycemia.
- Ryle's tube (for feeding purpose) and a urinary catheter should be passed.
- Skin care—frequent turning of patient to avoid pressure sores. Patient should be kept preferably in waterbed to prevent pressure sores.
- Oral hygiene—mouth washes, frequent suction.
- Eye care—taping of lids, prevention of corneal damage by applying lubricating eye drops and eye ointment.
- Nutrition and hydration—food and water may be given through Ryle's tube. I.V. fluids may also be used, if required.

Q. Enumerate the causes of headache.

- Headache is a very common complaint reported by patients. Most people experience headache at least once during their life.
- Most causes of headache are benign, but rarely headache can be due to potentially life-threatening central nervous system (CNS) diseases such as brain tumor, intracranial hemorrhage, etc.

Causes of Headache

Primary Headache Disorders (There is no Definite Cause)

- Migraine
- Tension headache
- Cluster headache

Secondary Headache Disorders (There is a Definite Cause)

- Subarachnoid hemorrhage
- Intracranial space occupying lesion (brain abscess, tumor, hematoma, AV malformation)
- Cortical vein thrombosis
- Severe hypertension
- Meningitis
- Temporal arteritis
- Glaucoma
- Sinusitis

Q. Describe the classification, pathophysiology, clinical features and treatment of migraine headache.

- Migraine is recurrent headache associated with visual and gastrointestinal disturbance. Though migraine is a benign headache, attacks of headache are usually severe.
- Migraine can be classified into three types:
  1. Migraine with aura (old term: Classic migraine)
  2. Migraine without aura (old term: Common migraine)
  3. Migraine variants (retinal migraine, ophthalmoplegic migraine, familial hemiplegic migraine, basilar migraine).

Epidemiology

The prevalence of migraine is high. It is three times more common in women than men. It tends to run in families, and more common in young females. Migraine without aura (common migraine) is the most common type (80% of all migraine cases).

Pathophysiology

- The exact cause of migraine is unknown. However, various theories have been put forward and various brain abnormalities have been found in patients with migraine.
- Migraine has a strong genetic component. Approximately 70% of migraine patients have a first-degree relative with a history of migraine.
- Migraine was previously thought to be a vascular phenomenon that resulted from intracranial vasoconstriction followed by rebound vasodilation. Currently, however, the neurovascular theory considers migraine as primarily a neurogenic process with secondary changes in cerebral perfusion associated with a sterile neurogenic inflammation.
- Migrainers have been found to have neuronal hyperexcitability in the cerebral cortex, especially in the occipital cortex.

Migraine Precipitants

Various precipitants of migraine have been identified, which are as follows:

- Stress
- Excessive or insufficient sleep
- Excessive exercise
- Eye strain or other visual triggers
- Exposure to bright or fluorescent lighting
- Loud noises
- Strong odors (e.g. perfumes, colognes, petroleum distillates)
- Certain food items (ice-cream, chocolate, cheese).

Clinical Features

Three phases of migraine can be recognized:

- *Premonitory symptoms:* precede an attack of migraine. These include fatigue, concentration difficulty, sensitivity to light or sound, nausea, blurred vision, yawning, etc.
- *Aura:* Migraine aura is a transient neurologic symptom due to transient focal neurological dysfunction. Auras typically occur before the onset of migraine headache, and the headache usually begins simultaneously with or just after the end of the aura phase. Most auras last for less than one hour. Auras can be visual disturbances (blurring of vision, fortification spectra, light flashes), sensory symptoms, motor weakness and speech disturbances.
- *Headache:* It is usually unilateral, severe and throbbing type. Headache is aggravated by routine physical activity such as walking or climbing stairs. It may be associated with nausea or vomiting. Patient prefers to lie down in a dark and silent room.

Investigations

- Migraine is a clinical diagnosis. Hence, investigations are ordered, only if an organic pathology is suspected or to rule out any comorbid illness.
- *Complete blood count:* To rule out anemia. High ESR is seen in giant cell arteritis (temporal arteritis) which can mimick migraine.
- *Neuroimaging (CT or MRI of head):* This is not routinely necessary. It is sometimes indicated to rule out intracranial pathology such as brain tumors.

Management

Treatment of an Acute Attack

- Paracetamol or any other simple analgesics should be given, with an antiemetic such as metoclopramide, if necessary. Analgesics are more effective, if started in the beginning of headache.
- Triptans (5-HT, agonists) can also abort an attack. These include sumatriptan, zolmitriptan, naratriptan and rizatriptan.
- During an attack, rest in a dark and quiet room.

Prophylaxis

- Avoid precipitating factors.
- The following drugs are used to prevent migraine attacks, if they are very frequent:

– *Beta-blockers* such as atenolol, metoprolol, and propranolol. Propranolol 10 mg three times daily, increasing to 40–80 mg three times daily.

– *Antidepressants*: Amitriptyline, clomipramine, mirtazapine.

– *Calcium channel blockers:* Verapamil, nifedipine

– *Antiepileptics:* Sodium valproate, topiramate.

Q. Enumerate the causes of facial pain.

Q. Discuss the etiology, clinical features and management of trigeminal neuralgia.

Causes of Facial Pain

- Trigeminal neuralgia
- Post-herpetic neuralgia
- Glossopharyngeal neuralgia
- Occipital neuralgia
- Superior laryngeal neuralgia
- Carotodynia
- Carotid artery dissection
- Post-traumatic facial pain
- Sinusitis
- Dental pain
- Cancer

TRIGEMINAL NEURALGIA (TIC DOULOUREUX)

Trigeminal neuralgia (TN) is sudden, usually unilateral, severe, brief, stabbing or lancinating, recurrent episodes of pain in the distribution of one or more branches of the trigeminal nerve.

Epidemiology

- The annual incidence of TN is 4 to 5 per lakh population.
- It is one of the most common cause of facial pain in the elderly. Most cases begin after age 50.
- It is slightly more common in women.

Etiopathogenesis

- Most cases of trigeminal neuralgia are caused by compression of the trigeminal nerve root.
- Compression by an aberrant loop of an artery or vein accounts for 80 to 90% of cases. Other causes of nerve compression include acoustic neuroma, meningioma, epidermoid cyst, saccular aneurysm or arteriovenous malformation.
- Compression leads to demyelination of the nerve in the area around the compression. Demyelination results in ectopic impulse generation and crossing of impulses between fibres. Touch sensation impulses may cross into fibers carrying pain sensation and lead to pain.
- Demyelination may also be caused by multiple sclerosis and lead to trigeminal neuralgia.

Clinical Features

- The pain of trigeminal neuralgia occurs in paroxysms and is maximal at the onset.
- The pain is described as 'electric shock-like' or 'stabbing' and is unilateral in most cases.
- It usually lasts from one to several seconds, and does not awaken the patient at night. Episodes may last weeks or months.
- Facial muscle spasms can be seen with severe pain. This finding gave rise to the older term for this disorder, 'tic douloureux.'
- Trigger zones in the distribution of the affected nerve may be present; lightly touching these areas often triggers an attack. Other triggers include chewing, talking, brushing teeth, cold air, smiling, and shaving.

Investigations

Magnetic resonance imaging/magnetic resonance angiography (MRI/MRA) can identify demyelinating lesions, a mass lesion in the cerebellopontine angle, or an ectatic blood vessel which may be responsible for trigeminal neuralgia.

Treatment

Medical Therapy

Pharmacological therapy is the initial treatment for most patients with trigeminal neuralgia that is not caused by a structural lesion. Treatment consists of drugs such as carbamazepine, sodium valproate, phenytoin, baclofen, or clonazepam. Newer antiepileptic drugs such as gabapentin, lamotrigine, and topiramate are also effective. Patients who fail to respond to medication should be considered for microvascular decompression surgery.

Surgical Therapy

A variety of surgical procedures may relieve symptoms in patients refractory to drug therapy. These include, microvascular decompression (involves the removal or separation of vascular structures from the trigeminal nerve). Percutaneous radiofrequency rhizotomy creates a lesion in the trigeminal ganglion by application of heat. The lesion is thought to selectively destroy pain impulses carried by unmyelinated or thinly myelinated fibers.

> **Q. Describe the course of facial nerve. Enumerate the causes and clinical features of facial nerve palsy at various levels.**

Facial nerve is a mixed nerve, but predominantly motor. It contains:

- Motor fibers to the facial muscles.
- Parasympathetic fibers to the lacrimal, submandibular, and sublingual salivary glands.
- Afferent fibers for taste from the anterior two-thirds of the tongue.
- Somatic afferents from the external auditory canal and pinna.

Course of Facial Nerve (Figs 8.1 and 8.2)

- Facial nerve arises from its motor nucleus in the pons. The part of nucleus which supplies upper face has bilateral hemispheric representation. Hence, in unilateral

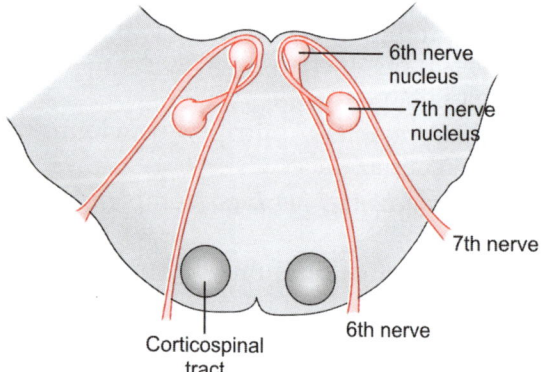

Fig. 8.1: Cross-section of pons showing origin of facial nerve

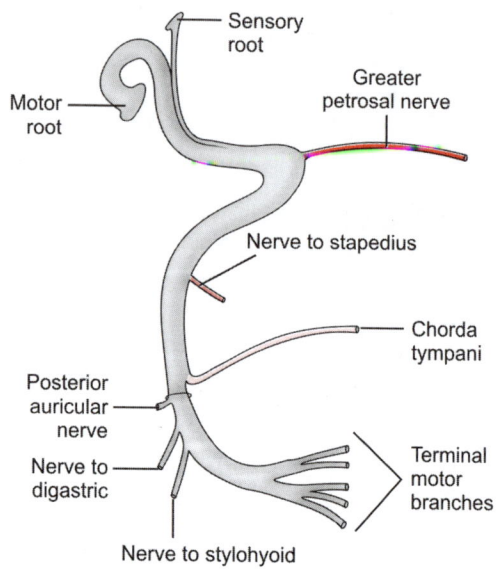

Fig. 8.2: Branches of facial nerve

UMN lesion of the facial nerve the upper part of the face is spared.

- Its fibers hook around the abducens nucleus (6th nerve) and then emerge from the lateral border of the pons.
- The nerve enters the internal auditory meatus along with eighth nerve and nervus intermedius.
- In the anterior part of inner ear, it bends downwards and anteriorly to enter facial canal.
- In the facial canal, it gives rise to greater petrosal nerve which supplies lacrimal

glands and a branch to the stapedius muscle and is later joined by the chorda tympani nerve. During its course through the facial canal of temporal bone, the nerve is related to the labyrinth, the ossicles and the mastoid air cells.

- It leaves the temporal bone through the stylomastoid foramen and passes anteriorly through the parotid gland to divide into its peripheral branches.
- Facial nerve has a small sensory component. Taste sensation from anterior two-thirds of the tongue and sensation of the external auditory canal are supplied by facial nerve. The taste fibres run through the lingual nerve and then join the chorda tympani which in turn joins the facial nerve in the facial canal distal to the geniculate ganglion. Finally, the tatse fibres enter the pons through the nervus intermedius to end in the nucleus tractus solitarius.

Clinical Features of LMN Facial Palsy

- Unilateral LMN lesion causes weakness of both upper and lower face on the same side of lesion.
- Drooping of angle of mouth, dribbling of saliva from the angle of mouth, deviation of mouth to normal side.
- There is weakness of frowning (frontalis) and of eye closure since upper facial muscles are weak.
- Corneal exposure and ulceration may occur due to inability of the eyes to close during sleep.
- The platysma muscle is also weak.

Clinical Features of UMN Facial Palsy

- In UMN lesions only the lower part of face is affected and upper part is spared because of bilateral hemispheric representation. Hence, raising eyebrows, wrinkling of

Table 8.1: Causes and clinical features of facial nerve lesions at various levels

Level	Causes	Clinical features
Supranuclear	tumors, abscess, vascular events (infarction and hemorrhage)	Contralateral UMN facial palsy
At the level of pons (nucleus)	Pontine tumors (e.g. glioma), demyelination, vascular lesions (hemorrhage, infarct), poliomyelitis, motor neurone disease.	Ipsilateral LMN facial palsy. Lesions in the pons also affect abduscent nerve producing lateral rectus palsy leading to convergent squint. Contralateral hemiparesis due to corticospinal tract involvement.
At cerebellopontine angle (CPA)	Acoustic neuroma, meningioma and secondary neoplasm.	Fifth, sixth, eighth and cerebellum are also affected with the facial nerve because all are close together in the CPA. Produces ipsilateral LMN facial palsy, sensorineural deafness, loss of corneal reflex, and ipsilateral cerebellar signs.
At petrous temporal bone	Bell's palsy, trauma, middle ear infection, herpes zoster (Ramsay Hunt syndrome), and tumors (e.g. glomus tumor).	Ipsilateral LMN facial palsy, loss of taste on the anterior two-thirds of the tongue and hyperacusis (loud noise distortion due to paralysis of stapedius)
At the level of skull base and parotid gland	Paget's disease of bone, parotid gland tumors, mumps, sarcoidosis, trauma, and Guillain-Barre syndrome.	Ipsilateral LMN facial palsy with intact taste sensation.

forehead, eye closure and blinking are all preserved.
- Clinical features in the lower part of the face are same as those described in LMN facial palsy.

Q. Discuss the etiology, clinical features, investigations and management of Bell's palsy.

Bell's palsy is an acute, LMN type facial palsy.

Etiology

- Exact cause is unknown.
- It is thought to be due to a viral (often herpes simplex) infection that causes swelling of the nerve within the petrous temporal bone and stylomastoid foramen leading to compression of the nerve.

Clinical Features

- Patient notices sudden unilateral facial weakness.
- Weakness is LMN type (see above for clinical features of LMN facial palsy). Bell's phenomenon is uprolling of eyeballs when patient tries to close the eyes.
- Weakness progresses over hours or several days. Spontaneous recovery usually starts in the second week. Complete recovery may take 12 months.
- Some patients may be left with residual weakness.

Investigations

- *Nerve conduction studies:* Such as electromyograph (EMG) and nerve conduction studies can be used to assess the severity of lesion and chances of recovery.
- *Imaging studies:* CT scanning and MRI can be used to rule out other causes of facial palsy such as tumors or vascular events. Pathological geniculate ganglion enhancement is seen in Bell's palsy.

Treatment

- Steroids (prednisolone 60 mg daily tapered over 10 days) with acyclovir have been shown to be more effective than either of these drugs alone.
- Eyes should be protected by applying artificial tears or tarsorrhaphy (suturing the upper to lower eyelid).
- Facial nerve stimulation is useful within 2 weeks, if surgical decompression is planned. Severe degeneration of the facial nerve is irreversible after 2 to 3 weeks.
- Surgical decompression of the facial nerve is not a currently recommended treatment. Decompression may be of benefit in patients with profound nerve dysfunction.

Q. Classify and enumerate the causes of meningitis.

Meningitis is an inflammatory disease of the arachnoid mater and the cerebrospinal fluid (Table 8.2).

Table 8.2: Causes of meningitis	
Bacteria	**Spirochetal**
• *Neisseria meningitidis*	• Leptospirosis
• *Streptococcus pneumoniae*	• Lyme disease
• *H. influenzae*	• Syphilis
• *Mycobacterium tuberculosis*	
Viruses	**Rickettsial**
• Herpes simplex	• Typhus fever
• Epstein-Barr virus	
Fungi	**Protozoal**
• *Cryptococcus neoformans*	• Naegleria
• Candida	

Q. Describe the etiology, clinical features, investigations and management of acute pyogenic meningitis (acute bacterial meningitis).

Q. Causes of neck stiffness.

Etiology

Common Organisms
- *Neisseria meningitidis*
- *Streptococcus pneumoniae*
- *H. influenzae.*

Uncommon Organisms
- *Staphylococcus aureus*
- *Listeria monocytogenes*
- *Klebsiella*
- *Pseudomonas*
- *Salmonella*
- *Neisseria gonorrhoeae*

Pathogenesis
- The organism responsible for meningitis can reach the CSF via three routes: (1) Colonization of the nasopharynx with subsequent bloodstream invasion and subsequent central nervous system (CNS) invasion, (2) invasion of the CNS following bacteremia due to a localized source, such as pneumonia, infective endocarditis or a urinary tract infection, (3) direct entry of organisms into the CNS from a contiguous infection (e.g. sinuses, mastoid), trauma, or neurosurgery.
- There are many steps involved before frank meningitis develops such as colonization of the host mucosal epithelium by pathogens, invasion into bloodstream, crossing of the blood–brain barrier, and multiplication within the CSF.
- Much of the damage from meningitis results from cytokines (interleukin-1, interleukin-6, and tumor necrosis factor-alpha) released within the CSF due to inflammatory response. Once inflammation is initiated, a series of injuries occur to the endothelium of the blood–brain barrier (e.g. separation of intercellular tight junctions) that result in vasogenic brain edema, loss of cerebrovascular autoregulation, and increased intracranial pressure. This results in localized areas of brain ischemia, cytotoxic injury, and neuronal apoptosis. All these pathologic changes manifest clinically as coma, seizures, deafness, and motor, sensory, and cognitive deficits.

Predisposing Factors
- Immunodeficient states: Asplenism, complement deficiency, corticosteroid excess, diabetes mellitus, chronic alcoholism and HIV infection.
- Acute otitis media.
- Recent exposure to someone with meningitis.
- Recent travel, particularly to areas with endemic meningococcal disease.
- Injection drug use.
- Recent head trauma with CSF otorrhea or rhinorrhea.

Clinical Features
- Patients with bacterial meningitis usually appear ill. The classic triad of acute bacterial meningitis consists of fever, neck rigidity, and altered mental status.
- Patients are usually febrile.
- Headache is also common and is diffuse and severe.
- *Neck stiffness:* Spasm of neck muscles on attempted flexion.
- *Kernig's sign:* Extension of knee from flexed thigh position causes passive resistance. This is due to the spasm of hamstring muscles due to the inflamed sciatic nerve as it passes through the spinal theca.
- Other manifestations include photophobia, seizures, focal neurologic deficits (including cranial nerve palsies), and papilledema.
- Certain bacteria, particularly *N. meningitidis*, can cause characteristic skin manifestations, such as petechiae and palpable purpura.

- Arthritis occurs in some patients with bacterial meningitis.

Investigations

- *Blood counts:* WBC count is often elevated with a left shift.
- *Blood cultures:* Blood cultures may be able to identify the causative organism in 50 to 75% of patients with bacterial meningitis.
- *Lumbar puncture and CSF analysis:* This is the test of choice to diagnose meningitis. Every patient with suspected meningitis should have LP done unless the procedure is contraindicated. CSF should be sent for protein, sugar, cell count, cell type, Gram's stain, India ink stain, culture sensitivity, AFB stain and culture and PCR studies. Opening pressure should be noted at the time of LP (Table 8.3).
- *CT scan head*: A contrast CT of brain shows meningeal enhancement in meningitis. It is also helpful to rule out other pathologies such as subarachnoid hemorrhage, cerebral abscess, mass lesion, middle ear and sinus disease.

Treatment

Bacterial meningitis is a medical emergency and treatment should be started as soon as it is suspected. The mortality rate of untreated disease approaches 100%.

Empiric Antibiotic Therapy

- Pending identification of the causative organism, empiric antibiotic therapy should be started. Antibiotics should be given intravenously.
- Third-generation cephalosporins, such as cefotaxime and ceftriaxone, are the drugs of choice for this purpose because they have good CSF penetration and also good activity against pathogens.
- Antibiotics can be changed later based on the specific organism causing meningitis.

Role of Steroids in Meningitis

- Trials have shown that dexamethasone given shortly before or at the same time as the first dose of antibiotics significantly improves outcomes in patients with meningitis.
- Dexamethasone reduces CSF synthesis of cytokines (such as tumor necrosis factor-alpha and interleukin-1), CSF inflammation, and cerebral edema which are responsible for much of the damage and sequelae.

Complications of Meningitis

- Obstructive hydrocephalus
- Seizures
- Intellectual impairment
- Deafness and cranial nerve palsies
- Subdural abscess.

	Normal	Viral meningitis	Pyogenic meningitis	Tuberculous meningitis
Appearance	Crystal-clear	Clear/turbid	Turbid/purulent	Turbid/viscous
Pressure	60 to 200 mm of CSF	Normal	Increased	Increased
WBC count	<5/mm^3, all lymphocytes	10–300/mm^3 Lymphocyte predominant	100–5000; >80% neutrophils	100–500/mm^3, most are lymphocytes
Protein	Less than 50 mg/dL	Increased	Increased	Increased >100
Glucose	40–60% of blood glucose	Normal	Low	Low

Table 8.3: CSF findings in meningitis of different etiology

- Septic shock
- ARDS
- DIC.

Q. Describe the etiology, clinical features, investigations and management of tuberculous meningitis (TBM).

Etiology

Mycobacterium tuberculosis.

Pathophysiology

- TBM develops in 2 steps. In the first step, *Mycobacterium tuberculosis* bacilli enter the host by droplet inhalation, and are phagocytosed by alveolar macrophages. Subsequently bacilli spread to regional lymph nodes to produce the primary complex. During this stage, bacteremia occurs and the tubercle bacilli seed many organs. In persons who develop TBM, bacilli seed to the meninges or brain parenchyma, resulting in the formation of subpial or subependymal foci of caseous lesions (tubercles).
- The second step in the development of TBM is an increase in size of a caseous lesions until it ruptures into the subarachnoid space. Tubercles (Rich focus) rupturing into the subarachnoid space cause meningitis. Those deeper in the brain or spinal cord parenchyma cause tuberculomas or abscesses. A severe inflammatory response is elicited by mycobacterial components. A thick exudate, phlebitis, arteritis, thrombosis, infarction and obstruction of CSF flow are common findings. Basal meningitis accounts for the frequent dysfunction of cranial nerves (CNs) III, VI, and VII, eventually leading to obstructive hydrocephalus from obstruction of basilar cisterns.

Clinical Features

- TBM presents as a subacute febrile illness which may progress through three phases:

1. *Prodromal phase:* Lasts 2 to 3 weeks. There is insidious onset of malaise, lassitude, headache, low-grade fever, and personality change.
2. *Meningitic phase:* Characterized by signs of meningeal irritation, headache, vomiting, lethargy, confusion, and cranial nerve palsies.
3. *Paralytic phase:* Confusion progresses to stupor and coma. Seizures and hemiparesis can occur.

- Fundoscopic examination often shows choroidal tubercles.
- If untreated, death occurs within 5 to 8 weeks of the onset of illness.

Diagnosis

- *CSF examination:* CSF shows elevated protein and decreased glucose concentration with predominant lymphocytosis. The demonstration of acid-fast bacilli (AFB) in the CSF remains the most rapid and effective means of reaching an early diagnosis. PCR for AFB should be sent in all suspectd cases of TB meningitis.
- *Brain imaging:* CT scan head may show meningeal enhancements especially basal meninges. Obstructive hydrocephalus may be present. MRI has more sensitivity in detecting the distribution of meningeal inflammatory exudates.
- *Montoux test:* It is usually positive.
- *Chest X-ray:* It may show evidence of pulmonary tuberculosis.
- *Other tests:* HIV test to rule out immunocomromised state, blood sugar, electrolytes, LFT, RFT, and CBP with ESR.

Treatment

- Antituberculous therapy should be started. Treatment involves initial two-month period of intensive therapy, with 4 drugs (isoniazid, rifampicin, pyrazinamide and ethambutol). This is followed by a continuation phase lasting 7 to 10 months, with two drugs (isoniazid, rifampicin).

- Steroids should be given to all patients with TB meningitis. Dexamethasone is given at a dose of 12 mg/day in divided doses or prednisone at a dose of 60 mg/day. Steroids should be given in full dose for 3 weeks, and then tapered off gradually over the following 3 weeks.
- *Surgery:* Patients with hydrocephalus may require surgical decompression to reduce raised intracranial pressure.

Q. Discuss the classification, etiology, clinical features, investigations and management of epilepsy.

Q. Discuss the etiology, clinical features, investigations and management of grand mal epilepsy (GTCS=generalized tonic clonic seizures).

- A seizure is a transient disturbance of cerebral function due to an abnormal paroxysmal neuronal discharge in the brain.
- Epilepsy is defined as a neurological condition characterized by recurrent epileptic seizures. Traditionally, the diagnosis of epilepsy requires the occurrence of at least two unprovoked seizures.
- Epilepsy is common and its prevalence is about 4 to 8%.

Etiology

The *etiology* of epilepsy is usually multifactorial. Both hereditary and environmental factors play a role. Following are the common causes of epilepsy.

- Idiopathic (commonest cause)
- Birth trauma
- Cerebral anoxia
- Developmental abnormalities (e.g. microcephaly, porencephaly)
- Metabolic abnormalities (e.g. hypocalcemia, hypoglycemia, hypomagnesemia, hyponatremia, uremia, hepatic encephalopathy)

- Infections (meningitis, tuberculosis, congenital syphilis, parasitic infestations)
- Head injury
- Neoplasm
- Cerebrovascular disease

Pathophysiology of a Seizure

- Seizures develop when the balance between excitatory and inhibitory mechanisms is disturbed at the cellular or the synaptic level. Glutamate is the most common excitatory neurotransmitter and gamma-aminobutyric acid (GABA) is the inhibitory neurotransmitter involved. Failure of inhibitory processes is thought to be the major mechanism leading to status epilepticus.
- Spread of electrical activity between neurons is normally restricted. During a seizure, large groups of neurons are activated repetitively and unrestrictedly. Inhibitory synaptic activity between neurons fails. This produces high-voltage spike-and-wave EEG activity, the electrophysiological hallmark of epilepsy.
- A focal (partial) seizure is epileptic activity confined to one area of cortex. Focal seizure can spread and involve all parts of the brain. This is called focal seizure with secondary generalization. Seizure can be generalized from the onset. This is called primary generalized seizure.
- Neuronal death occurs with prolonged seizures due to abnormal neuronal discharges. Neuronal death probably occurs due to the inability to handle large increases in intracellular calcium brought about by prolonged exposure to excitatory neurotransmitters.

Classification

There are various classifications of seizures. Following is the latest classification of seizures. In the new classification, the word 'focal' is used instead of 'partial'.

Focal onset seizures

- Simple focal seizures (consciousness preserved)
- Complex focal seizures (consciousness is impaired)
- Focal seizures evolving into secondarily generalized seizure

Generalized onset seizures

- Absence seizures
- Myoclonic seizures
- Clonic seizures
- Tonic seizures
- Primary generalized tonic-clonic seizures
- Atonic seizures

Status epilepticus

- Tonic-clonic status
- Focal status
- Absence status

Clinical Features

Focal Onset Seizures

Simple focal seizures

- Involve a part of the brain and consciousness is not lost.
- Simple focal seizure can be motor, sensory, psychic or associated with autonomic symptoms.
- A simple motor seizure may consist of jerking of one hand or twitching of one-half of the face.

Complex focal seizures

- These also involve a part of the brain but consciousness is impaired or lost. Most of these seizures arise in the temporal lobe.
- A motionless stare with altered consciousness followed by automatisms is the usual pattern. Automatisms are repetitive, purposeless, complex movements such as picking at clothes, smacking lips or swallowing. EEG usually shows abnormal spikes in the area where the seizures originate.

Focal seizures evolving into secondarily generalized seizures

- Here the seizures start in a focal area of the brain and then spread to involve the whole brain to become generalized seizure.
- *'Jacksonian march'* refers to orderly progression of focal seizure due to the spread of seizure in the cerebral cortex (e.g. from thumb to fingers to face to leg).

Generalized Onset Seizures (Non-focal Origin)

Absence seizures: Absence seizures involve brief, sudden lapses of consciousness. There is no aura or postictal confusion. Absence seizures are more common in children and there is significant inherited predisposition for absence seizures.

Myoclonic seizures: Myoclonic seizures consist of brief jerking motor movements that last less than 1 second and often cluster within a few minutes. It can involve any part of the body, but is mostly seen in limbs or facial muscles. If the seizures evolve into rhythmic jerking movements, they are classified as clonic seizure.

Clonic seizures: Clonic seizures consist of rhythmic jerking motor movements. They can be focal or generalized.

Tonic seizures: These are associated with intense stiffening of the body. There is no convulsive jerking. They occur most often during sleep, usually in children.

Generalized tonic-clonic seizures (earlier called grand mal seizures)

- These begin with sudden loss of consciousness.
- All muscles of the arms and legs as well as the chest and back become stiff which is called tonic phase. The patient may begin to appear cyanotic during this tonic phase. A loud cry may occur in the tonic phase as air is forcibly expelled across constricted vocal cords. Incontinence of urine and feces may occur.

- After approximately one minute, there is synchronous clonic muscle jerking.

Atonic seizures: Sudden loss of postural tone, with falling and loss of consciousness.

Investigations

CT or MRI scan of brain: CT or MRI scan should be done to exclude a structural brain lesion which could be the cause of seizures.

Electroencephalography (EEG): EEG is an essential study in the evaluation of epileptic seizures. It can help confirm the diagnosis and also differentiate between generalized and partial seizures. Use of provocation techniques such as sleep deprivation, hyperventilation and intermittent photic stimulation increases the sensitivity of EEG.

Prolactin levels: Serum prolactin concentration may rise and remain elevated for up to 6 hours after an epileptic attack.

Lumbar puncture

- This is helpful to exclude CNS infections such as meningitis, if there are clinical features suggestive of meningitis along with seizures.
- It should be done only after a space occupying brain lesion has been excluded by neuroimaging.

Treatment

During an Attack

- Put the patient in a safe place away from fire and sharp objects.
- Put the patient in lateral position and insert a padded mouth gag.
- Inj lorazepam 4 mg slow IV, or inj diazepam 10 mg slow IV.

Treatment of Underlying Condition

For example, correcting hypocalcemia or hypoglycemia; removal of a structural lesion such as brain tumor, vascular malformation, or brain abscess.

Antiepileptic Drug Therapy

- Antiepileptics are indicated in people with 2 or more episodes of seizures. Choice of antiepileptic drug depends on the type of epilepsy.
- Antiepileptics should be introduced slowly to minimize side effects, and gradually increased to achieve the therapeutic levels. If seizures continue to occur even after the maximum dose of first drug, then another antiepileptic drug should be added while keeping the patient on first drug. If seizures are controlled with the second drug, first drug can be gradually withdrawn.
- An attempt can be made to discontinue antiepileptic drugs, if the patient is seizure free for at least 2 years with a normal EEG. Drugs should be withdrawn gradually over 2 to 3 months.
- Examples of antiepileptic drugs are carbamazepine, phenytoin, lamotrigine, sodium valproate, levetiracetam, etc.

General Measures

- Avoid precipitating factors such as sleep deprivation, physical stress, blinking lights, loud noise, and alcohol intake.
- Advice the patient to avoid swimming, going to heights, fire and moving machinery.
- Avoid an occupation which puts the patient or public at risk such as driving a public transport vehicle.

Endocrinology

Q. Define diabetes mellitus. How do you classify diabetes mellitus?

- Diabetes mellitus is a clinical syndrome characterized by impaired insulin secretion and insulin resistance leading to hyperglycemia.
- Diabetes occurs worldwide and the incidence of both type 1 and type 2 diabetes is rising. Majority of diabetics have type 2 diabetes. Many factors such as greater longevity, obesity, unsatisfactory diet, sedentary lifestyle and increasing urbanization contribute to development of type 2 diabetes. Type 2 diabetes is now being observed in children and adolescents also.
- Type 1 diabetes was previously termed 'insulin-dependent diabetes mellitus' (IDDM) since it is associated with profound insulin deficiency requiring insulin injections. Type 2 diabetes was previously termed 'non-insulin-dependent diabetes mellitus' (NIDDM) because patients retain the capacity to secrete some insulin but exhibit impaired sensitivity to insulin (insulin resistance) and can usually be treated without insulin injections.

Classification of Diabetes Mellitus

I. Type 1 diabetes (insulin dependent diabetes mellitus)

II. Type 2 diabetes (non-insulin dependent diabetes mellitus)

III. Gestational diabetes mellitus (GDM)

IV. Other specific types of diabetes (Genetic defects of insulin action, pancreatitis, drug-induced)

Q. Discuss the etiology, clinical features, investigations and treatment of type 2 diabetes mellitus.

Etiology

In type 2 diabetes, there is a combination of insulin resistance and insulin deficiency. Insulin deficiency is due to impaired pancreatic β-cell function. But in the beginning of type 2 diabetes, there is actually increased insulin secretion to counteract insulin resistance. But as the disease progresses, there is progressive beta cell failure and insulin deficiency develops.

Insulin Resistance

- Resistance to the action of insulin in the liver and muscle leads to overproduction and underutilization of glucose respectively leading to hyperglycemia. Type 2 diabetes is often associated with central (visceral) obesity, hypertension and dyslipidemia (elevated LDL cholesterol and triglycerides, low HDL cholesterol). Coexistence of this cluster of conditions is called 'insulin resistance syndrome' or 'metabolic syndrome'. Metabolic syndrome predisposes to cardiovascular diseases.

- The exact cause of insulin resistance remains unclear. However, there are many factors which contribute to insulin resistance. Central obesity (especially intra-abdominal fat) causes insulin resistance because large quantities of free fatty acids (FFA) released by adipose tissue compete with glucose to be utilized by peripheral tissues. Adipose tissue also releases many hormones (e.g. cortisol, adipokines) which may decrease the sensitivity of insulin receptors.
- Lack of exercise increases insulin resistance by downregulation of insulin-sensitive kinases and by the accumulation of FFAs within skeletal muscle. Exercise allows non-insulin-dependent glucose uptake by muscles.

Pancreatic β-cell failure: There is progressive reduction in beta cell mass. There is deposition of amylin around beta cells which forms insoluble fibrils of amyloid leading to destruction of beta cells.

Genetic predisposition: Genetic factors are important in the etiology of type 2 diabetes. There is almost 100% concordance rate in monozygotic twins. Many susceptibility genes have been found which increase the risk of developing diabetes.

Obesity: Overeating increases the risk of type 2 diabetes, especially when combined with obesity and underactivity. The risk of developing type 2 diabetes increases tenfold in people with a body mass index of >30.

Aging: Type 2 diabetes usually affects middle-aged and elderly. Most of them are over 50 years of age.

Clinical Features

Asymptomatic: Many diabetics are asymptomatic and are detected during routine health checkups or when they are seen for some other illness. This is especially so in case of early type 2 diabetes.

Polyuria, nocturia: Occurs because of glucose in the urine which acts as an osmotic diuretic. This occurs only when there is very high blood glucose level.

Polyphagia: Though there is hyperglycemia, it cannot be used by cells due to lack of insulin or insulin resistance. Hence, a diabetic feels more hungry than usual.

Thirst, dry mouth: This happens because high blood glucose absorbs water from the tissues causing dehydration and thirst. Polyuria also leads to dehydration and increased thirst.

Easy fatigability: nability to properly utilize blood glucose leads to easy fatigability.

Delayed wound healing: Hyperglycemia inhibits inflammatory response, chemotaxis, decreased neutrophil function, etc. which lead to delayed wound healing.

Weight loss: Since there is loss of calories in the form of glucose in the urine, there is negative energy balance and weight loss. A person loses weight in spite of eating more.

Symptoms of peripheral neuropathy: Such as burning, tingling and numbness occur due to diabetic peripheral neuropathy. Initially these symptoms are felt in feet. Later on it may involve the legs and hands.

Blurring of vision: This is due to the change in refractory power of lens due to hyperglycemia. Diabetic retinopathy is also an other cause in advanced diabetes.

Recurrent infections: Uncontrolled diabetes is associated with an increased susceptibility to infection. Patients may present with skin sepsis (boils) and genital candidiasis, and complain of pruritus vulvae or balanitis.

Presenting as DKA and HHS: Some patients present for the first time with one of the acute complications of diabetes such as diabetic ketoacidosis (DKA) or HHS (hyperglycemic hyperosmolar syndrome). DKA is common in type 1 diabetes and HHS in type 2 diabetes.

Investigations

- Testing to detect type 2 diabetes in asymptomatic people should be considered in adults of any age who are overweight or obese (BMI >30 kg/m^2) and have one or more additional risk factors for diabetes such as physical inactivity, first-degree relative with diabetes, high-risk race/ethnicity. In those without these risk factors, testing should begin at age 45 years.
- If tests are normal, repeat testing at least at 3-year intervals is reasonable.

The American Diabetes Association (ADA) Criteria for the Diagnosis of Diabetes

A hemoglobin A1c (HbA1c) level of 6.5% or higher.

or

A fasting plasma glucose (FPG) level of 126 mg/dL or higher

or

A 2-hour plasma glucose level of 200 mg/dL or higher during a 75-g oral glucose tolerance test (OGTT),

or

A random plasma glucose of 200 mg/dL or higher in a patient with classic symptoms of hyperglycemia (i.e. polyuria, polydipsia, polyphagia, weight loss) or hyperglycemic crisis

Oral Glucose Tolerance Test (OGTT)

- OGTT is not recommended for routine clinical use but may be required in the evaluation of patients with IFG (impaired fasting glucose) or when diabetes is still suspected despite normal FBS. It is commonly done in the diagnosis of gestational diabetes mellitus.
- OGTT should be performed under controlled conditions to ensure its accuracy.

The following should be ensured before doing OGTT.

- o 3 days of unrestricted diet ((>150 g carbohydrates/day) and physical activity.
- o Patient should remain seated and not smoke during the test.
- o OGTT should be done after an overnight fast, using a glucose load containing 75 g of anhydrous glucose dissolved in water; 2 hr post load glucose levels of 200 mg/dL or greater establish the diagnosis of diabetes.
- Factors that decrease the value of OGTT include:
  - o Carbohydrate restriction (<150 g for 3 days)
  - o Bed rest or severe inactivity
  - o Medical or surgical stress
  - o Drugs (e.g. thiazides, steroids, β-blockers, phenytoin)
  - o Smoking
  - o Anxiety from repeated needle sticks.
- Hence, OGTT should not be performed in acutely ill patients (Table 9.1).
- Impaired glucose tolerance (IGT) and impaired fasting glucose (IFG) are now called 'pre-diabetes' states. People with these prediabetic states have a relatively high risk of developing diabetes and subsequent vascular disease. All patients with IFG and IGT should be treated with diet and exercise and should be followed up yearly for the progression to diabetes.

Urinalysis

- Glucosuria occurs when blood sugar goes more than 180 mg/dL (renal threshold for glucosuria). Glucosuria can be detected by Benedict's test or glucose strips.
- Proteinuria can occur due to development of diabetic nephropathy. Urine should be tested in all diabetics for the presence of proteinuria which can be treated with ACE inhibitors.
- Ketone bodies may be present in DKA.

Table 9.1: Interpretation of OGTT results

	FBS (mg/dL)	Two-hour PPBS (mg/dL)
Normal	<100	<140
IFG (impaired fasting glucose)	100–125	Normal (<140)
IGT (impaired glucose tolerance)	Normal (<100)	140–199
Diabetes	≥126	≥200 mg/dL

Glycated Hemoglobin (HbA1c)

- RBCs are freely permeable to glucose. As a result, glucose becomes irreversibly attached to hemoglobin (HbA1c) at a rate dependent upon the prevailing blood glucose. Since HbA1c circulates within RBCs whose lifespan lasts up to 120 days, its concentration reflects the average blood glucose level in the preceding 120 days.
- Its normal concentration is 4–6%. It is abnormally elevated in diabetic persons with chronic hyperglycemia.
- It should be measured every 3- to 4-month intervals so that adjustments in therapy can be made to optimize diabetes control.

Lipid Profile

Obese patients with diabetes may have abnormal lipid profile characterized by high triglyceride, high LDL and low HDL cholesterol. High LDL is atherogenic and may contribute to macrovascular complications of diabetes.

Renal Function Tests

Advanced diabetes is associated with diabetic nephropathy which may progress to renal failure. If renal failure develops, urea and creatinine will be elevated.

Treatment of Diabetes

Methods available for the treatment of type 2 diabetes are as follows:
- Diet
- Exercise
- Oral antidiabetic drugs
- Insulin
- Pancreas or islet cell transplantation

Early type 2 diabetes can be controlled by diet and lifestyle modification alone. Other patients will require drugs or insulin or both.

Diet (Medical Nutrition Therapy)

- A well-balanced, nutritious diet is important in the management of diabetes.
- The components of the diet should be as follows.
  - Carbohydrates: 45–65% of total daily calories
  - Protein: 10–35%
  - Fat: 25–35% (of which saturated fat is less than 7%)
- High protein intake may cause progression of renal disease in patients with diabetic nephropathy; for these individuals, protein intake should be restricted to 0.8 gm/kg/day.
- Dietary fibers such as cellulose, gum, and pectin are indigestible by humans. Dietary fiber increases intestinal transit and has beneficial effects on colonic function. It slows glucose absorption rate so that hyperglycemia is slightly diminished. Fiber has a favorable effect on blood cholesterol levels also. Diabetics should consume fiber rich foods such as oatmeal, cereals, and beans.
- Artificial and other sweeteners such as aspartame, saccharin, and sucralose can be used instead of sugar by diabetics. They are well tolerated and do not increase blood sugar.

- Patients should avoid sweets and other high calorie foods, reduce fats and oils and increase the intake of green leafy vegetables. Obese patients should consume fewer calories to reduce their weight. Vegetarian food is encouraged and non-vegetarian food is discouraged in diabetics as non-vegetarian food can contribute significantly in terms of calorie and fat content.
- Patients should reduce alcohol consumption and stop smoking.

Exercise

Regular exercise and healthy diet alone is enough for many patients with early type 2 diabetes. Regular exercise improves glycemic control and reduces insulin resistance. Exercise facilitates noninsulin dependent glucose entry into the cells.

Oral Antidiabetic Drugs

- Oral drugs are mainly effective in type 2 diabetes because most of them stimulate endogenous insulin secretion from beta cells of pancreas which are still able to secrete insulin. Oral drugs are not effective in type 1 diabetes as there is complete loss of insulin secreting ability of beta cells.
- The following are the groups of drugs available to treat diabetes mellitus.

- *Sulfonylureas*: Glibenclamide, gliclazide, glipizide, glimepiride
- *Biguanides*: Metformin
- *Thiazolidinediones:* Pioglitazone
- *Alpha-glucosidase inhibitors:* Voglibose, acarbose
- *Meglitinide derivatives:* Repaglinide, nateglinide
- *Dipeptidyl peptidase 4 (DPP-4) inhibitors:* Sitagliptin, vildagliptin
- *Selective sodium-glucose transporter-2 (SGLT-2) inhibitors:* Canagliflozin

Insulin

- Patients, whose sugar remains uncontrolled even after using a combination of all the oral drugs, require insulin.
- Oral drugs can be continued and insulin is added to oral drugs.
- Initially a single dose of intermediate- or long-acting insulin can be started at bedtime. Later on twice daily mixed insulin (short-acting plus intermediate-acting), or basal bolus type of insulin therapy (short-acting insulin before every meal and long-acting insulin as basal insulin) may be used.

Pancreas or Islet Cell Transplantation

- Both these procedures require suitable donors and long-term immunosuppression.
- Islet cell transplantation is a minimally invasive procedure, and easier than pancreas transplantation.

Q. Discuss the etiology, clinical features, investigations and treatment of type 1 diabetes mellitus.

Type 1 diabetes is also known as insulin-dependent diabetes mellitus (IDDM) because all these patients require insulin for blood glucose control. Type 1 diabetes starts at younger age.

Etiology of Type 1 Diabetes

Genetic Factors

Genetic factors account for about one-third of the susceptibility to type 1 diabetes. The HLA haplotypes DR3 and DR4 are associated with increased susceptibility to type 1 diabetes in Caucasians.

Autoimmunity

- Type 1 diabetes is a slowly progressive T cell-mediated autoimmune disease. Defective presentation of autoantigens derived from pancreatic beta cells probably leads to the development of autoimmunity. The pathological picture in type 1 diabetes is characterized by 'insulitis'—that is, infiltration of the islets with mononuclear cells (macrophages, T lymphocytes, natural killer cells and B lymphocytes).

- Islet cell antibodies can be detected even before the clinical development of type 1 diabetes.
- Type 1 diabetes may be associated with other autoimmune disorders such as thyroid disease, coeliac disease, Addison's disease, pernicious anemia and vitiligo.

Environmental Factors

- Along with genetic factors, environmental factors are important for the expression of type 1 diabetes.
- Reduced exposure to microorganisms in early childhood limits maturation of the immune system and may increase susceptibility to autoimmune diseases.
- Some viral infections (mumps, Coxsackie B4, retroviruses, rubella, CMV, EBV) may cause type 1 diabetes as evidenced by isolation of virus particles from the pancreas known to cause cytopathic or autoimmune damage to β cells.
- Dietary factors, such as cow's milk, have been implicated in triggering type 1 diabetes. Children who are given cow's milk early in infancy are more likely to develop type 1 diabetes than those who are breastfed.
- Stress may precipitate type 1 diabetes by increasing counter-regulatory hormones and immunomodulation.

Clinical Features

Same as type 2 diabetes.

Investigations

Same as type 2 diabetes.

Treatment

- Same as type 2 diabetes except that oral antidiabetic drugs do not work in type 2

diabetes mellitus. However, metformin can be used to increase insulin sensitivity.
- Almost all the patients with type 1 diabetes require insulin to control the blood sugar.

Q. Differences between type 1 and type 2 diabetes mellitus.

Table 9.2 describes differences between type 1 and type 2 diabetes mellitus.

Q. Enumerate the complications of diabetes. What are the factors associated with increased mortality and morbidity in people with diabetes?

Acute complications
- Diabetic ketoacidosis (DKA)
- Hyperosmolar hyperglycemic state (HHS)
- Hypoglycemia
- Lactic acidosis

Chronic (long-term) complications

Microvascular
- Diabetic retinopathy
- Diabetic neuropathy
- Diabetic nephropathy

Macrovascular
- Coronary artery disease
- Peripheral vascular disease
- Cerebrovascular disease

Others
- Gastrointestinal (gastroparesis, diarrhea)
- Genitourinary (uropathy/sexual dysfunction)
- Dermatological
- Infections
- Cataracts
- Glaucoma
- Periodontal disease

Factors Associated with Increased Mortality and Morbidity in People with Diabetes

- Long duration of diabetes
- Early age at onset of disease

Table 9.2: Differences between type 1 and type 2 diabetes

	Type 1	Type 2
Prevalence	Uncommon (5–10% of diabetes cases)	Common (>80% of diabetes cases)
Typical age at onset	<40 years	>40 years
Duration of symptoms	Weeks	Months to years
Body weight	Normal or low	Obese
Ketoacidosis	Common	Rarely
Rapid death without treatment with insulin	Yes	No
Autoantibodies	Yes	No
Diabetic complications at diagnosis	No	25% (because of late presentation)
Family history of diabetes	Uncommon	Common
Other autoimmune diseases	Common	Uncommon
HLA-DR3/4	Association present	No association
Insulin secretion	Absent or severely decreased	Increased or decreased
Insulin resistance	Absent	Present
Acanthosis nigricans	No	Common

- Uncontrolled blood sugars (as evidenced by high HbA1c)
- Associated hypertension
- Proteinuria; microalbuminuria
- Dyslipidemia (high LDL, low HDL)
- Obesity

Q. Discuss the pathogenesis, clinical features, investigations, management and complications of diabetic keto-acidosis (DKA).

- Diabetic ketoacidosis (DKA) is a major medical emergency and remains a serious cause of morbidity and mortality in people with diabetes. It is more likely to occur in type 1 diabetes because of complete dependence on insulin.
- Many undiagnosed diabetics may present for the first time with DKA.

Pathogenesis of DKA (Fig. 9.1)
- DKA usually evolves rapidly, over a 24-hour period.

- The cardinal biochemical features of diabetic ketoacidosis are: Hyperglycemia, hyperketonemia and metabolic acidosis.

- Two hormonal abnormalities are largely responsible for the development of hyperglycemia and ketoacidosis in patients with uncontrolled diabetes; insulin deficiency and glucagon excess. In addition to these factors, increased catecholamines and cortisol can contribute to the increase in glucose and ketoacid production.

- Hyperglycemia causes osmotic diuresis leading to dehydration and electrolyte loss, particularly of sodium and potassium. Average loss of fluid in DKA is 3–6 liters. Dehydration leads to hemoconcentration, hypovolemia, hypotension, decreased renal perfusion and oliguria.

- Ketosis results from insulin deficiency, exacerbated by elevated catecholamines and other stress hormones, resulting in unrestrained lipolysis and supply of free fatty acids for hepatic ketogenesis. Excess accumulation of acidic ketones (β-hydroxy

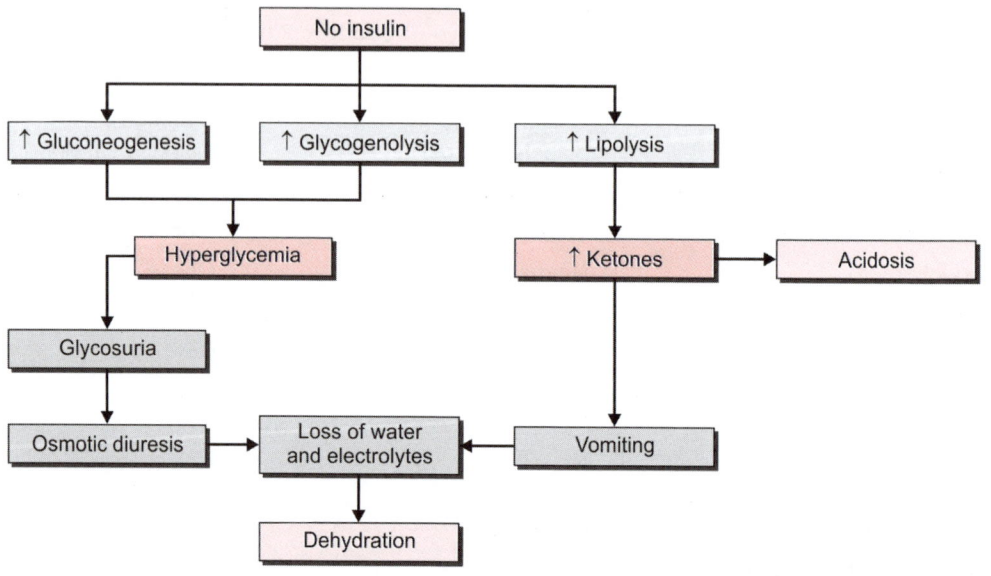

Fig. 9.1: Pathogenesis of DKA

butyric acid and acetoacetate) leads to metabolic acidosis.

- There are many precipitating factors which may trigger an attack of DKA due to increased insulin requirements.

Precipitating Factors for DKA

- Inadequate insulin treatment or noncompliance
- Infections (pneumonia, UTI, sepsis, etc.)
- Cerebrovascular accidents
- Myocardial infarction
- Acute pancreatitis
- Drugs (steroids, thiazides, clozapine or olanzapine, cocaine)

Clinical Features

Due to Hyperglycemia

Polyuria, polydipsia, and weight loss are the initial symptoms. As hyperglycemia worsens, serum osmolality increases leading to neurological signs and symptoms such as lethargy, focal deficits and obtundation which can progress to coma. Blurred vision may occur due to change in the refractory power of lens due to hyperglycemia.

Due to Dehydration

- Loss of skin turgor, dry tongue, cracked lips, sunken eyeballs, tachycardia, and hypotension.
- Cold extremities, peripheral cyanosis

Due to Metabolic Acidosis

- Deep and sighing breathing (Kussmaul breathing). Breath is usually fetid, and acetone smell may be present.
- Nausea, vomiting, and abdominal pain are common in DKA which may be related to acidosis. Abdominal pain is probably due to delayed gastric emptying and ileus induced by metabolic acidosis and electrolyte abnormalities.

Other Features

Signs of underlying precipitating illness may be present such as fever in infections, signs of consolidation in pneumonia, etc.

Investigations

- Urea and creatinine—may be elevated due to severe dehydration.
- Electrolytes—sodium level is variable depending on the hydration status. Potassium and bicarbonate are usually low.

- Blood glucose is often >250 mg/dL.
- Serum amylase and lipase are elevated in DKA. Sometimes acute pancreatitis can precipitate an attack of DKA in which case amylase and lipase are elevated.
- Arterial blood gas (ABG) shows presence of metabolic acidosis.
- Plasma ketone bodies are raised.
- Urinalysis shows presence of sugar and ketone bodies.
- ECG may show changes due to electrolyte abnormalities or MI which might have precipitated DKA.
- Infection screen: Full blood count, blood and urine culture, C-reactive protein, chest X-ray.

Diagnostic Criteria for DKA

- Blood glucose >250 mg/dL
- Arterial pH <7.3
- Serum bicarbonate <15 mEq/L
- Moderate degree of ketonemia and/or keto-nuria

Management of DKA

Principles of Treatment
- Correction of dehydration, hyperglycemia and electrolyte imbalance.
- Treatment of precipitating event.

Correction of Dehydration
The average fluid loss is 3 to 6 liters in DKA. Initially 1 to 2 liters of isotonic saline is given rapidly intravenously. Subsequent rate of fluid replacement depends on the hydration status and urine output. Patients who are able to drink can take some or all of their fluid replacement orally.

Correction of Hyperglycemia
- Intravenous insulin infusion should be started. Initially an intravenous bolus of regular insulin at 0.15 units/kg body weight is given, followed by a continuous infusion at a dose of 0.1 unit/kg/hour (5 to 7 units/hr in adults).
- Blood glucose should be monitored every hour. if necessary, the insulin infusion may be doubled every 2-hour until a steady glucose decline between 50 and 75 mg/h is achieved.

Potassium Replacement
If there is hypokalemia, potassium chloride should be given intravenously along with IV fluids.

Bicarbonate Replacement
Sodium bicarbonate is given intravenously, if pH is <7. Sodium bicarbonate should be diluted in distilled water and given.

Treatment of the Precipitating Event
Such as infection should be treated with antibiotics.

Q. Hyperosmolar hyperglycemic state (non-ketotic hyperosmolar syndrome).

- Hyperosmolar hyperglycemic state (HHS) is characterized by severe hyperglycemia, hyperosmolality and dehydration in the absence of ketosis.
- It is more common in type 2 diabetes, in middle-aged, and elderly.

Precipitating Factors
These are same as for DKA.

Pathogenesis
- Pathogenesis is same as DKA. In DKA, there is complete or severe deficiency of insulin which leads to formation of ketone bodies and acidosis. However, in HHS, some amount of insulin is present in the body which is enough to prevent fatty acid oxidation and formation of ketone bodies. Hence, in HHS, significant ketosis and acidosis is absent.
- Dehydration and hyperglycemia are more severe than DKA.

Clinical Features

- Onset may be insidious over a period of days or weeks, with weakness, polyuria, and polydipsia.
- Signs of dehydration are present.
- Acidotic breathing (Kussmaul respirations) is absent.
- Lethargy and confusion may be present which may progress to convulsions and deep coma.

Investigations

- Severe hyperglycemia is present (usually 600 mg/dL or more).
- Serum osmolality is markedly raised (>320 mOsm/kg).
- Ketosis and acidosis are usually absent.
- Serum sodium may be high (can exceed 140 mEq/L), contributing to increased serum osmolality.

- Urea and creatinine are usually elevated due to dehydration (prerenal azotemia).

Management

Management of HHS is same as that of DKA with following changes.
- Fluid deficit is more in HHS (average of 6 – 10 liters) than DKA, hence more fluid is required.
- There is no role for bicarbonate therapy as pH is not affected in HHS.

Prognosis

The overall mortality rate of HHS is more than ten times that of DKA. Prognosis is better when it is recognized early and prompt therapy is instituted.

Q. Enumerate the differences between DKA and HHS.

Table 9.3 describes the differences between DKA and HHS.

Table 9.3: Differences between DKA and HHS		
Features	*DKA*	*HHS*
• Common in	Type 1 diabetes	Type 2 diabetes
• Evolution	Over hours	Over days or weeks
• Alteration in sensorium	Variable	Stupor/coma
• Acetone smell in breath	Present	Absent
• Acidotic breathing (Kussmaul respirations)	Present	Absent
• Abdominal pain, vomiting	May be present	Usually absent
• Average fluid deficit	3–6 liters	6–9 liters
• Blood glucose	>250	>600
• Arterial pH	<7.3	>7.3
• Serum bicarbonate (mEq/L)	<15	>15
• Blood/urine ketones	Positive	Absent or trace
• Serum osmolality (mOsm/kg)	Variable	>320
• Mortality	5–10%	20–30%

Q. Define hypoglycemia. Discuss the causes, clinical features, diagnosis and treatment of hypoglycemia.

Hypoglycemia is low plasma glucose level (<50 mg/dL) *plus* simultaneous hypoglycemic symptoms that reverse with dextrose administration.

Causes

- Missed, delayed or inadequate meal
- Intense exercise
- Alcohol
- Drugs: Sulphonylureas, insulin, quinine, pentamidine.
- Malabsorption, e.g. celiac disease
- Critical illness: liver and renal failure, malaria
- Endocrine disorders; Addison's disease, insulinoma
- Malignancies: Sarcomas.
- Factitious (deliberately induced)
- Glycogen storage disorders
- Inborn errors of metabolism

Clinical Features

- Sweating
- Trembling
- Pounding heart
- Hunger
- Anxiety
- Confusion
- Drowsiness
- Speech difficulty
- Inability to concentrate
- In-coordination
- Focal neurological deficits
- Nausea
- Tiredness
- Headache

In most instances, patient can recognize the symptoms of hypoglycemia and take appropriate action which includes eating a snack or sugar, etc. However, in certain circumstances (e.g. during sleep, or when distracted by other activities), warning symptoms may not be perceived by the patient, so that appropriate action is not taken and drowsiness or unconsciousness occurs.

Complications of Severe Hypoglycemia

- Impaired cognitive function
- Intellectual decline
- Brain damage
- Coma
- Convulsions
- Focal neurological lesions
- Cardiac arrhythmias
- Myocardial ischemia
- Vitreous hemorrhage
- Hypothermia
- Accidents (including road traffic accidents) with injury

Measures to Prevent Hypoglycemia

- Do not skip meals after taking sulphonylurea or insulin.
- Use the correct dose of insulin and oral antidiabetic agents as prescribed.
- Avoid unaccustomed intense exercise especially on empty stomach.
- Take light snacks in between major meals and also at bedtime.
- Monitor blood sugar frequently.
- Carry supply of fast-acting carbohydrate (sweets, sugar, glucose tablets), and a glucagon injection while going for long travel.

Management of Hypoglycemia

- If the patient is conscious and able to swallow, glucose (50 g) or any other fast acting source of carbohydrate (sweets, honey, etc.) can be given orally.
- If the patient is in altered sensorium and unable to swallow, intravenous glucose (50 mL of 50% dextrose) is given. Inj glucagon (1 mg by intramuscular injection) can also be given, if IV access is a problem. As soon as the patient is able to swallow, glucose should be given orally.

- If hypoglycemia has occurred after the use of a long-acting insulin or drug such as glibenclamide, above treatment should be followed by an infusion of 10% dextrose for few hours, to prevent reccurence of hypoglycemia.

Q. Discuss the etiology, clinical features, investigations, and management of acromegaly.

- Acromegaly is the clinical syndrome that results from excessive secretion of growth hormone (GH).
- If GH hypersecretion occurs before epiphyses have fused, then gigantism will result. If GH excess occurs in adult life, after epiphyseal closure, then acromegaly occurs. If hypersecretion starts in adolescence and persists into adult life, then the two conditions may be combined.
- The mean age at diagnosis of acromegaly is 40 to 45 years.

Etiology

- The most common cause of acromegaly is a somatotroph (growth hormone-secreting) adenoma of the anterior pituitary. Most of these are macroadenomas.
- Other causes of acromegaly are:
  - o Excess secretion of growth hormone-releasing hormone (GHRH) by hypothalamic tumors, carcinoid tumors or small-cell lung cancers.
  - o Ectopic secretion of GH by nonendocrine tumors.

Clinical Features (Fig. 9.2)

- There is stimulation of growth of many tissues, such as skin, connective tissue, cartilage, bone, viscera, and many epithelial tissues.
- Findings include an enlarged jaw (macrognathia) and enlarged, swollen hands and feet. Facial features become coarse, with enlargement of the nose and frontal bones as well as the jaw. Teeth become spread apart. Macroglossia and enlargement of the

soft tissues of the pharynx and larynx lead to obstructive sleep apnea.
- Skin thickness is increased and hyperhidrosis is common. Hair growth increases, and some women have hirsutism.
- Enlargement of synovial tissue and cartilage causes hypertrophic arthropathy of the joints.
- Cardiovascular abnormalities include hypertension, left ventricular hypertrophy, and cardiomyopathy.
- Pituitary adenoma may cause local symptoms such as headache, visual field defects (classically bitemporal hemianopsia) and cranial nerve palsies. It may also cause decreased secretion of other pituitary hormones due to its mass effect, most commonly gonadotropins. Many women with acromegaly have menstrual dysfunction, hot flashes and vaginal atrophy.
- There is increased risk of colon cancer and uterine fibroids.
- Mortality is increased in acromegaly due to cardiovascular diseases and cancer.

Investigations

- Measurement of GH levels during an oral glucose tolerance test. In normal subjects, plasma GH suppresses to below 2 mU/L. In acromegaly, it does not suppress and there may be a paradoxical rise. This test may not be helpful in diabetes patients as inadequate insulin secretion may fail to suppress GH. However, in diabetic patients with acromegaly, IGF-1 levels are high and low in patients without acromegaly.
- Blood glucose levels may be high due to excess growth hormone causing insulin resistance.
- Prolactin concentrations are elevated in about 30% of patients due to co-secretion of prolactin from the pituitary adenoma.
- CT or MRI of brain demonstrates pituitary adenoma.
- Skull X-rays disclose cortical thickening, enlargement of the frontal sinuses, and enlargement and erosion of the sella

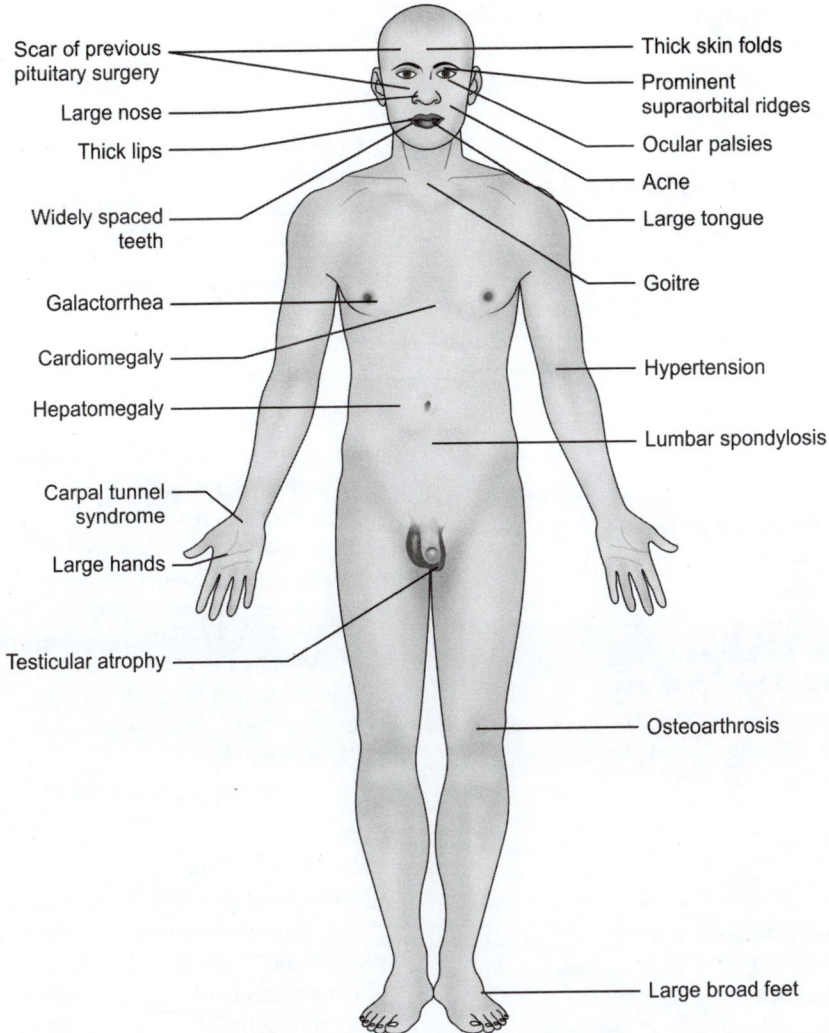

Scar of previous pituitary surgery

Large nose

Thick lips

Widely spaced teeth

Galactorrhea

Cardiomegaly

Hepatomegaly

Carpal tunnel syndrome

Large hands

Testicular atrophy

Thick skin folds

Prominent supraorbital ridges

Ocular palsies

Acne

Large tongue

Goitre

Hypertension

Lumbar spondylosis

Osteoarthrosis

Large broad feet

Fig. 9.2: Clinical features of acromegaly

turcica. X-rays of the hands show tufting of the terminal phalanges and soft-tissue thickening.

• Colonoscopy to screen for colonic neoplasms.

Management

Surgical

Trans-sphenoidal surgery to remove the adenoma is usually the first line of treatment and may result in cure. Surgery is also useful to debulk the tumor followed by second-line therapy.

Radiotherapy

External radiotherapy is usually employed as second-line treatment, if acromegaly persists after surgery.

Medical

This may be employed in patients with persisting acromegaly after surgery. Agents which can suppress GH secretion are somatostatin analogues (e.g. octreotide or lanreotide), dopamine agonists (bromocriptine, cabergoline) and GH receptor antagonist (pegvisomant).

Q. Discuss the etiology, clinical features, investigations and management of hyperthyroidism.

Hyperthyroidism is characterized by increased synthesis and secretion of thyroid hormones which leads to the hyper-metabolic state.

Causes of Hyperthyroidism

- Autoimmune thyroid disease
- Graves' disease
- Hashitoxicosis
- Toxic adenoma
- Toxic multinodular goiter
- TSH-mediated hyperthyroidism
- Struma ovarii
- Metastatic follicular thyroid cancer

Clinical Features

General
- Weight loss despite normal or increased appetite
- Heat intolerance
- Fatigue
- Goitre with bruit
- Single or multiple nodules may be present in the thyroid

GIT
- Diarrhea
- Anorexia
- Vomiting

CVS
- Systolic hypertension/increased pulse pressure
- Palpitations
- Sinus tachycardia
- Atrial fibrillation
- High output cardiac failure
- Angina

RS
- Exacerbation of asthma
- Dyspnea on exertion

Hematological
- Lymphadenopathy
- Normochromic normocytic anemia (due to increased plasma volume)

Nervous system
- Tremor
- Muscle weakness
- Periodic paralysis
- Hyper-reflexia

Skin
- Increased sweating
- Hair thinning, alopecia
- Palmar erythema
- Pretibial myxedema

Genitourinary system
- Amenorrhea/oligomenorrhea
- Infertility, spontaneous abortion
- Loss of libido, impotence
- Gynecomastia
- Urinary frequency and nocturia

Eyes
- Stare and lid lag
- Gritty feeling or pain in the eyes
- Excessive lacrimation
- Diplopia
- Loss of acuity
- Exophthalmos
- Periorbital and conjuctival edema
- Ophthalmoplegia
- Papilledema

Bone
- Osteoporosis (fracture, loss of height)

Psychiatric
- Anxiety, irritability, emotional lability, psychosis

Investigations

- Serum T_3 and T_4 are elevated.
- Serum TSH is low in primary thyrotoxicosis and high in TSH-induced thyrotoxicosis.
- TSH receptor antibodies (TRAb) are elevated in Graves' disease.

- Anti-thyroid peroxidase (anti-TPO) antibody titers are significantly elevated in Graves' disease, and usually are low or absent in toxic multinodular goiter and toxic adenoma.
- Isotope scanning may show increased uptake in Graves' disease.
- Thyroid ultrasound can identify nodules and distinguish solid from cystic lesions.
- FNAC (fine needle aspiration cytology) helps in obtaining cytologic material from nodules for histopathological examination.

Management

Antithyroid Drugs

- These drugs decrease the thyroid hormone synthesis and release from thyroid gland. The thionamide derivatives, propylthiouracil (PTU), methimazole and carbimazole are the drugs of first choice in Graves' disease.
- The most important side effect of antithyroid drugs is agranulocytosis. Patients should be told to discontinue their medication and contact their physician when fever occurs or infection develops, especially in the oropharynx.

Radioactive Iodine

- Radioactive iodine (^{131}I) is used to treat hyperthyroidism in older patients with moderate hyperthyroidism and thyroid enlargement, for patients with a prior allergic or toxic reaction to the antithyroid medication, poor compliance with antithyroid drugs and after antithyroid drugs have failed to induce a long-term euthyroid state.
- Radioiodine treatment is contraindicated during pregnancy and pregnancy should be avoided for 6 to 12 months after radioiodine treatment.

Surgical Therapy

Subtotal thyroidectomy can be used to treat hyperthyroidism in patients with large goiter, malignant thyroid nodule, and pregnant women with severe hyperthyroidism, which is difficult to control with antithyroid drugs.

Symptomatic Treatment

In all patients with thyrotoxicosis, a nonselective beta-blocker such as propranolol should be used to control symptoms such as tachycardia, palpitations and tremors.

> **Q. Discuss the etiology, pathogenesis, clinical features, investigations and management of Graves' disease.**

Graves' disease, first described by Robert Graves, is a syndrome that consists of hyperthyroidism, goiter, ophthalmopathy and occasionally infiltrative dermopathy (pretibial myxedema).

Etiology and Pathogenesis

- Graves' disease is an autoimmune disorder caused by autoantibodies to the TSH receptors (TSHR-Ab) that activate the receptor, thereby stimulating thyroid hormone synthesis and secretion as well as thyroid growth (causing goiter). These antibodies are produced by B lymphocytes.
- Infliltrative ophthalmopathy and dermopathy are specific to Graves' disease and are due to immunologically mediated activation of fibroblasts in extraocular muscles and skin, with accumulation of glycosaminoglycans leading to water trapping and edema.
- There is a genetic predisposition for Graves' disease as evidenced by strong association of Graves' disease with HLA-B8, DR3 and DR2, and high concordance rate in monozygotic twins. Viral and bacterial infections have been suspected to trigger the development of thyrotoxicosis in genetically susceptible individuals. *Escherichia coli* and *Yersinia enterocolitica* possess cell membrane antigens resembling TSH receptors; antibodies to these microbial antigens may cross-react with the TSH receptors on the host thyroid follicular cell.

- Iodine supplementation in iodine deficient areas can trigger the development of thyrotoxicosis in those with pre-existing subclinical Graves' disease.
- Histologic examination of the thyroid gland shows follicular hyperplasia, and patchy lymphocytic infiltration.

Clinical Features

- Are same as that discussed under hyperthyroidism.
- Features specific to Graves' disease are ophthalmopathy and infiltrative dermopathy (pretibial myxedema).
- Ophthalmopathy leads to proptosis and lid retraction preventing complete eye closure, resulting in exposure keratitis and corneal ulceration. Compression of the optic nerve by enlarged muscles may lead to impaired visual acuity, visual field defects, impairment of color vision, and papilledema.
- Treatment of ophthalmopathy involves prevention of drying and infection of the cornea by applying artificial tears and antibiotic drops. Surgical decompression may be required in severe proptosis with optic nerve compression.

Investigations and management of Graves' disease are same as that discussed under hyperthyroidism.

Q. Enumerate the causes of hypothyroidism.

Q. Discuss the clinical features, diagnosis, and management of primary hypothyroidism.

Etiology of Hypothyroidism

Primary hypothyroidism
- Chronic autoimmune (Hashimoto's) thyroiditis
- Iatrogenic (thyroidectomy, radioiodine therapy or external irradiation)
- Iodine deficiency or excess
- Drugs (thionamides, lithium, amiodarone)

- Infiltrative diseases (fibrous thyroiditis, hemochromatosis, sarcoidosis)
- Congenital causes (thyroid agenesis, dysgenesis)

Secondary (central) hypothyroidism
- TSH deficiency
- TRH deficiency

Primary Hypothyroidism

Primary hypothyroidism refers to hypothyroidism caused by disease of the thyroid gland itself. Decreased secretion of T_3 and T_4 leads to a compensatory increase in TSH secretion. Thus, the combination of a low serum T_3, T_4 and a high serum TSH concentration indicates primary hypothyroidism.

Clinical Features

General
- Weight gain, fatigue, somnolence, cold intolerance, hoarseness of voice, slurred speech, puffy face and loss of eyebrows.

Skin
- Dry, cold and pale skin, decreased sweating, nonpitting edema (myxedema), carotenemia, coarse hair and hair loss, xanthelasma.

Hematologic
- Anemia, macrocytosis.

CVS
- Diastolic hypertension, bradycardia, reduced cardiac output.

RS
- Hypoventilation, sleep apnea, exertional dyspnea, pleural effusion.

GIT
- Enlargement of the tongue, constipation (due to decreased gut motility).

Reproductive system.
- Oligomenorrhea, amenorrhea or menorrhagia, decreased fertility, increased risk of abortion, decreased libido, erectile dysfunction.

Neuropsychiatric
- Encephalopathy, myxedema coma, mental retardation in children, carpal tunnel syndrome,

cerebellar ataxia, depression, psychosis, myotonia, delayed relaxation of tendon reflexes.

Musculoskeletal
- Slow movement, myalgia, arthralgia, aches and stiffness.

Metabolic
- Hyperuricemia, hyponatremia, hyperlipidemia.

Investigations
- Serum T_3, T_4 is low and TSH elevated (>5).
- Serum cholesterol, triglycerides, lactate dehydrogenase (LDH), creatinine kinase (CK) and AST may be raised.
- Serum sodium levels may be low.
- Chest X-ray may show cardiomegaly.
- ECG may show sinus bradycardia with low voltage complexes.

Treatment
- Hypothyroidism is treated with levo-thyroxine (T_4), with doses ranging from 50 to 200 µg/day. It is given once a day. Most patients require lifelong treatment and periodic evaluations should be done.
- A starting dose of 50 µg/day can be used and then increased every 4 weeks to reach the final replacement level. In elderly patients and those with coronary artery disease, the initial dose should be 25 µg/day and then increased every 4 weeks.
- The aim is to achieve a euthyroid status with TSH, T_4, and T_3 levels in the normal range. TSH is the most sensitive indicator and treatment should be aimed at normalizing TSH level.

Q. Enumerate the causes of hypercalcemia. Discuss the management of hypercalcemia.

Q. Hypercalcemic crisis.

- Normal calcium level in the body is 8–10 mg/dL. Out of this, 4 to 5 mg/dL is ionized calcium and the remaining is bound to albumin.
- Calcium level of 10–12 mg/dL is mild hypercalcemia and level above 14 mg/dL indicates severe hypercalcemia.

Etiology of Hypercalcemia

Increased bone resorption
- Hyperparathyroidism
- Malignancy
- Thyrotoxicosis
- Immobilization

Increased calcium absorption
- Increased calcium intake
- Milk alkali syndrome
- Hypervitaminosis D

Clinical Features

Renal
- Polyuria
- Polydipsia
- Nephrolithiasis
- Nephrocalcinosis
- Distal renal tubular acidosis
- Nephrogenic diabetes insipidus
- Acute and chronic renal insufficiency

Gastrointestinal
- Nausea, vomiting
- Constipation
- Pancreatitis
- Peptic ulcer disease

Musculoskeletal
- Muscle weakness
- Bone pain
- Osteopenia/osteoporosis

Neuropsychiatric
- Anxiety, depression
- Decreased concentration
- Confusion, stupor, coma

Cardiovascular
- Shortening of the QT interval
- Bradycardia
- Hypertension

Eye
- Calcium may precipitate in the cornea (band keratopathy)

Hypercalcemic Crisis

- Often seen in elderly patients with primary hyperparathyroidism.
- Clinical features are dehydration, hypotension, abdominal pain, vomiting, and altered sensorium.

Investigations

- ECG may show shortened QT interval, AV block, bundle branch block, and prolonged PR and QRS.
- In hyperparathyroidism, PTH level is elevated.
- Serum concentration of PTH-related protein (PTHrp) is elevated in malignancy-related hypercalcemia.
- Serum concentration of the vitamin D metabolites, 25-hydroxyvitamin D (calcidiol) and 1,25-dihydroxyvitamin D (calcitriol) should be measured.
- Serum uric acid and LDH are elevated in malignancy.
- Plasma protein electrophoresis, urine for Bence-Jones protein and bone marrow examination are useful to rule out multiple myeloma.
- Chest X-ray, ultrasound abdomen and CT scan to rule out malignancy.
- Bone scan to rule out bone metastases.

Management

Mild to Moderate Hypercalcemia

Patients with mild hypercalcemia do not require immediate treatment. Factors which aggravate hypercalcemia should be avoided. These are drugs such as thiazide diuretics and lithium, volume depletion, prolonged bed rest, and high calcium diet (>1000 mg/day). Adequate hydration is recommended. Symptomatic patients are treated with bisphosphonates.

Severe Hypercalcemia (Calcium >14 mg/dL; Hypercalcemic Crisis).

- Rehydration with isotonic saline.
- Administration of calcitonin.

- Bisphosphonates: Zoledronic acid or pamidronate.
- Steroids: Prednisolone or hydrocortisone. Steroids inhibit vit-D conversion to calcitriol. They are helpful in vit-D intoxication, malignancies and granulomatous diseases.
- Calcitonin plus saline reduces calcium concentration within 12 to 48 hours whereas bisphosphonates will be effective by the second to fourth day.
- Hemodialysis should be considered, if serum calcium is above 18 mg/dL.

Treatment of the Underlying Cause

Such as malignancy, hyperparathyroidism, etc.

Q. Discuss the etiology, clinical features, investigations and management of hypocalcemia.

Q. Enumerate the causes of tetany. Discuss the clinical features and management of tetany.

Q. Trousseau's sign; Chvostek's sign.

Hypocalcemia is an abnormal reduction in serum ionized calcium concentration(< 9 mg/dL). Only ionized, free serum calcium affects neuromuscular function and is clinically important.

Etiology of Hypocalcemia (Tetany)

- Hypoparathyroidism
- Vit-D deficiency (nutritional deficiency, intestinal malabsorption, CKD)
- Acute pancreatitis
- Vitamin D resistance
- Massive blood transfusion (citrate-anticoagulated blood can decrease the concentration of ionized Ca)
- Alkalosis (hyperventilation, excessive vomiting)

Clinical Features

- *Neuromuscular manifestations (tetany):* Hypocalcemia leads to neuromuscular irritability leading to tetany. Tetany is uncommon unless the serum ionized calcium concentration falls below 4.3 mg/dL. Other factors that worsen tetany are alkalosis and hypomagnesemia. Tetany is characterized by both sensory and motor features. Initially sensory symptoms such as circumoral numbness, paresthesias of the hands and feet are seen. Motor symptoms are stiffness and clumsiness, myalgia, and muscle spasms. Hand muscle spasm leads to adduction of the thumb, flexion of the metacarpophalangeal joints and wrists, and extension of the fingers. Spasm of the respiratory muscles and of the glottis can cause cyanosis. Autonomic manifestations include diaphoresis, bronchospasm, and biliary colic. Latent tetany may be present when signs of overt tetany are lacking. It can be demonstrated by Trousseau's and Chvostek's signs. *Trousseau sign* is the induction of carpal spasm by inflation of a sphygmomanometer above systolic blood pressure for three minutes. It can also be induced by hyperventilation for one to two minutes after release of the cuff. Trousseau's sign is due to the ischemia of the nerve trunk under the cuff which increases excitability. *Chvostek's sign* is contraction of the ipsilateral facial muscles when facial nerve is tapped anterior to the ear. This leads to contraction of corner of the mouth, the nose and the eye.
- Other neurological features are seizures and intellectual impairment.
- Psychiatric manifestations—emotional instability, anxiety, depression, confusion, hallucinations, and frank psychosis. All are reversible with treatment.
- Skin manifestations—dry skin, hyperpigmentation, dermatitis and psoriasis.
- Eye—cataracts.
- Dental—dental abnormalities occur when hypocalcemia is present during early development. They include dental hypoplasia, failure of tooth eruption, defective enamel and root formation, and abraded carious teeth.
- Cardiovascular—hypotension (in acute hypocalcemia), decreased myocardial contractility, and congestive heart failure.
- Gastrointestinal—steatorrhea due to impaired pancreatic secretion, gastric achlorhydria.
- Skeletal—hypocalcemia associated with hypophosphatemia, as in vitamin D deficiency, causes rickets in children and osteomalacia in adults.
- Endocrine manifestations—impaired insulin release.

Investigations

- Serum calcium level is low.
- Serum PTH level is low in hypoparathyroidism.
- Serum vitamin D level is low in vitamin D deficiency.
- ECG shows prolonged QT interval.

Management

- Tetany can be treated by rebreathing expired air in a paper bag or administering 5% CO_2 in oxygen. This increases arterial carbon dioxide which increases ionized calcium.
- Injection of 20 mL of a 10% calcium gluconate intravenously raises the serum calcium concentration immediately. An intramuscular injection of 10 mL may be given to obtain a more prolonged effect.
- Treatment of underlying cause.

Q. Hypoparathyroidism.

Hypoparathyroidism is characterized by deficiency of PTH, and hypocalcemia.

Causes

- After thyroid surgery (parathyroids are accidentally removed).
- Autoimmune

- Autosomal dominant hypoparathyroidism
- Pseudohypoparathyroidism (resistance to PTH)

Clinical Features

Features of hypocalcemia are seen. (See under hypocalcemia).

Treatment

- In acute manifestations of hypocalcemia (such as tetany), intravenous calcium gluconate is given.
- Vitamin D supplementation—vitamin D (in the form of vitamin D_2, or ergocalciferol), or calcitriol (1,25-dihydroxyvitamin D) are given orally daily to maintain normal calcium levels.

Q. Discuss the etiology, clinical features, investigations and management of Cushing syndrome (glucocorticoid excess).

Cushing syndrome is due to chronic glucocorticoid excess. The most common cause is iatrogenic, due to prolonged administration of glucocorticoids such as prednisolone.

Etiology

ACTH-dependent Cushing syndrome
- Pituitary adenoma secreting ACTH (i.e. Cushing's disease)
- Ectopic ACTH syndrome
- Ectopic CRH syndrome
- ACTH therapy

ACTH-independent Cushing syndrome
- Adrenal adenoma
- Adrenal carcinoma
- Steroid therapy

Clinical Features (Fig. 9.3)

- The typical patient with Cushing syndrome is a middle-aged plethoric woman with truncal obesity and hypertension.
- Obesity is central (centripetal obesity) with sparing of limbs which gives 'lemon on stick appearance'. There is accentuation of normal fat over the upper part of the back, giving a 'buffalo hump' appearance. The neck is thick and short. The supraclavicular fat pads are enlarged.
- Skin manifestations include skin atrophy, easy bruisability, and purple striae in the trunk, breasts, and abdomen. In pituitary tumors secreting ACTH, and in ectopic ACTH syndrome, hyperpigmentation can occur.
- Menstrual irregularities—oligomenorrhea, amenorrhea, etc.
- Signs of adrenal androgen excess—women with Cushing syndrome often have signs of androgen excess. These include hirsutism, thinning of scalp hair, deepening of voice, and clitoral enlargement.
- Proximal muscle wasting and weakness.
- Osteoporosis is common and may lead to pathologic fractures and vertebral collapse. Low back pain is a common presenting feature.
- Neuropsychiatric symptoms—emotional lability, depression, irritability, anxiety and panic attacks.
- Diabetes mellitus may develop due to increased hepatic gluconeogenesis and insulin resistance.
- Hypertension and cardiovascular risk is a major cause of morbidity and mortality.

Investigations

Investigations are useful to confirm the diagnosis of Cushing syndrome and to find out the etiology.

To Confirm the Presence of Cushing's Syndrome

- Serum cortisol level—serum cortisol level is normally lowest at 12 midnight. There is loss of diurnal variation in Cushing syndrome, and midnight level is high.
- 24-hour urinary cortisol excretion—is high in patients with Cushing syndrome (normal <90 µg/24 hours).
- Overnight dexamethasone suppression test—1 mg of dexamethasone is given at 11

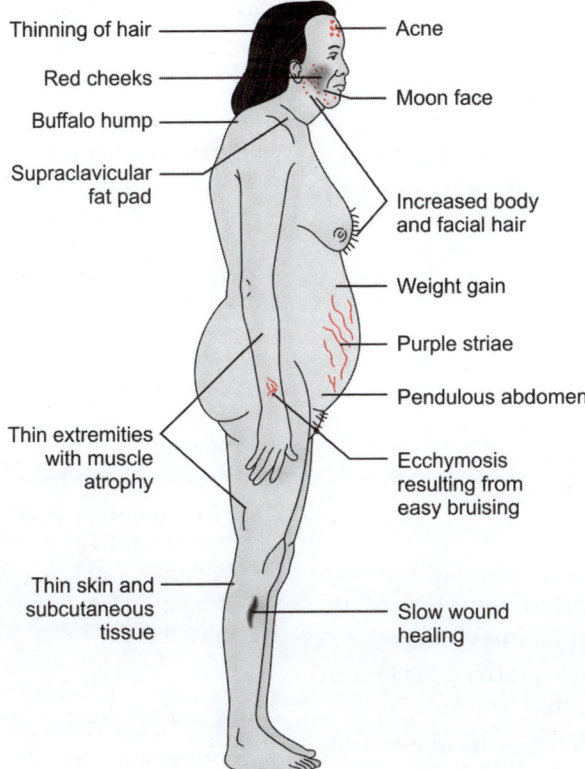

Thinning of hair

Red cheeks

Buffalo hump

Supraclavicular fat pad

Acne

Moon face

Increased body and facial hair

Weight gain

Purple striae

Pendulous abdomen

Thin extremities with muscle atrophy

Ecchymosis resulting from easy bruising

Thin skin and subcutaneous tissue

Slow wound healing

Fig. 9.3: Clinical features of Cushing syndrome

PM to 12 AM, and serum cortisol is measured at 8 AM the next morning. In most normal patients, this drug suppresses morning serum cortisol to <1.8 µg/mL, whereas patients with Cushing syndrome have a higher level.

- Low dose dexamethasone suppression test—this is an alternative to overnight dexamethasone suppression test. 0.5 mg dexamethasone is given 6th hourly for 2 days. 24-hr urine cortisol on second day and 8 AM serum cortisol after 48 hours are measured. Urine cortisol <36 µg/day or serum cortisol <1.8 µg/dL excludes Cushing's syndrome.

To Establish the Cause of Cushing Syndrome

- Once the presence of Cushing syndrome is confirmed, measurement of plasma ACTH is the key to establishing the differential diagnosis.

- Increased cortisol level and an undetectable ACTH indicates an adrenal pathology. Increased cortisol level with increased ACTH level indicates either pituitary source or an ectopic source of ACTH.
- MRI can localize the tumors secreting ACTH or cortisol.
- CT or MRI detects most adrenal adenomas.

Additional Tests

Serum electrolytes (usually high sodium and low potassium), glucose (elevated), glycosylated hemoglobin and bone mineral density measurement.

Management

Most patients are treated surgically with medical therapy given for a few weeks prior to operation.

Medical Therapy

It includes the following drugs:

- *Somatostatin analogs:* Pasireotide is a somatostatin analog which inhibits ACTH secretion and thereby cortisol secretion. It is indicated for treatment of Cushing disease in which pituitary surgery is not an option.
- *Adrenal steroid inhibitors:* Metyrapone, ketoconazole, etomidate
- *Glucocorticoid receptor antagonist:* Mifepristone
- *Adrenolytic agents:* Mitotane. This drug causes adrenal cortical necrosis.

Surgery

- In Cushing's disease, trans-sphenoidal surgery with selective removal of the adenoma is the treatment of choice.
- Adrenal adenomas are removed via laparoscopy or a loin incision.
- Ectopic ACTH syndrome—localized tumors (e.g. bronchial carcinoid) should be removed. Unresectable malignancies may be treated by radiotherapy and chemotherapy. Medical therapy can be used for recurrences.

> **Q. Discuss the etiology, clinical features, investigations and management of adrenal insufficiency.**

> **Q. Discuss the etiology, clinical features, investigations and management of Addison disease.**

- Adrenal insufficiency results from destruction or dysfunction of the entire adrenal cortex. It affects glucocorticoid and mineralocorticoid function.
- It is of two types: Primary (inability of the adrenals to produce hormones), and secondary (due to pituitary or hypothalamic disease leading to ACTH and CRH deficiency). Primary adrenal insufficiency is also known as Addison disease.

- Adrenal insufficiency can be acute or chronic. Acute adrenal insufficiency (acute adrenal crisis) is a medical emergency.

Etiology

- Idiopathic
- Genetic
- Infections (tuberculosis, HIV/AIDS, histoplasmosis)
- Carcinoma (metastatic carcinoma, lymphoma)
- Infiltrative diseases (hemochromatosis, sarcoidosis, amyloidosis)
- Iatrogenic (bilateral adrenalectomy, postradiotherapy)
- Adrenal hemorrhage
- Hypothalamic or pituitary disease (due to decreased CRH or ACTH)
- Withdrawal of glucocorticoid therapy
- Drugs: Aminoglutethimide, metyrapone, ketoconazole

Clinical Features

- Symptoms and signs are due to low glucocorticoid, low mineralocorticoid, and low adrenal androgen levels.
- Glucocorticoid deficiency causes malaise, fatigue, generalized weakness, nausea, vomiting, anorexia, weight loss, postural hypotension and hypoglycemia.
- Mineralocorticoid deficiency causes hyponatremia and hyperkalemia. Salt craving may be present in some patients.
- ACTH excess in primary adrenal deficiency (Addison disease) causes skin hyperpigmentation. Hyperpigmentation is not seen in secondary adrenal insufficiency as ACTH is low.

Investigations

- *Serum cortisol level:* An early morning (between 8 and 9 AM) serum cortisol concentration less than 3 µg/dL suggests adrenal insufficiency and a value above 19 µg/dL excludes it.
- *ACTH stimulation test (Synacthen test):* 250 µg of ACTH (Synacthen) is given by IM injection at any time of day. Blood samples

are drawn at 0 and 30 minutes for plasma cortisol. In normal subjects, plasma cortisol is >17 µg/dL either at baseline or at 30 minutes. Cortisol levels fail to increase in primary adrenal insufficiency.

- *Serum ACTH level:* Primary and secondary adrenal insufficiency can be distinguished by measurement of ACTH which is low in ACTH deficiency and high in Addison's disease.
- *Serum electrolytes:* Hyponatremia and hyperkalemia are seen.
- *HIV test*, if risk factors for infection are present.
- *Plain X-ray abdomen* may show adrenal calcification in tuberculosis.
- *Ultrasound abdomen* is useful to assess the size of adrenals and also to detect any tumors.
- *CT or MRI* of adrenals to look for size of adrenals and metastatic malignancy.
- *Adrenal and other organ specific antibodies* may be present in autoimmune adrenalitis.

Management

- Patients should receive lifelong steroid replacement therapy. Cortisol 15 mg in the morning and 5 mg in the evening should be given daily.
- During intercurrent illness, the dose of steroid should be doubled.
- Patient should carry a steroid card all the time which should give information regarding diagnosis, steroid, dose and doctor. Patients should be encouraged to wear a bracelet engraved with the diagnosis all the time. All these can help in emergencies.
- Underlying cause should be treated.

Q. Acute adrenal crisis (acute adrenal insufficiency; Addisonian crisis).

- Acute adrenal crisis can occur in the following situations.
- Serious infection or other major stress in a previously undiagnosed patient with adrenal insufficiency.

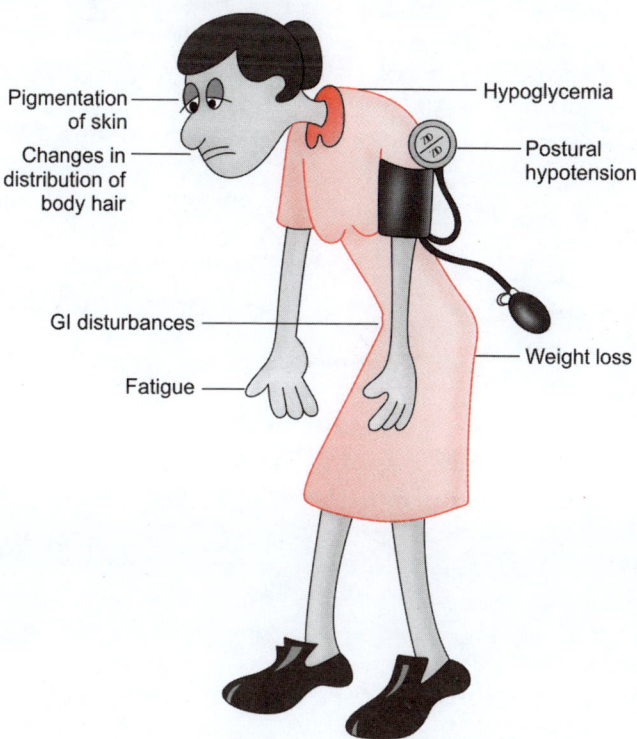

Fig. 9.4: Clinical features of adrenal insufficiency

- Skipping of steroid or failure to increase the dose in a patient with known adrenal insufficiency during major illness or stress.
- Bilateral adrenal hemorrhage (Waterhouse-Friderichsen syndrome, anticoagulant therapy)
- Pituitary apoplexy
- Rapid withdrawal of steroids in a patient who is taking them for a long time.

Clinical Features (Fig. 9.4)

- Hypotension or shock
- Dehydration
- Nausea, vomiting and abdominal pain. Abdominal rigidity or rebound tenderness may be present mimicking acute abdomen.
- Confusion or disorientation
- Fever may be present due to underlying infection.

- There may be hyperkalemia, hyponatremia, and hypoglycemia.

Management

- It is a medical emergency.
- Rapid replacement of steroid, sodium and water deficits are the primary goals of therapy.
- IV fluid (DNS) is started immediately.
- Inj hydrocortisone 100 mg is given intravenously and repeated every 6 hours thereafter. Hydrocortisoncan be given intramuscularly, if there is problem with IV access.
- Once the patient's condition improves, he is put on oral steroids and oral fluids and the dose of steroids is slowly tapered to the maintenance dose.
- The precipitating cause should be identified and treated.

Critical Care

- Syncope is transient loss of consciousness and postural tone with spontaneous recovery. This definition excludes seizures, coma, shock, or other states of altered consciousness.
- Loss of consciousness happens due to a reduction of blood flow to the reticular activating system of the brainstem. It happens within 10 seconds of cessation of cerebral blood flow. Patient usually recovers consciousness as soon as he is flat on the ground.
- Though most cases of syncope are benign, there can be serious underlying problems such as cardiac disorders.

Causes of Syncope

Vascular (Loss of Vascular Tone)

- Vasovagal syncope
- Autonomic neuropathy
- Volume depletion
- Carotid sinus hypersensitivity
- Reflex mediated (cough, micturition)
- Drugs (alpha blockers, nitrates)

Cardiac Disorders

- Valvular heart diseases (AS, MS)
- Aortic dissection
- Atrial myxoma
- Cardiac tamponade
- Hypertrophic obstructive cardiomyopathy
- Myocardial ischemia, infarction
- Pulmonary embolism
- Pulmonary hypertension
- Arrhythmias

Neurological

- Vertebrobasilar insufficiency
- Transient ischemic attack

Metabolic

- Hyperventilation
- Hypoglycemia
- Hypoxemia

Psychogenic Syncope

- Anxiety
- Conversion disorders

APPROACH TO A CASE OF SYNCOPE

History

- Elicit a detailed history of the event from the patient or bystanders.
- Ask the following questions:
  - Was loss of consciousness complete?
  - Was loss of consciousness with rapid onset and of short duration?

o Was recovery spontaneous, complete, and without sequelae?

o Was postural tone lost?

- If the answers are yes, syncope is likely; if one, or more answers are negative, other causes of loss of consciousness should be considered.
- *Precipitating factors:* They include fatigue, sleep or food deprivation, hot weather, alcohol consumption, pain, and strong emotions such as fear or apprehension.
- *Details of patient activity before the event:* Activity prior to syncope may give a clue to the etiology of symptoms. Syncope occurring during specific situations such as shaving, coughing, voiding indicates situational syncope (reflex syncope). Syncope occurring within 2 minutes of standing suggests orthostatic hypotension. Syncope while seated or lying is more likely to be cardiac origin.
- *Symptoms prior to the onset of syncope:* Faintness, dizziness, or light-headedness occurs prior to true syncope. An aura prior to loss of consciousness may suggest seizure. Presence of chest pain, dyspnea, and palpitations may suggest cardiac cause. Severe headache, focal neurologic deficits, diplopia, ataxia, or dysarthria prior to the syncopal event suggests neurological cause such as intracranial bleed or vertebrobasilar insufficiency.
- Duration of loss of consciousness (LOC) can indicate the cause. In syncope, LOC lasts for only a few seconds to a few minutes. In neurological problems, LOC usually lasts longer, a few minutes to hours.
- Confusion after syncope, tongue bite, urinary and fecal incontinence, and convulsive activity indicate seizure as the cause of LOC.
- Obtain drug history, because many drugs cause postural hypotension and syncope. These are calcium channel blockers, alpha-blockers, diuretics, etc.
- Past history of cardiac disease, seizure disorder, diabetes (hypoglycemia), etc. should be asked. History of pregnancy should be asked because ectopic rupture can cause syncope.

Physical Examination

- *Vital signs:* Fever indicates underlying infection as the cause of syncope. Tachycardia may be an indicator of pulmonary embolism, hypovolemia, tachyarrhythmia, or acute coronary syndrome. Bradycardia may point toward a cardiac conduction defect, or acute coronary syndrome. Postural changes in blood pressure (BP), hypotension, and increased heart rate may point toward an orthostatic cause of syncope.
- *CVS:* Look for murmurs, signs of cardiac failure such as basal crepitations of lung, presence of S3 and presence of arrhythmias.
- *CNS:* Look for any signs of head injury, pupillary abnormalities, cranial nerve deficits, motor deficits, abnormal deep tendon reflexes, and sensory deficits.
- *RS/abdomen:* Look for any abnormalities.

Investigations

- *Check blood glucose* immediately using glucometer to rule out hypoglycemia. Other tests include complete blood count, serum electrolytes, cardiac enzymes, LFT and renal function tests.
- *ECG:* To rule out acute myocardial infarction or myocardial ischemia, arrhythmias, conduction defects.
- *Stool* for occult blood to rule out any GI bleed.
- *Urine pregnancy test* in women to rule out ectopic rupture.
- *Computed tomography (CT) of the head:* To rule out any intracranial pathology such as hemorrhage or infarction in patients with neurologic deficits or in patients with head trauma secondary to syncope.
- *Echocardiography:* Test of choice for evaluating cardiac causes of syncope such as heart failure, valvular heart diseases, etc.

- *Head-up tilt-table test:* Useful for confirming autonomic dysfunction and postural hypotension causing syncope.
- *Electroencephalography (EEG):* Indicated, if seizure is a likely diagnosis.
- *Stress test:* A cardiac stress test is appropriate for patients in whom cardiac syncope is suspected and who have risk factors for coronary atherosclerosis.

Management

Treatment depends on the underlying cause.

- *Situational syncope:* Patient education regarding the condition.
- *Orthostatic syncope:* Patient education; wearing elastic compression stocking to lower limbs, mineralocorticoids, and other drugs (e.g. midodrine); elimination of drugs associated with hypotension; increasing oral fluid intake.
- *Cardiac arrhythmias*: Antiarrhythmic drugs or pacemaker placement.
- *Valvular heart disease*: Surgical correction.

Q. Write briefly about vasovagal syncope.

- Vasovagal syncope is due to a reduction of venous return to heart due to prolonged standing, hot weather or after meals.
- Decreased venous return leads to underfilling of ventricles which causes Bezold-Jarisch reflex characterized by initial sympathetic activation leading to vigorous ventricular contraction. This stimulates ventricular mechanoreceptors which produces parasympathetic (vagal) activation and sympathetic withdrawal causing bradycardia, vasodilatation or both leading to syncope.
- Vasovagal syncope can be confirmed by head-up tilt testing, where patient is put on a table which is then tilted to an angle of 70° for up to 45 minutes while the ECG and blood pressure are monitored.
- Treatment is not necessary but in severe cases β-blockers (which inhibit the initial sympathetic activation) or disopyramide (a

vagolytic agent) can be used. A dual-chamber pacemaker is useful, if the symptoms are predominantly due to bradycardia.

Q. Shock.

Shock is defined as multifactorial syndrome resulting in inadequate tissue perfusion and cellular oxygenation affecting multiple organ systems.

Classification and Causes

- *Hypovolemic shock:* It occurs due to inadequate circulating volume (e.g. hemorrhage).
- *Obstructive shock:* This is caused by extracardiac obstruction of blood flow. Examples: Cardiac tamponade, pulmonary embolism, tension pneumothorax.
- *Cardiogenic shock:* This occurs due to cardiac failure. Examples: Myocardial infarction, myocarditis, etc.
- *Distributive shock:* This is due to widespread vasodilatation leading to hypotension. Examples: Septic shock, anaphylactic shock, neurogenic shock.
- *Endocrine shock:* This results from hormonal pathology. Examples: Acute adrenal insufficiency, myxedema coma.

Pathophysiology (Fig. 10.1)

- The fundamental defect in shock is reduced perfusion of vital tissues. Reduced perfusion leads to tissue hypoxia leading to anaerobic metabolism with increased production of CO_2 and accumulation of lactic acid. Cellular function declines, and if shock persists, irreversible cell damage and death occur.
- During shock, both the inflammatory and clotting cascades may be triggered in areas of hypoperfusion. There is widespread endothelial dysfunction with increased capillary permeability leading to leakage of fluid and plasma proteins into the interstitial space. In the GI tract, increased

permeability may allow the enteric bacteria to enter into the bloodstream, potentially leading to sepsis or metastatic infection. Inflammatory cascade also releases vasodilator substances such as nitric oxide (NO) leading to vasodilatation and hypotension. BP may be normal in the early stages of shock. (Although hypotension eventually occurs, if shock is not reversed.)

- In septic shock, blood flow to capillaries is reduced due to fibrin deposition even though large-vessel blood flow is preserved.
- Compensatory measures occur to counteract tissue hypoxia and hypotension. Cells extract more oxygen from the blood and there is sympathetic system activation due to hypotension leading to tachycardia and peripheral vasoconstriction. There is selective vasoconstriction (splanchnic circulation, skin) shunting blood to vital organs such as heart and brain.
- Ultimately, because of all these changes, multiple organ dysfunction syndrome (MODS) which is defined as the progressive dysfunction of 2 or more organs sets in leading to death.

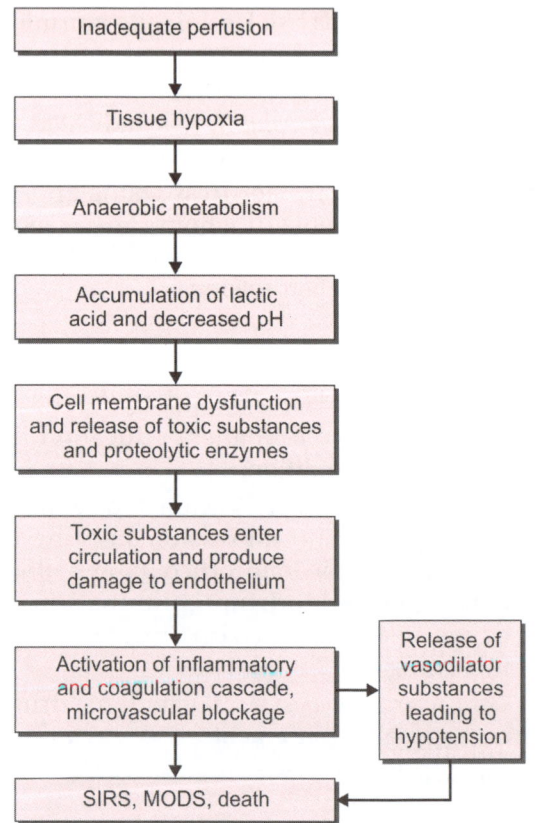

Fig. 10.1: Pathophysiology of shock

Clinical Features

- Lethargy, confusion, and somnolence are common.
- The hands and feet are pale, cool, and clammy.
- Cyanosis may be present.
- Capillary filling time is prolonged.
- Peripheral pulses are weak, tachypnea and tachycardia may be present.
- BP is low (<90 mm Hg systolic) or not recordable. However, it may be normal in early stages of shock.
- In septic shock, skin may be warm, or fever may be present. Some patients with anaphylactic shock have urticaria or wheezing.
- Chest pain and dyspnea may be present in cardiogenic shock due to myocardial infarction.

- Evidence of multiorgan dysfunction (MODS) such as decreased urine output (kidney involvement), jaundice (liver involvement), dyspnea (ARDS), etc. may be present.

Investigations

- Complete blood count
- LFT, RFT
- Serum electrolytes
- PT, aPTT
- Serum cortisol (if suspecting adrenal insuficiency)
- ABG
- ECG, echocardiogram
- Monitoring of central venous pressure (CVP)
- Chest X-ray, ultrasound abdomen to identify any chest (pneumonia, ARDS) or abdominal pathology

Treatment

- Admit the patient in ICU and monitor vital signs.
- Supplemental oxygen by face mask.
- Intubation and mechanical ventilation, if shock is severe or if ventilation is inadequate.
- Intravenous fluids: Initially 1 liter of 0.9% saline is infused over 15 min. Further fluid therapy is based on the underlying condition and may require monitoring of CVP.
- If BP remains low even after giving fluid challenge, intravenous infusion of noradrenaline or dopamine is started. Dobutamine is preferred in cardiogenic shock.
- Cardiogenic shock is treated by percutaneous coronary interventions, intra-aortic balloon pump, etc.
- Parenteral antibiotics (meropenem or piperacillin tazobactum) are started, if there is suspicion of septic shock.
- Intravenous steroids (hydrocortisone or dexamethasone) are given for adrenal insufficiency.

Q. Acute respiratory distress syndrome (ARDS).

Q. Acute lung injury (ALI).

- ARDS was earlier defined as the acute onset of respiratory failure, bilateral infiltrates on chest X-ray, hypoxemia (PaO_2/FiO_2 ratio <200 mm Hg), and pulmonary capillary pressure <18 mm Hg (if measured) to rule out cardiogenic edema. In addition, acute lung injury (ALI) was defined as PaO_2/FiO_2 of 200 to <300 mm Hg.
- However, the above definition of ARDS was found to be inadequate and hence, the definition was further refined in 2011 by a panel of experts who met at Berlin and is termed the Berlin definition of ARDS. In the Berlin definition, there is no use of the term acute lung injury (ALI).

ARDS Berlin Definition

Timing	Within 1 week of a known clinical insult or new or worsening respiratory symptoms
Chest imaging (X-ray or CT scan)	Bilateral opacities—not fully explained by effusions, lobar/lung collapse, or nodules
Origin of edema	Respiratory failure not fully explained by cardiac failure or fluid overload.
Oxygenation (with PEEP or CPAP ≥5 cm H$_2$O	Mild ARDS: PaO_2/FiO_2 200 to ≤300 mm Hg. Moderate ARDS: PaO_2/FiO_2 100 to ≤200 mm Hg. Severe ARDS: PaO_2/FiO_2 ≤100 mm Hg

Causes of ARDS

ARDS is caused by diffuse lung injury due to many medical and surgical disorders.

Direct lung injury	Indirect lung injury
Pneumonia	Anaphylaxis (drugs, wasp, bee sting)
Aspiration of gastric contents	
	Drug overdose (heroin, barbiturates)
Lung contusion	
Smoke inhalation	Pancreatitis
Amniotic fluid embolism	Sepsis
	Shock
Fat embolism	Severe trauma
Near-drowning	Multiple bone fractures
Diffuse alveolar hemorrhage	Multiple blood transfusions
	Burns

Pathogenesis

- Inflammatory cells collect in the lungs because of direct or indirect lung injury listed above. Cytokines are released from inflammatory cells which cause damage to capillary endothelial cells and alveolar epithelial cells. Damage to these cells causes increased vascular permeability and decreased production of surfactant which result in interstitial and alveolar pulmonary edema, alveolar collapse, and hypoxemia.

- Three stages can be recognized in the evolution of ARDS; exudative, proliferative, and fibrotic stages.
- The exudative phase is characterized by alveolar edema, neutrophil-rich leukocytic infiltration and hyaline membrane formation.
- Proliferative phase occurs within 7 days and is characterized by interstitial inflammation and early fibrotic changes. Some patients enter the fibrotic phase approximately 3 weeks after the initial lung injury which is characterized by substantial fibrosis and bullae formation.

Clinical Features

- ARDS is marked by the rapid onset of dyspnea that usually occurs 12–48 hours after the initiating event.
- Physical examination reveals labored breathing, tachypnea, intercostal retractions, and diffuse crepitations.
- Many patients with ARDS have multiple organ failure.

Investigations

- *Chest X-ray* shows diffuse or patchy bilateral infiltrates which become confluent with sparing of costophrenic angles. Air bronchograms may be seen. Heart size is normal, and pleural effusions are nil or minimal.
- *ABG* analysis shows marked hypoxemia that is refractory to supplemental oxygen.
- *Bronchoscopy and lung biopsy* can be considered in patients in whom the cause of ARDS is not clear.

Treatment

- Treatment of ARDS must include identification and treatment of the underlying precipitating condition (e.g. sepsis, aspiration, trauma).

- Treatment of hypoxemia usually requires mechanical ventilation. Prone positioning may improve oxygenation by recruiting atelectatic alveoli. A variety of mechanical ventilation strategies like using volume-cycled ventilation with small tidal volumes have shown benefit in trials.
- Fluid administration should be restricted and enough to maintain pulmonary capillary wedge pressure at the lowest level compatible with adequate cardiac output. Crystalloid solutions should be used when intravascular volume expansion is necessary. Diuretics should be used to reduce intravascular volume, if pulmonary capillary wedge pressure is elevated.
- Systemic corticosteroids have been studied extensively with variable results. Though steroids cannot be recommended routinely for all patients, studies have shown benefit in late-phase ARDS.
- Supportive care should be provided to minimize venous thromboembolism, gastrointestinal bleeding, and central venous catheter infections. Adequate nutrition should be provided for a good outcome.

Course and Prognosis

- Mortality rate associated with ARDS is 30–40%. Median survival is about 2 weeks.
- Most survivors of ARDS are left with some pulmonary symptoms (cough, dyspnea, sputum production), which tend to improve over time.

Q. Define cardiac arrest. Discuss the causes and management of cardiac arrest.

Q. Cardiopulmonary resuscitation (CPR).

- Cardiac arrest is defined as sudden loss of pumping ability of the heart. This leads to abrupt loss of consciousness due to lack of cerebral blood flow. It leads to death in the absence of an active intervention, although spontaneous reversions occur rarely.

- Cardiac arrest occurring in hospital has better chances of survival than out of hospital arrest. Similarly cardiac arrest due to VT or VF has better chances of survival than cardiac arrest due to asystole and pulseless electrical activity.
- The onset of irreversible brain damage usually begins within 4 to 6 minutes after loss of cerebral circulation.

Causes of Cardiac Arrest

- Myocardial infarction
- VF (ventricular fibrillation)
- VT (ventricular tachycardia)
- Asystole
- Pulseless electrical activity
- Rupture of the ventricle
- Cardiac tamponade
- Massive pulmonary embolism
- Electrolyte imbalance (hypokalemia and hyperkalemia)
- Drugs

Management of Cardiac Arrest (Cardiopulmonary Resuscitation)

- The most important thing which increases the survival after cardiac arrest is immediate CPR. The sooner it is initiated the better is the prognosis.
- The goals of CPR in cardiac arrest are: (1) Restoring a spontaneous circulation as quickly as possible; and (2) maintaining continuous artificial circulatory support until return of a spontaneous circulation has been achieved.
- The keys to survival from sudden cardiac arrest are early recognition, early CPR, early defibrillation and early transfer to hospital.
- *CPR consists of 4 main parts:*
  1. Circulation (C)
  2. Airway (A)
  3. Breathing (B)
  4. Defibrillation (D)
- Note that as per new American heart Association guidelines, the sequence of CPR is CAB and not ABC. The management strategy for cardiac arrest can be divided into five steps:
  1. Initial assessment and activation of emergency medical services
  2. Basic life support (BLS)
  3. Early defibrillation by a first responder (if available)
  4. Advanced life support (ALS)
  5. Post-resuscitation care.

Initial Assessment and Activation of Emergency Medical Services

Assess the victim for response. If no response, call for help. If you are alone, activate emergency services and get an automatic external defibrillator, if available.

BLS

- Check for pulse. This is best done by feeling for carotid pulse at the neck. You should take at least 5 seconds and no more than 10 seconds to assess pulse.
- If there is no carotid pulse, chest compressions should be started at a rate of 100/minute. Chest should be compressed in the middle of chest at the level of nipple line.
- Open the victim's airway and check for breathing. Airway can be opened by head tilt-chin lift maneuver.
- If there is no breathing, give 2 breaths (either mouth-to-mouth or by using a face mask). The breaths should make the chest rise and fall.
- This cycle of 30 compressions and 2 breaths should be continued until the return of spontaneous circulation and breathing or till the patient is declared dead. Breaths can be given by mouth-to-mouth breathing or by using bag and mask device. Patient can also be intubated using endotracheal tube for more effective ventilations.

Early Defibrillation by a First Responder

Since the terminal event in most cases of cardiac arrest is ventricular fibrillation, defibrillation as early as possible is very important for successful resuscitation of the victim. For this purpose, automated external defibrillators (AED) can be made use of in a setting outside the hospital. Such AEDs are kept at public places such as airports, railway stations, shopping malls, etc. AED can be used even by lay people.

Advanced Life Support (ALS)

This involves use of various drugs during CPR such as injection adrenaline and atropine. These drugs are given intravenously. Other drugs which are useful in cardiac arrest are calcium gluconate, sodium bicarbonate, magnesium sulfate, and amiodarone. Bag mask ventilation or endotracheal intubation is done for maintaining airway and breathing.

Post-Resuscitation Care

After revival, patient should be kept in recovery position and monitored in ICU. The cause of cardiac arrest should be established and treated.

Q. Left heart failure.

Definition

- Heart failure is a clinical syndrome that results from any structural or functional cardiac disorder that impairs the ability of the ventricle to fill with or eject blood.
- It is a common health problem especially in industrialized countries.

Causes of Left Heart Failure

There are many causes of heart failure. However, 5 causes account for most of the cases of heart failure. These are:

1. Ischemic heart disease: (myocardial infarction, myocardial ischemia).
2. Cardiomyopathies
3. Congenital heart disease
4. Valvular heart disease
5. Hypertensive heart disease

Clinical Features

Dyspnea: *Exertional dyspnea* is seen in early heart failure. As heart failure advances, dyspnea occurs with progressively less strenuous activity and ultimately it is present even at rest.

- *Orthopnea* is dyspnea in lying down position and is a later manifestation than exertional dyspnea. Orthopnea is due to redistribution of fluid from the abdomen and lower extremities into the chest in lying position, which increases the pulmonary capillary pressure, combined with elevation of the diaphragm.
- *Paroxysmal nocturnal dyspnea (PND)* is sudden onset dyspnea and cough occurring usually 1 to 3 hours after the patient retires. Symptoms usually resolve over 10 to 30 minutes after the patient arises, often gasping for fresh air from an open window. PND happens due to accumulation of excessive blood in the lungs during sleep causing pulmonary edema, depression of the respiratory center and decreased sympathetic activity during sleep. The patient gets up suddenly feeling excessively breathless and choked and longs for fresh air. He may bring out pink frothy sputum.
- *Acute pulmonary edema* results from transudation of fluid into the alveolar spaces because of acute rise in capillary hydrostatic pressures due to sudden decrease in cardiac function. Patient may present with cough or progressive dyspnea. Wheezing is common due to bronchospasm. If acute pulmonary edema is not treated earlier, patient may begin coughing up pink (or blood-tinged), frothy fluid and become cyanotic and acidotic. Some patients may present with Cheyne-Stokes respiration (periodic respiration or cyclic respiration) which is characterized by periods of apnea, hypoventilation and hyperventilation.

Fatigue: This is due to reduced perfusion of skeletal muscles.

Cerebral symptoms: They are due to reduced cerebral perfusion and include altered mental status, confusion, lack of concentration, memory impairment, headache, anxiety and insomnia.

Oliguria, nocturia: Reduced renal perfusion during day causes sodium and water retention and oliguria. Renal perfusion increases at night due to shift of fluid from the extravascular to the intravascular compartment, resulting in increased excretion of sodium and water and nocturia.

NYHA Classification of Heart Failure

The New York Heart Association (NYHA) classification system is the simplest and most widely used method to gauge symptom severity. The classification system is a well-established predictor of mortality and can be used at diagnosis and to monitor treatment response.

Functional capacity	Description
I	No limitations of physical activity No heart failure symptoms (fatigue, palpitation, dyspnea)
II	Mild limitation of physical activity Heart failure symptoms with significant exertion; comfortable at rest or with mild activity
III	Marked limitation of physical activity Heart failure symptoms with mild exertion; only comfortable at rest
IV	Discomfort with any activity Heart failure symptoms occur at rest

Physical Signs

Vital signs
- Pulse is fast and of low volume. Pulsus alternans may be seen in LVF.
- BP is low in severe heart failure.
- Respiratory rate may be high due to pulmonary edema.

General examination: Patient is dyspneic and orthopnic. Peripheries are cold and may be cyanosed. In chronic, severe heart failure, weight loss may occur, leading to a syndrome of cardiac cachexia. Cardiac cachexia is due to elevated levels of cytokines.

CVS: Cardiac enlargement (apex beat shifted down and out) may be seen. S_1 may be diminished in intensity. Third and fourth heart sounds are often audible. Pansystolic murmur may be heard due to incompetence of mitral and tricuspid valve due to dilatation of ventricles.

RS: Tachypnea may be present due to pulmonary edema. Bilateral fine basal crepitations and ronchi may be heard due to pulmonary edema. Sometimes signs of pleural effusion may be present.

NS: Confusion, memory disturbances may be seen.

Investigations

- *Chest X-ray:* The presence of cardiomegaly is a strong indicator of heart failure. Pulmonary edema may be seen as bilateral batwing hilar haziness, generalized haze (due to interstitial oedema), and Kerley's B lines (due to prominent interlobular lymphatics) at the lung base. Bilateral pleural effusion may be seen which is usually more on right side.
- *Electrocardiogram (ECG):* It can show cardiac rhythm, identify ischemia, prior or recent MI, and detect evidence of left ventricular hypertrophy. It also shows conduction defects and electrolyte disturbances.
- *Echocardiogrphy:* Transthoracic echo can confirm the presence of heart failure and also quantify it. It also provides information on left and right ventricular size, regional wall motion abnormality (as an indicator ischemia or infarction), condition of the heart valves, and ventricular hypertrophy.
- *Natriuretic peptide measurements:* Elevated serum levels ANP (atrial natriuretic peptide) and BNP (brain natriuretic peptide) are seen in heart failure.
- *Cardiac catheterization:* In heart failure, there is increased end-diastolic ventricular pressure, reduced cardiac output and reduced

ventricular ejection fraction. Coronary angiogram can identify the extent of coronary artery disease.

Treatment of Heart Failure

The ideal approach would be to treat both the underlying and precipitating causes. Correction of underlying cause (e.g. surgical correction of valvular defects) may dramatically improve heart failure. Correction of underlying cause may not always be possible (e.g. old myocardial infarction). Precipitating causes like infections, severe anemia, hyperthyroidism, etc. should be looked for and corrected.

Control of Excessive Fluid

- *Low salt diet and fluid restriction:* Can help in decreasing many of the clinical manifestations of heart failure.
- *Diuretics:* These agents reduce preload and pulmonary congestion. These agents include frusemide, torsemide, thiazides, spironolactone and amiloride.

Prevention of Deterioration of Myocardial Function

- *Angiotensin-converting enzyme (ACE) inhibitors:* ACE inhibitors slow the maladaptive remodeling of ventricles, and reduce the afterload by causing vasodilatation. ACE inhibitors have been shown to improve survival in patients with heart failure. Examples of ACE inhibitors are captopril, enalapril, lisinopril, ramipril, perindopril, etc.
- *Angiotensin receptor blockers (ARB):* These agents have similar effects as ACE inhibitors. They are used when patients cannot tolerate ACE inhibitors due to cough, angioneurotic edema, and leukopenia.

Examples of ARBs are losartan, telmisartan, olmesartan, etc.
- *Aldosterone antagonist:* In heart failure, there is increased secretion of aldosterone, which causes Na^+ retention (hence fluid retention) and vasoconstriction. Spironolactone is an antagonist of aldosterone and when given to heart failure patients on long-term basis reduces mortality and sudden death.
- *Beta-blockers:* Beta-blockers have been shown to improve the symptoms of heart failure, and to reduce long-term mortality, and sudden death. Examples are atenolol, metoprolol, bisoprolol, and carvedilol.
- *Vasodilators:* Direct vasodilators are helpful in patients with severe heart failure who have systemic vasoconstriction despite ACE inhibitor therapy. Decrease in peripheral resistance enhances cardiac output by decreasing afterload. Examples are hydralazine and isosorbide dinitrate.
- *Digoxin:* It enhances myocardial contractility and hence improve symptoms of heart failure.
- When patients do not respond to all the above measures, have class IV heart failure, and are unlikely to survive one year, they should be considered for assisted circulation and/or cardiac transplantation.

Non-Pharmacological Measures

- *Rest:* Rest reduces the demand on the heart. Adequate rest reduces venous pressure and pulmonary congestion. Absolute bed rest is not required even for patients with severe heart failure.
- *Diet:* The diet should provide adequate calories to maintain ideal weight. Obese patients should have a low-calorie diet. Oils and fats should be cut down. The sodium intake should not exceed 6 g of salt per day.

Multiple Choice Questions

INFECTIONS

1. Which statement is true about fever:
A. Fever results when the hypothalamic set point for temperature is set to a higher level.
B. Infections are the most common cause
C. Endogenous pyrogens cause fever
D. All of the above   *Ans.* D

2. Typhoid fever is caused by:
A. *Salmonella typhi*
B. *Shigella*
C. *Campylobacter jejuni*
D. *Helicobacter pylori*   *Ans.* A

3. Typhoid bacilli in chronic carriers reside in:
A. Gallbladder
B. Pancreas
C. Bone marrow
D. Lymph nodes   *Ans.* A

4. Pea soup appearance of stools is seen in:
A. Malaria
B. Dengue
C. Typhoid
D. Amebic dysentery   *Ans.* C

5. Relative bradycardia is a feature of:
A. Malaria
B. Cholera   C. Typhoid
D. Amebic dysentery   *Ans.* C

6 Intestinal perforation in typhoid fever usually occurs in:
A. 1st week of illness
B. 2nd week of illness
C. 3rd week of illness
D. 4th week of illness   *Ans.* C

7. Typhoid vaccines provide protection for:
A. 3 to 5 years   B. 10 to 15 years
C. 20 to 30 years
D. Lifelong   *Ans.* A

8. The diagnostic 'gold standard' for enteric fever is:
A. Widal test   B. Blood culture
C. Stool culture
D. Peripheral blood smear   *Ans.* B

9. Chronic typhoid carrier is one who excretes *salmonella* organism in stool for:
A. 1 to 2 months after the acute infection
B. 6 to 12 months after the acute infection
C. More than 12 months after the acute infection
D. None of the above   *Ans.* C

10. **Characteristic pseudomembrane at the site of infection is caused by:**
    A. Diphtheri
    B. Enteric fever
    C. Malaria
    D. Tetanus   *Ans.* A

11. **Most common form of diphtheria is:**
    A. Faucial (pharyngeal)
    B. Nasal
    C. Laryngeal
    D. Cutaneous   *Ans.* A

12. **Drug of choice for diphtheria:**
    A. Metronidazole
    B. Erythromycin
    C. Quinolones
    D. Sulphonamides   *Ans.* B

13. **Which of the following is also known as glandular fever?**
    A. CML
    B. Typhoid
    C. Kala-azar
    D. Infectious mononucleosis   *Ans.* D

14. **Which of the following can cause generalized lymphadenopathy?**
    A. HIV infection
    B. Hepatitis-B infection
    C. Vit-D deficiency
    D. Doxycycline   *Ans.* A

15. **Which of the following diphtheria strain causes most severe disease?**
    A. Mitis
    B. Intermedius
    C. Gravis
    D. Cutis   *Ans.* C

16. **Which of the following bacteria produces Chinese letter patterns on Albert's stain?**
    A. *Corynebacterium diphtheriae*
    B. *Salmonella typhi*
    C. *Clostridium tetani*
    D. *Campylobacter jejuni*   *Ans.* A

17. **Syphilis is caused by:**
    A. *Treponema pallidum*
    B. HIV 1   C. *Clostridium tetani*
    D. Hepatitis B   *Ans.* A

18. **Primary syphilis is characterized by:**
    A. Painless chancre
    B. Generalized lymphadenopathy
    C. Gumma
    D. All of the above   *Ans.* A

19. **Tabes dorsalis is caused by:**
    A. Syphilis
    B. Hepatitis B
    C. HIV infection
    D. Tuberculosis   *Ans.* A

20. **Hutchinson's teeth and "mulberry" molars are seen in:**
    A. Primary syphilis
    B. Secondary syphilis
    C. Congenital syphilis
    D. Tertiary syphilis   *Ans.* C

21. **Dark-field microscopy is used in the diagnosis of:**
    A. HIV infection
    B. Syphilis
    C. Malaria
    D. Tuberculosis   *Ans.* B

22. **VDRL test is used in the diagnosis of:**
    A. HIV infection
    B. Syphilis   C. Malaria
    D. Tuberculosis   *Ans.* B

23. **HIV is a:**
    A. Single-stranded RNA virus
    B. Double-stranded RNA virus
    C. Single-stranded DNA virus
    D. Double-stranded DNA virus   *Ans.* A

24. **Immunodeficiency in HIV infection is mainly due to:**
    A. Destruction of neutrophils
    B. Destruction of CD4 lymphocytes
    C. Destruction of macrophages
    D. Decreased production of antibodies   *Ans.* B

25. **Acute seroconversion phase is characterized by all, EXCEPT:**
    A. Rapid viral replication
    B. Drop in CD4 cell count
    C. Flu-like illness
    D. Kaposi sarcoma   *Ans.* D

26. Which of the following drug is used for prophylaxis against *Pneumocystis jirovecii* pneumonia in HIV patinets?
    A. Trimethoprim-sulfamethoxazole
    B. Azithromycin
    C. Ganciclovir
    D. Fluconazole   *Ans.* A

27. Herpes zoster (shingles) is caused by:
    A. Varicella-zoster virus
    B. Herpes simplex virus-1
    C. Epstein-Barr virus
    D. Cytomegalovirus   *Ans.* A

28. Which of the following is true about chickenpox?
    A. Caused by varicella-zoster virus
    B. Mainly affects elderly
    C. Incubation period is 1 to 2 days
    D. Characterized by monomorphic macular rash   *Ans.* A

29. Which of the following is NOT TRUE about herpes zoster (shingles)?
    A. It is due to reactivation of latent VZV from the dorsal root ganglia
    B. Dermatomes from T_3 to L_3 are commonly affected
    C. Complications of herpes zoster are postherpetic neuralgia and CNS involvement
    D. Antiviral drugs are of no use.   *Ans.* D

30. Infectious mononucleosis is caused by:
    A. Cytomegalovirus
    B. Epstien-Barr virus
    C. Herpes simplex
    D. *Helicobacter pylori*   *Ans.* B

31. Which of the following is also known as glandular fever or kissing disease?
    A. Infectious mononucleosis
    B. HIV infection
    C. Herpes zoster
    D. Enteric fever   *Ans.* A

32. Triad of fever, pharyngitis, and lymphadenopathy is seen in:
    A. Infectious mononucleosis
    B. HIV infection
    C. Herpes zoster
    D. Enteric fever   *Ans.* A

33. Paul-Bunnell test is used to diagnose:
    A. Infectious mononucleosis
    B. HIV infection
    C. Hepatitis-B
    D. Enteric fever   *Ans.* A

34. Koplik's spots are seen in
    A. Typhoid fever
    B. Infectious mononucleosis
    C. Measles
    D. Rubella   *Ans.* C

35. Subacute sclerosing panen-cephalitis is a complication of:
    A. Typhoid fever
    B. Infectious mononucleosis
    C. Measles
    D. Rubella   *Ans.* C

36. Parotid swelling is seen in:
    A. Infectious mononucleosis
    B. Measles
    C. Rubella
    D. Mumps   *Ans.* D

37. Malaria is caused by:
    A. *Plasmodium* species of protozoa
    B. *Entamoeba histolytica*
    C. *Giardia*
    D. *Nocardia*   *Ans.* A

38. Which of the following causes most severe malaria?
    A. *Plasmodium vivax*
    B. *P. falciparum*
    C. *P. ovale*
    D. *P. malariae*   *Ans.* B

39. Malaria is transmitted by:
    A. Anopheles mosquitoes
    B. Culex mosquitoes
    C. Aedes egypti
    D. Ticks   *Ans.* A

40. Which of the following causes tertian malaria?
A. *Plasmodium vivax*
B. *P. falciparum*
C. *P. ovale*
D. *P. malariae*   *Ans.* A

41. All of the following drugs are used to treat malaria, EXCEPT:
A. Chloroquine
B. Quinine
C. Artesunate
D. Digoxin   *Ans.* D

RESPIRATORY SYSTEM

1. Airway hyperresponsiveness is seen in:
A. Tuberculosis
B. Asthma
C. Bronchiectasis
D. Pneumonia   *Ans.* B

2. Curschmann's spirals are seen in:
A. Tuberculosis
B. Asthma
C. Bronchiectasis
D. COPD   *Ans.* B

3. High-pitched polyphonic rhonchi are heard in:
A. Asthma
B. Bronchiectasis
C. Pneumonia
D. Fibrocavity   *Ans.* A

4. Which of the following drugs is not used in asthma?
A. Salbutamol
B. Ipratropium bromide
C. Propranolol
D. Theophylline   *Ans.* C

5. Montelukast in asthma acts by:
A. Inhibit the synthesis of leukotrienes
B. Inhibit the degranulation of mast cells
C. Relaxation of bronchial smooth muscle
D. Inhibit phosphodiesterase enzyme   *Ans.* A

6. Salbutamol in asthma acts by:
A. Inhibit the synthesis of leukotrienes
B. Inhibit the degranulation of mast cells
C. Relaxation of bronchial smooth muscle
D. Inhibit phosphodiesterase enzyme   *Ans.* C

7. Most important risk factor for COPD is:
A. Smoking
B. Air pollution
C. Genetic factors
D. Occupational exposures   *Ans.* A

8. Pneumonia is:
A. Infection of the lung parenchyma
B. Infection of pleural space
C. Infection of larynx
D. All of the above   *Ans.* A

9. Most common organism causing community-acquired pneumonia is:
A. *Streptococcus pneumoniae*
B. *H. influenzae*
C. *Mycoplasma pneumoniae*
D. *Legionella*   *Ans.* A

10. All of the following are stages of lobar pneumonia, EXCEPT:
A. Stage of congestion
B. Stage of red hepatization
C. Stage of gray hepatization
A. Stage of bronchitis   *Ans.* D

11. Bronchial breath sound is heard in:
A. Pneumonic consolidation
B. Bronchiectasis
C. Pneumothorax
D. COPD   *Ans.* A

12. Clinical features of pneumonia include:
A. Fever
B. Cough
C. Breathlessness
D. All of the above   *Ans.* D

13. **Bronchiectasis refers to:**
    A. Abnormal and permanent dilatation of bronchi
    B. Hyper-reactive airways
    C. Infection of airways
    D. Bronchospasm   *Ans.* A

14. **Hemoptysis is:**
    A. Vomiting of blood
    B. Coughing of blood
    C. Blood in stools
    D. Bleeding from nose   *Ans.* D

15. **Montoux test is used in the diagnosis of:**
    A. Tuberculosis
    B. Typhoid
    C. Malaria
    D. HIV   *Ans.* A

16. **Clinical features of pulmonary TB include:**
    A. Evening rise of temperature
    B. Night sweats
    C. Weight loss
    D. All of the above   *Ans.* D

17. **Number of sputum samples to be tested to diagnose pulmonary TB:**
    A. At least one sample
    B. Two samples
    C. Minimum 3 samples
    D. Minimum 5 samples   *Ans.* C

18. **Which of the following is a second-line anti-TB drug?**
    A. Isoniazid
    B. Rifampicin
    C. Ethambutol
    D. Ethionamide   *Ans.* D

19. **Multidrug-resistant tuberculosis (MDR-TB) refers to tuberculosis resistant to:**
    A. At least isoniazid and rifampicin, and possibly more drugs
    B. Isoniazid and ethionamide
    C. Isoniazid, streptomycin and ofloxacin
    D. All of the above   *Ans.* A

20. **Which of the following is NOT TRUE about DOTS (directly observed therapy short course)?**
    A. DOTS is the most effective strategy available for controlling TB.
    B. Patients are given anti-TB drugs under the direct observation of the health care provider/community DOT provider
    C. In DOTS, the responsibility of ensuring regular and complete treatment of the patient lies with the health system
    D. In DOTS, the duration of treatment is 12 months   *Ans.* D

21. **Pleural effusion is an abnormal collection of:**
    A. Fluid in the pleural space
    B. Air in the pleural space
    C. Blood in the pleural space
    D. All of the above   *Ans.* A

22. **Transudative pleural effusion is seen in:**
    A. Congestive heart failure
    B. Pneumonia   C. Malignancy
    D. Empyema   *Ans.* A

23. **Exudative pleural effusion is seen in:**
    A. Congestive heart failure
    B. Cirrhosis of liver with portal HTN
    C. Nephrotic syndrome
    D. Pneumonia   *Ans.* D

24. **Stony dull percussion note is seen in:**
    A. Pneumonia
    B. Pneumothorax
    C. Pleural effusion
    D. Cavity   *Ans.* C

25. **Which of the following causes bronchial breath sound?**
    A. Acute asthma   B. COPD
    C. Pneumonic consolidation
    D. Pneumothorax   *Ans.* B

26. Pneumothorax refers to:
A. Fluid in the pleural space
B. Air in the pleural space
C. Pus in the pleural space
D. Blood in the pleural space   *Ans. B*

GASTROINTESTINAL TRACT

1. Which of the following can cause gum hypertrophy?
A. Phenytoin sodium
B. CML
C. Vit-D deficiency
D. Doxycycline   *Ans. A*

2. Which of the following is NOT TRUE about stomatitis?
A. It refers to oral inflammation and formation of ulcers
B. It is a painless condition
C. Swelling and redness of mouth is seen
D. Treatment should be directed towards underlying cause   *Ans. B*

3. Gingival hyperplasia is seen in all, EXCEPT:
A. Phenytoin use
B. Acute myeloid leukemia
C. Vitamin C deficiency
D. Iron deficiency   *Ans. D*

4. Which of the following is NOT TRUE of aphthous ulcers:
A. These are painful oral ulcers
B. Common in childhood and adolescence
C. Healing occurs with scarring
D. Exact cause is unknown   *Ans. C*

5. Dysphagia refers to:
A. Difficulty in swallowing
B. Pain while swallowing
C. Difficulty in chewing
D. Difficulty in digestion   *Ans. A*

6. Which of the following can lead to peptic ulcer:
A. *H. pylori* infection
B. NSAIDs and aspirin

C. Gastrinoma (Zollinger-Ellison syndrome)
D. All of the above   *Ans. D*

7. Complications of peptic ulcer include all, ECXEPT:
A. Hemorrhage
B. Perforation
C. Pneumonia
D. Gastric outlet obstruction due to scarring.   *Ans. C*

8. Most common complaint in malabsorption syndrome is:
A. Diarrhea
B. Fever
C. Pain abdomen
D. Weight loss   *Ans. A*

9. Steatorrhea is due to:
A. Fat malabsorption
B. Protein malabsorption
C. Carbohydrate malabsorption
D. Vitamin A malabsorption   *Ans. A*

10. Which of the following causes dysentery?
A. *Entamoeba histolytica*
B. Hepatitis A
C. *Vibrio cholerae*
D. *Giardiasis*   *Ans. A*

11. All of the following cause dysentery (blood in stool), EXCEPT:
A. *Cholera*
B. *Shigella*   C. *Salmonella*
D. *Entamoeba histolytica*   *Ans. A*

12. Treatment of acute diarrhea involves all, EXCEPT:
A. Oral rehydration salt
B. Intravenous hydration in severe dehydration
C. Antibiotics in case of infective diarrhea
D. Laxatives   *Ans. D*

13. Which of the following is a prehepatic cause of jaundice?
A. Acute hepatitis
B. Liver abscess   C. Cirrhosis
D. Hemolysis   *Ans. D*

14. Which of the following causes cirrhosis of liver?
A. Hepatitis B infection
B. Vitamin D deficiency
C. COPD
D. Enteric fever   *Ans.* A

15. Which of the following causes massive splenomegaly?
A. Viral hepatitis
B. Enteric fever (typhoid)
C. Malaria
D. Chronic myeloid leukemia   *Ans.* D

16. Which of the following spreads by feco-oral route?
A. Hepatitis A
B. Hepatitis B
C. Hepatitis C
D. HIV   *Ans.* A

17. Which of the following does not lead to chronic hepatitis?
A. Hepatitis A
B. Hepatitis B
C. Hepatitis C
D. Autoimmune hepatitis   *Ans.* A

18. Hepatitis A spreads by:
A. Feco-oral route
B. Parenteral route
C. Respiratory droplets
D. Needle prick   *Ans.* A

19. Hepatitis E spreads by:
A. Feco-oral route
B. Droplet infection
C. Blood transfusion
D. All of the above   *Ans.* A

20. Complications of cirrhosis of liver include all, EXCEPT:
A. Variceal bleeding
B. Hepatic encephalopathy
C. Hepatorenal syndrome
D. Intestinal perforation   *Ans.* D

21. Ascites refers to the accumulation of excess fluid in the:
A. Peritoneal cavity
B. Pleural cavity
C. Pericardial space
D. Subarachnoid space   *Ans.* A

22. Shifting dullness is a sign which is positive in:
A. Ascites
B. Pericardial effusion
C. Splenomegaly
D. Hepatomegaly   *Ans.* A

CARDIOVASCULAR SYSTEM

1. Rheumatic fever is caused by:
A. Group-A beta-hemolytic *Streptococcus*
B. *Staphylococcus*
C. *Campylobacter jejuni*
D. *Plasmodium vivax*   *Ans.* A

2. Which of the following statements is FALSE regarding rheumatic fever?
A. Major health problem in the developing countries
B. Most common among children in the 5- to 15-year age group
C. Caused by group A beta-hemolytic *Streptococcus*
D. Causes permanent joint deformities   *Ans.* D

3. Jones criteria is used in the diagnosis of:
A. Rheumatic fever
B. Infective endocarditis
C. Rheumatoid arthritis
D. Myocarditis   *Ans.* A

4. Most common cause of mitral stenosis is:
A. Rheumatic heart disease (RHD)
B. Congenital mitral stenosis
C. Carcinoid tumors
D. Systemic lupus erythematosus *Ans.* A

5. Most common valve lesion in rheumatic fever is:
A. Mitral stenosis
B. Aortic stenosis
C. Tricuspid stenosis
D. Aortic regurgitation   *Ans.* A

6. Clinical features of mitral stenosis include all, EXCEPT:
A. Cardiac apex is tapping in nature

B. Loud first heart sound
C. Mid-diastolic 'rumbling' murmur over the apex
D. Ejection systolic murmur in mitral area   *Ans.* D

7. **Complications of mitral stenosis include all, EXCEPT:**
   A. Atrial fibrillation
   B. Pulmonary hypertension
   C. Recurrent chest infections
   D. Aortic aneurysm   *Ans.* D

8. **Which of the following does not cause aortic stenosis?**
   A. Congenital bicuspid valve
   B. Age-related aortic sclerosis
   C. Rheumatic heart disease
   D. Marfan's syndrome   *Ans.* D

9. **Which of the following is NOT a feature of aortic stenosis?**
   A. Collapsing pulse
   B. Heaving apex
   C. Systolic thrill in the aortic area
   D. Ejection systolic murmur in aortic area   *Ans.* A

10. **Slow rising pulse is seen in:**
    A. Aortic regurgitation
    B. Aortic stenosis
    C. Mitral regurgitation
    D. Mitral stenosis   *Ans.* B

11. **Which of the following is not an antihypertensive drug?**
    A. Amlodipine
    B. Metoprolol   C. Salbutamol
    D. Enalapril   *Ans.* C

12. **Which of the following statements about hypertension is FALSE?**
    A. Hypertension leads to left ventricular hypertrophy
    B. Hypertension is a risk factor for stroke
    C. Most cases of hypertension are due to lomerulonephritis
    D. High sodium intake is associated with hypertension   *Ans.* C

13. **Angina pectoris is:**
    A. Pain due to spasm of pectoralis muscles
    B. Discomfort in the chest due to myocardial ischemia
    C. Pain in the epigastric region due to gastritis
    D. Bluish swelling under the tongue   *Ans.* B

14. **Which of the following is FALSE regarding stable angina?**
    A. It is precipitated by effort, and relieved by rest
    B. Stable angina is caused by fixed stenosis in coronary arteries
    C. Most commonly felt in the mid-sternal region and radiates to the neck, left shoulder, and left arm.
    D. Usually lasts for more than 30 minutes   *Ans.* D

15. **Which of the following is used in the treatment of angina?**
    A. Salbutamol
    B. Noradrenaline
    C. Dopamine
    D. Nitrates   *Ans.* D

16. **Which of the following is not an acute coronary syndrome (ACS)?**
    A. Stable angina
    B. Unstable angina
    C. Non-ST-elevation myocardial infarction (NSTEMI)
    D. ST-elevation myocardial infarction (STEMI)   *Ans.* A

17. **Features of unstable angina include:**
    A. It occurs at rest or with minimal exertion
    B. It is severe and of new onset
    C. It occurs with a crescendo pattern
    D. All of the above   *Ans.* D

18. Which of the following is the drug of choice in hypertensive emergencies?
    A. Enalapril
    B. Sodium nitroprusside
    C. Nifedipine
    D. Nebivolol   *Ans.* B

19. Which of the following is true about myocardial infarction?
    A. Is the irreversible necrosis of heart muscle secondary to prolonged ischemia.
    B. It is usually caused by coronary vasospasm
    C. Troponins are usually in the normal range
    D. All of the above   *Ans.* A

20. Which of the following is not a complication of myocardial infarction?
    A. Heart failure
    B. Ventricular septal defect (VSD)
    C. Mitral stenosis
    D. Cardiac arrhythmias   *Ans.* C

21. Infective endocarditis (IE) is the infection of:
    A. Endocardial surface of the heart
    B. Pericardium
    C. Myocardium
    D. All of the above   *Ans.* A

22. Which of the following causes acute infective endocarditis?
    A. *Staphylococcus*
    B. *Streptococcus viridans*
    C. *Enterococcus fecalis*
    D. HACEK group   *Ans.* A

23. Janeway lesions are seen in:
    A. Myocardial infarction
    B. Infective endocarditis
    C. Rheumatic fever
    D. Atrial septal defect   *Ans.* B

24. Which of the following is not a feature of infective endocarditis?
    A. Roth's spots   B. Osler's nodes
    C. Janeway lesions
    D. Rose spots   *Ans.* D

25. Duke criteria is used in the diagnosis of:
    A. Rheumatic fever
    B. Infective endocarditis
    C. Rheumatoid arthritis
    D. Myocardial infarction   *Ans.* B

26. Which of the following is NOT TRUE about paroxysmal supraventricular tachycardia (PSVT)?
    A. PSVT is paroxysmal and recurrent
    B. Often seen in young patients with no structural heart disease
    C. Heart rate is usually 100 to 120 per minute
    D. Most common symptom of PSVT is rapid regular palpitations   *Ans.* C

27. Drug of choice in paroxysmal supraventricular tachycardia (PSVT) is:
    A. Atenolol
    B. Digoxin   C. Atropine
    D. Adenosine   *Ans.* D

28. Which of the following is NOT a cyanotic congenital heart disease?
    A. Fallot's tetralogy
    B. Transposition of the great vessels
    C. Severe Ebstein's anomaly
    D. Atrial septal defect (ASD)   *Ans.* D

29. Which of the following is associated with cyanosis?
    A. Atrial septal defect (ASD)
    B. Ventricular septal defect (VSD)
    C. Patent ductus arteriosus (PDA)
    D. Fallot's tetralogy   *Ans.* D

30. Fallot's tetralogy is characterized by:
    A. Pulmonary stenosis, VSD, overriding aorta, and right ventricular hypertrophy
    B. Aortic stenosis, ASD, overriding aorta and left ventricular hypertrophy

C. Aortic stenosis, ASD, transposition of great vessels and overriding aorta
D. Pulmonary stenosis, patent ductus arteriosus, overriding aorta and left ventricular hypertrophy   *Ans.* A

31. **Paroxysmal nocturnal dyspnea (PND) is:**
   A. Sudden onset dyspnea and cough occurring usually 1 to 3 hours after the patient retires
   B. Dyspnea in lying down position
   C. Dyspnea in standing position
   D. Is dyspnea at night seen in bronchial asthma   *Ans.* A

32. **Infective endocarditis refers to infection of:**
   A. Pericardium of the heart
   B. Myocardium of the heart
   C. Endocardium of the heart
   D. All three layers of the heart   *Ans.* C

33. **Which of the following causes acute left ventricular failure?**
   A. Acute myocardial infarction
   B. Congenital heart disease
   C. Mitral stenosis
   D. Diabetes mellitus   *Ans.* A

34. **Pulsus alternans is seen in:**
   A. Left ventricular failure
   B. Hypertension
   C. Hypothyroidism
   D. Hypovolemic shock   *Ans.* A

35. **Paroxysmal nocturnal dyspnea is seen in:**
   A. Left ventricular failure
   B. Hypertension
   C. Hypothyroidism
   D. Hypovolemic shock   *Ans.* A

36. **While performing single rescuer adult CPR, the ratio of chest compressions and breaths is:**
   A. 15:2
   B. 30:2

   C. 20:2
   D. 40:3   *Ans.* B

37. **Features of congestive cardiac failure are all, EXCEPT:**
   A. Pedal edema
   B. Raised JVP
   C. Basal crepitations over the lungs
   D. Normal echocardiogram   *Ans.* D

HEMATOLOGY

1. **Thrombocytopenia refers to:**
   A. Decrease in RBC count
   B. Decrease in WBC count
   C. Decrease in platelet count
   D. Increase in eosinophil count   *Ans.* C

2. **Microcytic anemia is seen in:**
   A. Vitamin B_{12} deficiency
   B. Folic acid deficiency
   C. Acute blood loss
   D. Iron deficiency   *Ans.* D

3. **Megaloblastic anemia is seen in:**
   A. Vitamin B_{12} deficiency
   B. Thalassemia
   C. Acute blood loss
   D. Iron deficiency   *Ans.* A

4. **Which of the following causes normocytic anemia?**
   A. Vit amin B_{12} deficiency
   B. Folic acid deficiency
   C. Acute blood loss
   D. Iron deficiency   *Ans.* C

5. **Pica is:**
   A. Persistent eating of substances such as dirt or paint that have no nutritional value.
   B. Persistent drinking of cold water to relieve thirst
   C. Seen in vit-B_{12} deficiency
   D. Seen in diabetes mellitus   *Ans.* A

6. **Pica is seen in:**
   A. Iron deficiency
   B. Vitamin B_{12} deficiency
   C. Vitamin D deficiency
   D. Diabetes mellitus   *Ans.* A

7. **Koilonychia refers to:**
   A. Flattening of nails
   B. Spooning of nails
   C. Clubbing of fingers
   D. Onycholysis   *Ans.* B

8. **Koilonychia is seen in:**
   A. Iron deficiency
   B. Vitamin B_{12} deficiency
   C. Vitamin D deficiency
   D. Folic acid deficiency   *Ans.* A

9. **Normal recommended dietary allowance for vitamin B_{12} is:**
   A. 2 µg/day   B. 10 µg/day
   C. 50 to 100 µg/day
   D. 25 µg/day   *Ans.* A

10. **Vitamin B_{12} is mainly stored in:**
    A. Liver
    B. Spleen   C. Kidneys
    D. Fat tissue   *Ans.* A

11. **Vitamin B_{12} is mainly found in:**
    A. Milk and meat
    B. Green leafy vegetables
    C. Citrus fruits
    D. Pulses   *Ans.* A

12. **Which of the following causes peripheral neuropathy?**
    A. Iron deficiency
    B. Vitamin B_{12} deficiency
    C. Vitamin D deficiency
    D. Folic acid deficiency   *Ans.* B

13. **Hypersegmented neutrophils are seen in:**
    A. Iron deficiency
    B. Vitamin B_{12} deficiency
    C. Vitamin D deficiency
    D. Folic acid deficiency   *Ans.* B

14. **Pernicious anemia is due to:**
    A. Iron deficiency
    B. Vitamin B_{12} deficiency
    C. Vitamin D deficiency
    D. Folic acid deficiency   *Ans.* B

15. **Which of the following is NOT a cause of hemolytic anemia?**
    A. Hereditary spherocytosis
    B. Thalassemias

C. Sickle cell anemia
D. Aplastic anemia   *Ans.* D

16. **Which of the following is an acquired cause of hemolytic anemia?**
    A. Hereditary spherocytosis
    B. Thalassemias
    C. Sickle cell anemia
    D. Autoimmune hemolytic anemia   *Ans.* D

17. **Agranulocytosis refers to:**
    A. Decrease in RBC count
    B. Decrease in WBC count
    C. Decrease in platelet count
    D. Increase in eosinophil count   *Ans.* B

18. **Massive splenomegaly is all, EXCEPT:**
    A. CML
    B. Typhoid
    C. Kala-azar
    D. Myelofibrosis   *Ans.* B

19. **Which of the following causes splenic infarcts?**
    A. Hereditary spherocytosis
    B. Thalassemias
    C. Sickle cell anemia
    D. Autoimmune hemolytic anemia   *Ans.* C

20. **Which of the following is true about thalassemias?**
    A. A group of inherited hemolytic anemias
    B. Characterized by reduced or absent production of one or more globin chains of hemoglobin
    C. Common in the Mediterranean region
    D. All of the above   *Ans.* D

21. **Which of the following causes massive splenomegaly:**
    A. Enteric fever
    B. Hepatitis A
    C. Chronic myeloid leukemia
    D. Thalassemia   *Ans.* C

22. **Which of the following is the drug of choice for chronic myeloid leukemia?**
    A. Hydroxyurea
    B. Busulphan
    C. Imatinib mesylate
    D. Cytarabine   *Ans.* C

23. **Which of the following is true about primary hemostasis?**
    A. It is due to platelet plug formation at sites of injury.
    B. It occurs within seconds of injury
    C. It is important in stopping blood loss from capillaries, small arterioles, and venules.
    D. All of the above   *Ans.* D

24. **Which of the following is true about secondary hemostasis?**
    A. It occurs due tofibrin plug formation
    B. Requires several minutes for completion
    C. Important to prevent bleeding in larger vessels
    D. All of the above   *Ans.* D

25. **Thrombocytopenia refers to:**
    A. Decreased platelet count
    B. Decreased RBC count
    C. Decreased WBC count
    D. Decreased neutrophil count   *Ans.* A

26. **Which of the following does not cause thrombocytopenia?**
    A. Aplastic anemia
    B. Marrow infiltration (leukemia, myeloma, carcinoma, myelofibrosis, osteopetrosis)
    C. Myelodysplasia
    D. Acute blood loss   *Ans.* D

27. **Hemophilia A is due to:**
    A. Facto V deficiency
    B. Factor VII deficiency
    C. Factor VIII deficiency
    D. Factor IX deficiency   *Ans.* C

28. **Hemophilia A is a:**
    A. X-linked recessive disease
    B. X-linked dominant disease
    C. Autosomal recessive disease
    D. Autosomal dominant disease   *Ans.* A

29. **Which of the following is true about hemophilia A?**
    A. Factor VIII levels are reduced
    B. X-linked dominant disease
    C. Family history is usually absent
    D. Usually females suffer from the disease   *Ans.* A

30. **Which of the following is not used in the treatment of hemophilia?**
    A. Factor VIII concentrates
    B. Epsilon-aminocaproic acid
    C. Desmopressin
    D. Heparin   *Ans.* D

31. **Which of the following causes generalized lymphadenopathy?**
    A. Disseminated tuberculosis
    B. HIV   C. Lymphoma
    D. All of the above   *Ans.* D

32. **Oral manifestations of iron deficiency include:**
    A. Pale and bald tongue
    B. Pale mucous membrane
    C. Angular stomatitis
    D. All of the above   *Ans.* D

RENAL SYSTEM

1. **Which of the following does not lead to acute renal failure?**
    A. Heart failure
    B. Septic shock
    C. Hemorrhage
    D. Acute glomerulonephritis
    E. Diabetes mellitus   *Ans.* E

2. **Which of the following can cause acute kidney injury?**
    A. Diarrhea
    B. Diabetes mellitus
    C. NSAID abuse
    D. COPD   *Ans.* A

3. **All of the following are pre-renal causes of renal failure, EXCEPT:**
   A. Heart failure
   B. Septic shock
   C. Hemorrhage
   D. Acute diarrhea
   E. Prostate enlargement   *Ans.* E

4. **Which of the following is an indication for hemodialysis?**
   A. Urea >180 mg/dL and creatinine >8 mg/dL
   B. Refractory fluid overload with pulmonary edema
   C. Resistant hyperkalemia
   D. Severe metabolic acidosis (pH less than 7.1)
   E. All of the above   *Ans.* E

5. **Urea to creatinine ratio of more than >20:1 indicates:**
   A. Prerenal failure
   B. Intrarenal cause of renal failure
   C. Postrenal cause of renal failure
   D. All of the above   *Ans.* A

6. **Which of the following is not a feature of chronic kidney disease?**
   A. Anemia
   B. Hyperkalemia
   C. Hypercalcemia
   D. Hyperphosphatemia   *Ans.* C

7. **Anemia in chronic kidney disease is due to:**
   A. Decreased iron levels
   B. Decreased erythropoietin
   C. Decreased vitamin B_{12}
   D. Loss of iron binding protein in urine   *Ans.* B

8. **Nephrotic syndrome is characterized by:**
   A. Proteinuria
   B. Hypoalbuminemia
   C. Peripheral edema
   D. All of the above   *Ans.* D

9. **Nephrotic syndrome is more prevalent in:**
   A. Children
   B. Adolescents

   C. 20 to 50 years
   D. Old age   *Ans.* A

10. **Which of the following drugs is used in the treatment of nephrotic syndrome?**
    A. Chloramphenicol
    B. Prednisolone
    C. Danazol
    D. All of the above   *Ans.* B

11. **Which of the following is not a feature of acute glomerulonephritis?**
    A. Hematuria
    B. Hypertension   C. Oliguria
    D. Edema   *Ans.* B

12. **RBC casts in the urine are seen in:**
    A. Nephrotic syndrome
    B. Glomerulonephritis
    C. Urinary tract infection
    D. All of the above   *Ans.* B

13. **Massive proteinuria (>3 g/day) is a feature of:**
    A. Nephrotic syndrome
    B. Glomerulonephritis
    C. Urinary tract infection
    D. All of the above   *Ans.* A

14. **Poststreptococcal glomerulonephritis is due to:**
    A. Group A beta hemolytic streptococci
    B. Group B beta hemolytic streptococci
    C. *Streptococcus viridans*
    D. Any of the above   *Ans.* A

15. **Which of the following is a water-soluble vitamin?**
    A. Vitamin A
    B. Vitamin E
    C. Vitamin C
    D. Vitamin D   *Ans.* C

16. **Which of the following is a fat-soluble vitamin?**
    A. Vitamin A
    B. Vitamin D
    C. Vitamin E
    D. Vitamin K
    E. All of the above   *Ans.* E

17. Night blindness is a feature of:
A. Vitamin A deficiency
B. Niacin deficiency
C. Vitamin C deficiency
D. Vitamin K deficiency   *Ans.* A

18. Bitot's spots are seen in:
A. Vitamin A deficiency
B. Niacin deficiency
C. Vitamin C deficiency
D. Vitamin K deficiency   *Ans.* A

19. Beriberi is due to:
A. Thiamine deficiency
B. Niacin deficiency
C. Folate deficiency
D. Vitamin K deficiency   *Ans.* A

20. Pellagra is due to:
A. Thiamine deficiency
B. Niacin deficiency
C. Folate deficiency
D. Vitamin K deficiency   *Ans.* B

21. Scurvy is caused by the deficiency of:
A. Vitamin A deficiency
B. Niacin deficiency
C. Vitamin C deficiency
D. Vitamin K deficiency   *Ans.* C

22. Rickets is due to:
A. Vitamin A deficiency
B. Vitamin-D deficiency
C. Vitamin C deficiency
D. Vitamin K deficiency   *Ans.* B

23. Osteomalacia is due to:
A. Vitamin A deficiency
B. Vitamin D deficiency
C. Vitamin C deficiency
D. Vitamin K deficiency   *Ans.* B

24. Which of the following vitamins is very important for blood clotting?
A. Vitamin A
B. Vitamin K
C. Vitamin C
D. Vitamin D   *Ans.* B

NERVOUS SYSTEM

1. Trigeminal neuralgia affects:
A. 3rd cranial nerve
B. 5th cranial nerve
C. 7the cranial nerve
D. 9th cranial nerve   *Ans.* B

2. Drugs used in the prophylaxis of migraine headache include:
A. Propranolol
B. Sodium valproate
C. Amitryptaline
D. All of the above   *Ans.* D

3. Which of the following drugs is used in the treatment of trigeminal neuralgia?
A. Paracetamol
B. Carbamazepine C. Propranolol
D. Verapamil   *Ans.* B

4. Bell's palsy is a type of:
A. LMN facial palsy
B. UMN facial palsy
C. Trigeminal nerve palsy
D. Oculomotor palsy   *Ans.* A

5. Neck stiffness is seen in:
A. Trigeminal neuralgia
B. LMN type facial nerve palsy
C. Meningitis
D. Pharyngitis   *Ans.* C

6. Bell's phenomenon is seen in:
A. Facial nerve palsy
B. Trigeminal palsy
C. Oculomotor nerve palsy
D. All of the above   *Ans.* A

7. Electroencephalogram (EEG) is used in the evaluation of:
A. Epilepsy
B. Trigeminal neuralgia
C. Meningitis
D. Facial palsy   *Ans.* A

8. During an attack of generalized tonic clonic seizures, which of the following SHOULD NOT be done?
A. Put the patient in a safe place away from fire and sharp objects

B. Put the patient in lateral position and insert a padded mouth gag

C. Inj lorazpam 4 mg slow IV OR inj diazepam 10 mg slow IV

D. Hydrate the patient by pouring water into the mouth *Ans.* D

ENDOCRINOLOGY

1. Clinical features of diabetes mellitus include:
   A. Polyuria
   B. Polydipsia
   C. Polyphagia
   D. Delayed wound healing
   E. All of the above *Ans.* E

2. Which of the following requires lifelong insulin therapy?
   A. Type 1 diabetes
   B. Gestational diabetes
   C. Type 2 diabetes
   D. All of the above *Ans.* A

3. Which of the following is not an antidiabetic drug?
   A. Glimepiride
   B. Metformin
   C. Pioglitazone
   D. Verapamil *Ans.* D

4. Which of the following is an acute medical emergency?
   A. Diabetic retinopathy
   B. Diabetic neuropathy
   C. Diabetic Nephropathy
   D. Diabetic ketoacidosis *Ans.* D

5. Tetany is due to:
   A. *Clostridium tetanus*
   B. *Closridium perfringens*
   C. Hypocalcemia
   D. Hypercalcemia *Ans.* C

6. Features of hypoglycemia include all, EXCEPT?
   A. Sweating
   B. Trembling
   C. Pounding heart
   D. Polyuria *Ans.* D

7. Which of the following is not a cause of hypoglycemia?
   A. Malabsorption
   B. Addison's disease
   C. Insulinoma
   D. Hypothyroidism *Ans.* D

8. Acromegaly is due to increased secretion of:
   A. Throxine
   B. Adrenaline
   C. Growth hormone
   D. Cortisol *Ans.* C

9. Which is not a feature of acromegaly?
   A. Macrognathia
   B. Macroglossia
   C. Large hands
   D. Weight loss *Ans.* D

10. Which is not a feature of hyperthyroidism?
    A. Weight loss
    B. Heat intolerance
    C. Palpitations
    D. Constipation *Ans.* D

11. Which is not an antithyroid drug?
    A. Propylthiouracil
    B. Methimazole
    C. Carbimazole
    D. Tinidazole *Ans.* D

12. Which is not a feature of hypothyroidism?
    A. Weight gain
    B. Cold intolerance
    C. Hoarseness of voice
    D. Diarrhea *Ans.* D

13. Low T_3, low T_4, and high TSH indicate:
    A. Primary hypothyroidism
    B. Secondary (pituitary) hypothyroidism
    C. Primary hyperthyroidism
    D. Secondary hyperthyroidism *Ans.* A

14. **Features of Cushing's syndrome include:**
    A. Obesity   B. Buffalo hump
    C. Proximal muscle wasting
    D. Hypertension
    E. All of the above   *Ans.* E

15. **Centripetal obesity (lemon on stick appearance) is a feature of:**
    A. Addison's disease
    B. Hypothyroidism
    C. Cushing's disease
    D. Graves' disease   *Ans.* C

16. **Weight loss, hypoglycemia, hyponatremia, and hyperkalemia are seen in:**
    A. Addison's disease
    B. Hypothyroidism
    C. Cushing's disease
    D. Graves' disease   *Ans.* A

Index

Abdominal distention 56
Acid peptic disease 53
Acute adrenal crisis 199
Acute adrenal insufficiency 199
Acute blood loss 120
Acute coronary syndromes 91
Acute diarrhea 69
Acute HIV infection 12
Acute kidney injury 147
Acute leukemia 127
Acute lung injury 205
Acute myeloblastic leukemia 128
Acute myocardial infarction 92
Acute pyogenic meningitis 170
Acute respiratory distress syndrome 205
Acute rheumatic fever 75
Acute severe asthma 30
Acute viral hepatitis 61
Addison disease 198
Addisonian crisis 199
Adrenal insufficiency 198
Agranulocytosis 144
AIDS 11
AIDS stage 13
Alpha thalassemias 126
Anemia 56, 115
Anemia of chronic disease 120
Antihemophilic factor 142
Antituberculous drugs 39, 41
Aortic regurgitation 83
Aortic stenosis 81
Aphthous ulcers 51
Aplastic anemia 122, 145
Approach to a case of fever 2
Arrhythmias 100
Aschoff nodule 75
Assessment of dehydration 71
Atrial fibrillation 100
Atrial septal defect 106
Autoimmune hemolytic anemia 122

Balanced diet 156
Bell's palsy 170
Beriberi 157
Beta thalassemias 126

Blast crisis in CML 132
Bleeding and clotting disorders 56, 138, 146
Blood loss anemia 120
Bronchial asthma 26
Bronchiectasis 36
Bronchogenic carcinoma 46
Bronchopneumonia 34
Brudginski's sign 171
Burkitt lymphoma 137

Capillary resistance test 140
Cardiac arrest 206
Cardiopulmonary resuscitation 206
Cardiovascular syphilis 9
CDC classification system for HIV-infected 13
Chickenpox 17
Child-Turcotte-Pugh scoring system 65, 68
Christmas disease 143
Chronic hepatitis 64
Chronic kidney disease 148
Chronic myeloid leukemia 130
Chronic obstructive pulmonary disease 30
Chvostek's sign 194
Cirrhosis of liver 65
Classification of asthma 27
Clinical categories of HIV infection 13
CNS infection 17
Coagulation cascade 137
Coma 163
Community-acquired pneumonia 33
Congenital heart diseases 104
Congenital hyperbilrubinemic disorders 59
Congenital rubella 22
Congenital syphilis 9
Congestive cardiac failure 109
Coronary angioplasty 91
Coronary artery bypass grafting (CABG) 91
Cushing syndrome 196

Dark-field microscopy 10
Diabetes mellitus 177, 181
Diabetic ketoacidosis 183
Diarrhea 56, 69
Differences between Hodgkin's and
    non-Hodgkin's lymphoma 136

Diphtheria 5
Diphtheria antitoxin 6
Diphtheria toxoid 7
Disorders of luminal phase 55
Disorders of mucosal phase 55
DOTS 43
Duke criteria 95, 97
Dysentery 73
Dysphagia 52
Dyspnea 44

Ebstein's anomaly 104
Edema 56
Eisenmenger's syndrome 105
Enteric fever 3
Epilepsy 174
Erythema marginatum 75, 77
Essential hypertension 85
Exudative pleural effusion 44

Facial nerve palsy 168
Facial pain 167
Fallot's tetralogy 104, 108
Febrile neutropenia 144
Fecal incontinence 69
Fever 1
Flatulence 56
Fluorosis 159

Generalized lymphadenopathy 144
Generalized tonic clonic seizures 174
Genital herpes 17
German measles 22
Gingival hyperplasia 50
Glandular fever 18
Glomerulonephritis 153
Glucocorticoid excess 196
Gram's stain 6
Grand mal epilepsy 174
Graves' disease 191
Gummatous syphilis 9

H. pylori eradication 55
Headache 165
Heart failure 109
Hematologic disease 145
Hemodialysis 148
Hemoglobin S 124
Hemolytic anemias 121
Hemophilia A 142
Hemophilia B 143
Hemorrhagic disorders 138
Hemostasis 137
Hepatitis A 61, 62
Hepatitis B 63
Hepatomegaly 61

Herpes labialis 16
Herpes simplex 16
Herpes simplex keratitis 17
Herpes zoster 17, 18
Herpetic gingivostomatitis 16
Herpetic whitlow 17
Hess test 140
HIV 11
Hodgkin's lymphoma 132
Human immunodeficiency virus 11
Hyperosmolar hyperglycemic state 185
Hypertension 85
Hypertensive emergeny 88
Hypertensive urgency 88
Hyperthyroidism 190
Hypocalcemia 194
Hypoglycemia 187, 188
Hypoparathyroidism 195
Hypothyroidism 192

Iatrogenic pneumothorax 48
Idiopathic thrombocytopenic purpura 140
Infectious mononucleosis 18
Infective endocarditis 94
Infective endocarditis prophylaxis 98
Interstitial pneumonia 35
Iron deficiency anemia 115, 116, 145
Ischemic heart disease 88

Janeway leisons 100
Jaundice 58
Jones criteria 75, 77

Kernig's sign 171

Laboratory differentiation of
    different types of jaundice 61
Latent syphilis 8
Leukemias 127, 146
Life cycle of malarial parasite 23
Light's criteria 44
Lipoid nephrosis 153
Lobar pneumonia 34
Lung abscess 38
Lung cancer 46
Lymphomas 132
Macrocytic anemia 117
Malabsorption syndrome 55
Malaria 22
Malaria vaccine 25
Management of HIV infection 14
MDR tuberculosis 43
Measles 19
Mechanism of coagulation 137
Meningitis 170
Microcytic anemia 115

Migraine headache 165
Miliary pneumonia 35
Minimal change disease 153
Mitral regurgitation 80
Mitral stenosis 78
Mumps 20
Myocardial infarction 92

Neck stiffness 170
Neonatal herpes simplex 17
nephritic syndrome 151, 153
Neurosyphilis 9
Neutropenia 144
Niacin deficiency 158
Nil disease 153
Non-Hodgkin's lymphomas 135
Non-ketotic hyperosmolar syndrome 185
Non-ST-elevation myocardial infarction 91
Non-treponemal tests 10
Nutrient malabsorption 56
NYHA classification of heart failure 112

Opportunistic infections 11
Oral glucose tolerance test 179
Oral iron therapy 115
Osler's nodes 100

Parenteral iron therapy 115
Paroxysmal supraventricular tachycardia 101
Patent ductus arteriosus 107
Paterson-Kelly syndrome 115
Pathogenesis 75
Pea soup appearance 4
Pellagra 158
Peptic ulcer 53
Pernicious anemia 119
Philadelphia chromosome 130
Pica 115
Pleural effusion 44
Plummer-Vinson syndrome 115
Pneumococcus 33
Pneumonia 33
Pneumothorax 48
Polycythemia 145
Post primary (reactivation) pulmonary
    tuberculosis 39
Post-exposure prophylaxis for HIV 16
Post-streptococcal glomerulonephritis 155
Primary syphilis 7, 8
Prinzmetal's angina 89
Pseudo-diarrhea 69
Pulmonary tuberculosis 39
Reduction of HIV transmission 15
Reed-Sternberg cells 134
Revised national TB control programme 43
Rheumatic fever prophylaxis 78

Rickets 160
Risk factors involved in asthma 26
Roth's spots 100
Rubella 22
Rubeola 19

Scurvy 159
Secondary hypertension 88
Secondary syphilis 8
Sequelae of pulmonary tuberculosis 42
Sequelae of tuberculosis 39
Severe falciparum malaria 25
Shingles 17, 18
Shock 203
Sickle cell anemia 124
Sickle cell crisis 124
Splenomegaly 144
Spontaneous pneumothorax 48
Stable angina 89
Status asthmaticus 30
Steatorrhea 56
Stomatitis 50
Syncope 201
Syphilis 7

Tertiary or late syphilis 8, 9
Tests for *H. pylori* 54
Tetany 194
Thalassemias 126, 146
Thrombocytopenia 140
Thrombocytopenic purpura 140
Tic douloureux 167
Torsades de pointes 103
Tourniquet test 140
Transmission of HIV 12
Transudative pleural effusion 44
Traumatic pneumothorax 48
Traveler's diarrhea 72
Treponemal-specific tests 10
Trigeminal neuralgia 167
Trousseau's sign 194
Tuberculous meningitis 173
Type 1 diabetes mellitus 181
Type 2 diabetes mellitus 177
Typhoid carrier 5
Typhoid fever 3

Unstable angina 89, 91
Urinalysis 179

Varicella 17
Vasovagal syncope 203
Venereal disease research laboratory test 11
Ventricular fibrillation 103

Ventricular septal defect 105
Ventricular tachycardia 102
Vitamin A (retinol) deficiency 156
Vitamin B_1 (thiamine) deficiency 157
Vitamin B_{12} defficiency 117, 118
Vitamin B_{12} deficiency anemia 145
Vitamin C (ascorbic acid) deficiency 159
Vitamin D deficiency 160
Vitamin K 162

von Willebrand disease 141
von Willebrand factor 142

Weight loss and fatigue 56
Wernicke-Korsakoff syndrome 157
WHO guidelines for the treatment of
    tuberculosis 42

XDR tuberculosis 43